Assessment & Intervention for Communication Disorders in Culturally & Linguistically Diverse Populations

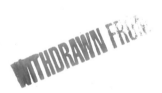

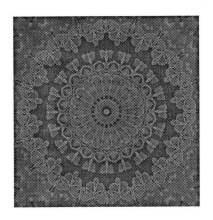

ASSESSMENT & INTERVENTION FOR COMMUNICATION DISORDERS IN CULTURALLY & LINGUISTICALLY DIVERSE POPULATIONS

HENRIETTE W. LANGDON, ED.D., F-CCC-SLP

Professor Communicative Disorders and Sciences
San José State University, San José, California

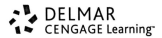
DELMAR
CENGAGE Learning

Australia • Brazil • Japan • Korea • Mexico • Singapore • Spain • United Kingdom • United States

**DELMAR
CENGAGE Learning™**

Assessment & Intervention for Communication Disorders in Culturally & Linguistically Diverse Populations
Henriette W. Langdon

Vice President, Health Care Business Unit: William Brottmiller

Director of Learning Solutions: Matthew Kane

Senior Acquisitions Editor: Sherry Dickinson

Senior Product Manager: Juliet Steiner

Editorial Assistant: Angela Doolin

Marketing Director: Jennifer McAvey

Marketing Manager: Chris Manion

Marketing Coordinator: Vanessa Carlson

Production Director: Carolyn Miller

Content Project Manager: Katie Wachtl

Senior Art Director: Jack Pendleton

For product information and technology assistance, contact us at
Cengage Learning Customer & Sales Support, 1-800-354-9706

For permission to use material from this text or product, submit all requests online at **www.cengage.com/permissions**
Further permissions questions can be emailed to
permissionrequest@cengage.com

Library of Congress Control Number: 2007019331

ISBN-13: 978-1-4180-0139-1

ISBN-10: 1-4180-0139-2

Delmar
Executive Woods
5 Maxwell Drive
Clifton Park, NY 12065
USA

Cengage Learning is a leading provider of customized learning solutions with office locations around the globe, including Singapore, the United Kingdom, Australia, Mexico, Brazil, and Japan. Locate your local office at **www.cengage.com/global**

Cengage Learning products are represented in Canada by Nelson Education, Ltd.

To learn more about Delmar, visit **www.cengage.com/delmar**

Purchase any of our products at your local bookstore or at our preferred online store **www.cengagebrain.com**

Printed in the United States of America
3 4 5 6 7   16 15 14 13 12

FD233

Dedication

To my brother Leon, who shares very similar childhood and early adolescence experiences, and to the memory of our parents, Dr. Samuel Wyszewianski (1916–2005) and Camila S. Wyszewianski (1920–2005), who strongly believed in raising their children to appreciate a multilingual and multicultural world.

Contents

CHAPTER 1

CULTURALLY AND LINGUISTICALLY DIVERSE (CLD) POPULATIONS: FACTS AND FIGURES 1

CHAPTER 2

SECOND-LANGUAGE DEVELOPMENT AND DUAL LANGUAGE PROCESSES 23

CHAPTER 3

OPTIMAL SECOND-LANGUAGE LEARNING FOR CLD POPULATIONS 50

CHAPTER 4

CLD POPULATIONS' CONNECTIONS TO SCHOOLS, HEALTH CARE, AND OTHER AGENCIES IN THE COMMUNITY 78

CHAPTER 5

ASSESSMENT PROCEDURES FOR CLD CHILDREN: INFANCY THROUGH ADOLESCENCE 108

CHAPTER 6

ARRIVING AT A FINAL DIAGNOSIS FOR LANGUAGE PROBLEMS IN CLD POPULATIONS: INFANCY THROUGH ADOLESCENCE 143

CHAPTER 7

INTERVENTION ISSUES FOR CLD CHILDREN: INFANCY THROUGH ADOLESCENCE 177

CHAPTER 8

CLD/ADULT POPULATIONS: ASSESSMENT AND INTERVENTION ISSUES 209

LIST OF TABLES

LIST OF FIGURES

PREFACE

The requirements for competency in the field of speech and language pathology are complex. Today, speech-language pathologists (SLPs) provide services to clients of all ages whose proficiency in English and their native language is highly variable. This variability is due to factors such as the clients' length of residency in the United States; opportunity to interact with native speakers of English; level of formal education; and cognitive abilities, personality, and experiences. This variability is also common in the other parts of the world where the field of speech-language pathology is recognized as a profession.

When SLPs cannot communicate directly with their clients, they need to collaborate with trained interpreters and translators. Working with the assistance of an interpreter adds one additional layer of complexity to the SLPs' multiple responsibilities. In any interaction with a monolingual or bilingual client, SLPs must monitor and adjust their own communication skills to convey clear messages, and this is also true when the SLP is working with clients who are in a similar age group, or who have disabilities. Assessing and working with a preschool-age child who has articulation disorders requires different skills and discourse strategies than those necessary for assessing and working with a school-age child or adolescent who has similar difficulties or language-learning disabilities. When communicating with a client who has suffered from a stroke or is a victim of a traumatic brain injury, SLPs need to make other types of modifications in order to be able to assess these patients and offer them strategies that will allow them to compensate for their various communication deficits.

Additionally, the process of interviewing and reporting findings may vary depending on certain factors—such as the reason for administering any given test item, or the particular client/family involved. Some clients and families respond differently to the very same question or comments, because responses depend on an individual's interpretation of the question—as well as on his or her personality, knowledge base, and experiences. Some families need to have more details about a given assessment or intervention procedure than other families do. Decisions about intervention may vary depending on a family's personal beliefs, culture, and background, and there may be differences among members of a single family. These complexities are multiplied when clients come from diverse linguistic and cultural backgrounds.

Even though many SLPs are bilingual, they may not be able to provide services to bilingual clients because the language they know does not match that of their client. The ranking of the 10 languages most frequently spoken by CLD families does not consistently match the ranking of languages that are taught in higher education. This is illustrated in Table P-1. Perhaps society at large has not taken sufficient time to consider that there is a demand for learning languages other than Spanish. As can be seen from the data presented in the table, there is a critical need for serving individuals who speak Asian languages other than Japanese and Chinese—languages such as Tagalog, Vietnamese, and Korean. Therefore, although the SLP's being bilingual may be advantageous in situations where there is a match between the SLP's and the client's language, when there is no match, being bilingual may present the same kinds of challenges as those encountered by a monolingual clinician. It is evident that there are many barriers that prevent today's monolingual or bilingual SLPs from feeling confident in conducting assessments and interventions for communication disorders in CLD populations.

TABLE P-1   Rank Order of Languages Spoken by Immigrants versus Rank Order of Language Instruction in Higher Education

Immigrants' Language		Taught in Higher Education	
Language	Rank order	Language	Rank order
Spanish	1	Spanish	1
French	2	French	2
Chinese	3	German	3
German	4	Italian	4
Tagalog	5	Sign language	5
Vietnamese and Italian	6	Japanese	6
Korean	7	Chinese	7
Russian	8	Latin	8
Polish	9	Russian	9
Arabic	10	Greek	10

Source: Adapted from the National Virtual Translation Center, 2006, and Welles, 2004.

PURPOSE OF THE TEXT

Assessment and Intervention for Communication Disorders in Culturally and Linguistically Diverse Populations is written for both undergraduate and graduate students who are taking a course in this subject. It is also written for the practicing SLP who wishes to review any of the specific issues relating to these populations. A book of this nature cannot answer all questions concerning the multitude of linguistic and cultural groups currently living in the United States. Therefore, additional resources are given within the various chapters.

In working with CLD populations, it is necessary to integrate knowledge from various disciplines that include linguistics, cognition, sociology, and education. Even though information on the various aspects of bilingualism and biculturalism that are related to these disciplines may be available, the information is far from complete. As Bialystok (2001) states, "[P]artly, the research is difficult to conduct because it requires interdisciplinary perspectives that are not common in most developmental studies. Meaningful studies of bilingual children often require intersecting skills in cognition, linguistics, sociology, and education, a combination not usually enlisted by most researchers" (p. 248). De Bot and Makoni (2005) make similar remarks regarding older populations: "The intersection between multilingualism and aging, particularly in situations of decline, is an important area of study because the population of the aging is growing and living longer. The aging population also happens to be multilingual. Although there is a growing elderly population that is bilingual, there are relatively few studies that have focused on multilingual aging" (p. 136). Therefore, the focus of this book is to offer the student and practicing clinician information and strategies that can be used when planning and carrying out assessments of, and drafting treatment plans for, any client considered to be culturally and/or linguistically diverse.

ORGANIZATION OF TEXT

Language development and learning are part of the life of an individual and result from the interaction of various factors: rearing practices; amount and type of contact with the native and second languages; age of acquisition of each language; general experiences; number of years and consistency of formal schooling; and personal characteristics such as sociability, motivation, and attitude toward each language and its culture. The assessment of a CLD individual is quite complex and cannot be successfully completed by only administering tests—even if they exist in the individual's primary language and normative data are available. The process requires first a careful consideration and analysis of the individual's background that will shape the direction in which the assessment will take place. The steps to be taken mirror those of an investigation. Selecting the necessary pieces for the construction of the puzzle is very important.

When the SLP speaks the same language as the client, it is much easier to provide services without having to collaborate with an interpreter. However, the process of initiating and carrying out an assessment—as well as the process of evaluating and interpreting the findings—is challenging regardless of the SLP's knowledge of another language. First of all, the SLP must keep in mind general information about bilingualism and about the factors that affect bilingualism. Second, the SLP should not only be aware of the process of bilingual language acquisition and development, but be aware of the issues that apply to specific bilingual language combinations, as well. The language acquisition and development process of a French-Spanish speaker will, for example, necessarily be different than that of a French-Arabic speaker. Accordingly, the SLP should be aware of the phenomena that occur as a consequence of the interaction of two languages—and understand the resulting implications for language processing and cognitive development.

As can be noted from the following outline of this book, a great deal of material in the text focuses on providing information that will assist the SLP in planning the assessment. My philosophy is that assessment preparation is at the core of a successful diagnosis of, and intervention plan for, any client. Preparation is especially important when working with those clients for whom English is the second language. The strategies and information presented in this text apply to any client who may be living in an environment where a new second language is prevalent. To assist the student, practicing SLP, and interested reader of this topic, the cases of five individuals (three children and two adults) will be followed throughout the book and will illustrate the various concepts developed in each of the eight chapters. These cases are designated "Our Clients."

Chapter 1, "Culturally and Linguistically Diverse (CLD) Populations: Facts and Figures," discusses data related to CLD children and adults, including those who have been identified as having various speech, language, and communication impairments. The discussion centers on the larger identified language and cultural minority groups that include Hispanics, African-Americans, Asian-Americans and Pacific Islanders, and Native Americans and Alaskan Natives.

Chapter 2, "Second-Language Development and Dual Language Processes," discusses issues related to dual language development, including the use of and interaction between two languages. Issues such as language proficiency, dominance, interference, and loss are discussed. In addition, the text explores the implications for cognitive development and language processing that relate to bilingualism.

Chapter 3, "Optimal Second-Language Learning for CLD Populations," discusses the various facets of language learning in a classroom environment. Following a review of the history of bilingual education in the United States, selected models of bilingual instruction, and research findings that support the efficacy of specific programs, are described. In addition, the best strategies for second-language teaching are outlined.

Chapter 4, "CLD Populations' Connections to Schools, Health Care, and Other Agencies in the Community," provides general guidelines for understanding cross-cultural differences in the attitudes and experiences of the various populations with regard to schools, health care, and other agencies in the community. The chapter describes childrearing, communication patterns occurring within families, and children's experiences in attaining literacy and accessing formal education. A variety of supportive health care and community agencies are referenced. The chapter also discusses CLD families' attitudes toward various educational and medical disabilities.

Chapter 5, "Assessment Procedures for CLD Children: Infancy through Adolescence," discusses topics such as the process of conducting an assessment in two languages, and how to decide whether to use one or two languages when carrying out an assessment. Another section of the chapter outlines procedures for obtaining a language sample and for analyzing all aspects of language (form, content, use) when there are tests available in the child's language. Procedures are also outlined for those situations in which tests are not available in the child's language, and the discussion includes some strategies for collaborating with an interpreter in those instances. The chapter ends with a suggested protocol for reporting test results and assessment findings.

Chapter 6, "Arriving at a Final Diagnosis for Language Problems in CLD Populations: Infancy through Adolescence," includes a discussion about the connections between oral and written language and explores that relationship with regard to both monolingual and bilingual students. The chapter offers a definition of the concept "language disorder" as it might relate to CLD students whose bilingual backgrounds are quite diverse—and offers suggestions for how to describe the nature of such a disorder. A protocol for what to include in an assessment report is included at the end of the chapter, together with a complete assessment report for each of the three youngest clients we have been following throughout the book.

Chapter 7, "Intervention Issues for CLD Children: Infancy through Adolescence," suggests specific strategies for effectively meeting the needs of CLD children who have a variety of language-learning disabilities (LLD). Examples of interventions for students at different grade levels are presented. The process of choosing the language of intervention is discussed in two sections: the first one pertains to the school setting and the second to the home setting. Suggestions for parents whose proficiency in English may be quite variable are included. Preferred service delivery models for this population are also described. The end of the chapter offers specific intervention strategies for each of the three young clients whose reports appeared in Chapter 6.

Chapter 8, "CLD/Adult Populations: Assessment and Intervention Issues," discusses the unique challenges facing this population. Topics include an assessment protocol, a review of the available research concerning bilingual patients' recovery from stroke, and a discussion of the best intervention practices for clients with various acquired neurological disorders. Detailed assessment reports and intervention strategies for the two adult clients whose cases we have been following are presented at the end of the chapter.

ABOUT THE AUTHOR

Henriette W. Langdon, Ed.D., F-CCC-SLP, is a professor in the Communicative Disorders and Sciences Department at San José State University in San José, California. For the past 33 years, Dr. Langdon's work has centered on researching and designing assessment strategies and intervention programs for English-language learners who are also experiencing language and learning difficulties. She has written other books on this subject as well as several articles, and she has lectured locally, nationally, and internationally on these topics. Dr. Langdon is fluent in English, French, Polish, and Spanish. She is a Fellow of the American Speech-Language-Hearing Association (ASHA) and a recipient of the Certificate of Recognition for Special Contributions in the area of Multicultural Affairs. In 2006 she was awarded the Honors of the California Speech-Language-Hearing Association.

ACKNOWLEDGEMENTS

Writing a book is an undertaking that requires a great deal of dedication as well as encouragement. I could not have taken the time to accomplish such a task without the award of a sabbatical from my full-time job as Professor of Communicative Disorders and Sciences at San José State University. Therefore, I would like to thank the committee from the College of Education who selected my project as a worthwhile task to complete during a sabbatical. In addition to supplemental time for working, the author of a book needs support from family, colleagues, and friends in order to carry out the project. Unfortunately, while writing this book I experienced something we all need to expect: the death of one's parents. Indeed, shortly after I began writing the book, the project was interrupted as both of my parents passed on within only six weeks of each other. I am very saddened because both my parents were supportive of my work, and my father particularly was very interested in the progress of this project. However, because I had the support of my husband, daughter, brother, friends and colleagues, and Juliet Steiner, Senior Product Manager at Delmar, Cengage Learning, I was able to "collect myself" and complete the project within expected deadlines.

This work is a revision of a book that I edited 15 years ago (1992) entitled *Hispanic Children and Adults with Communication Disorders: Assessment and Intervention,* originally published by Aspen Publishers under the editorship of Dr. Katharine Butler. The original book was an edited version, and I want to thank the authors who contributed to that version, because in writing the chapters of this book I relied on the information they provided in the 1992 text and often reiterated what they wrote. My gratitude goes to Gustavo Arámbula, Carol Beaumont, Lilly Cheng, and Barbara Merino. In addition, Lilly Cheng's assistance and support at the time that I was working on the 1992 text was invaluable and is still greatly appreciated.

"It takes a village to raise a child" is a very appropriate phrase to use to describe my process of writing this revised version of the 1992 book. There are many people who were and are in that village, and without their help, support, and encouragement, I could not have completed this work. My heartfelt thanks go out to:

Kalen Conerly, Acquisition Editor at Delmar, Cengage Learning, who thought I could do anything.

Juliet Steiner, Senior Product Manager at Delmar, Cengage Learning, who always believed in me and was there to coach, listen, and counsel.

Katie Wachtl, Content Project Manager, and Jack Pendleton, Senior Art Director (both at Delmar, Cengage Learning), for all their work on this book.

The book would not have been as clear and polished if it were not for the very careful work and helpful edits of Michelle Gaudreau, copyeditor at ICC MacMillan. I am most grateful for her patience and attention to detail. And of course, Gunjan Chandola, Project Manager at ICC MacMillan, made sure we all remained focused on our work and respected our deadlines, something of which I am most appreciative.

Friends and colleagues who were there to cheer and encourage me, and who maintained faith in my ability to complete the project, include John Consalvi, Nancy Flores-Castilleja, Dr. Hortencia Kayser, Margaret and Thomas Knowlton, Ellen Lamberth, Dean Susan Meyers, Dr. Marion Meyerson, Dr. Barbara Morrill, Brendan O'Connor Webster, Char Rau, Carrie Slymaker, Dr. Elise Trumbull, Sharen Valles, and Dr. Gloria Weddington. I also thank my family, who were kind enough to listen to my eternal "Do you think I will ever complete this?" They include my ever-supportive husband Carl and my daughter Maxine, who helped with some of the charts and graphics. Leon, my brother and friend, is on that very important list as well.

However, this book would not have really been completed without the direct interest, editorial comments, and support of someone I have always admired and looked up to, my teacher and mentor, Dr. Elisabeth H. Wiig.

Thank you, all my friends and supporters, for your encouragement!

With great appreciation,
Henriette W. Langdon
April, 2007

C H A P T E R   1

CULTURALLY AND LINGUISTICALLY DIVERSE (CLD) POPULATIONS: FACTS AND FIGURES

"The U.S. represents a confluence of voluntary immigrants, involuntary immigrants and indigenous peoples—each with its own cultural history and roots."
(Trumbull, Rothstein-Fish, Greenfield, & Quiroz, 2001, p. 2)

CHAPTER OUTLINE

INTRODUCTION

The population of the United States has changed dramatically in the past 35 years. Despite local and international criticism, over the last decade the United States has opened its doors to more immigrants than any other country in the world (Camarota, 2001).

Today the cultural and linguistic diversity of the United States is the result of three significant waves of immigration. The first wave occurred between 1830 and 1890; immigrants came from Scandinavia, Ireland (immigrants escaping the potato famine), China, Latin America (immigrants participating in the 1848 gold rush), and Germany. As many as 20 million more people emigrated from Austria, Hungary, Italy, and Russia during the second wave of immigration, which occurred between 1890 and the onset of World War I. Thereafter, immigration ceased almost completely, and did not resume until the 1950s when Cuban refugees fleeing Castro's regime settled in Florida. The flow of immigration into the U.S. has escalated in the last 30 years, bringing newcomers from all corners of the world. Whereas earlier immigrants came from Europe, the more recent immigrants, forced to emigrate for political or economic reasons, came from Asia (after the Vietnam War), different parts of Latin America (in particular Mexico and Central America), and Africa. In addition, 15 to 20 million illegal immigrants (one in 14 people) reside in the United States.

According to the 2000 Census, 56 million U.S. residents were either foreign-born or first-generation. They had emigrated from a multitude of countries—primarily Latin America, followed by Asia and Europe. As many as 18% of the total U.S. population aged 5 and over, or 47 million people, reported speaking a language other than English at home (Shin & Bruno, 2003). This number represents a 47% increase over the numbers reported by the 1990 Census. In the last 30 years, changes in procedures for classifying the U.S. population have occurred as well. In 1970, the Census Bureau designated only two classifications: White or Black, or "Other," which included Native American, Eskimo or Aleut, Asian-American, and Pacific Islander. In the 2000 Census, "Other" referred to Alaskan Native, Asian-American, and Native Hawaiian American. In responding to the 2000 Census, individuals also had the option of marking more than one race (Singer, 2004). Hispanic and Latino statistics were collected separately from race. Table 1-1 lists changes in U.S. racial composition over the last 30 years. Results of the 2000 Census indicated that, for the first time, Hispanics outnumbered any other cultural/ethnic minority (12.5%) as compared with Black and "Other" (11.4%). Additionally, the number of children and adults reported as being "Other" racial minorities has increased dramatically—from 1.5% to 14.8% for children and 1.4% to 9.9% for adults.

It is predicted that by the year 2050 the Hispanic group will constitute almost 25% of the total U.S. population. The number of Pacific Islanders and individuals with Asian backgrounds will increase twofold, from 3.8% to 8%. In contrast, the proportion of blacks is estimated to remain fairly constant during this 50-year period, with only a slight increase from 12.7% to 14.6%. The white population, on the other hand, will go from 69.4% in 2000 to only 50.1% by 2050; and the

TABLE 1-1 U.S. Population by Race and Age 1970–2000

RACE	1970	1980	1990	2000	Difference between 1970–2000
Total					
White	87.4	83.2	80.3	75.1	−12.3
Black	11.1	11.7	12.0	12.3	1.2
Other	1.4	5.2	7.6	12.5	11.1
Children					
White	84.8	78.6	75.1	68.6	−16.2
Black	13.7	14.7	15.0	15.1	1.4
Other	1.5	6.7	9.9	16.3	14.8
Adults					
White	88.9	84.9	82.2	77.4	−11.5
Black	9.8	10.5	11.0	11.4	1.6
Other	1.4	4.5	6.8	11.2	9.9
Hispanic Ethnicity	...	6.4	9.0	12.5	6.1

Source: "The Changing Face of America," by A. Singer, 2004, *e-Journal USA: Society & Values*, 9(2).

Native American, Eskimo, Aleut, and other population groups will increase from 2.5% in 2000 to 5.3% (U.S. Census Bureau, 2004).

The changes reflected in the demographics of the nation have had an impact on the role and responsibilities of speech-language pathologists (SLPs). The American Speech-Language-Hearing Association (ASHA), the accreditation agency for all university training institutions in speech and language pathology and audiology, has made a commitment to focus on best practices in serving Culturally and Linguistically Diverse (CLD) populations. The latest published document on the professional responsibilities of SLPs is titled Background Information and Standards and Implementation for the Certificate of Clinical Competence in Speech-Language Pathology *(ASHA, 2005a), and highlights two important areas that relate to the topic discussed in this book. The first area pertains to the "knowledge of the principles and methods of prevention, assessment, and intervention for people with communication and swallowing disorders, including consideration of anatomical/physiological, psychological, developmental, and linguistic and cultural correlates of the disorders." The second area is under the section of "interaction and personal qualities" and states that "the SLP needs to be an effective communicator who is capable of recognizing the needs, values, preferred mode of communication, and cultural/linguistic background of the client/patient, family, caregivers, and relevant others, and who can provide counseling regarding communication and swallowing disorders to clients/patients, family, and caregivers" (ASHA, 2005a).*

The number of SLPs who can serve clients in their primary language has increased in the last 20 years, but not at the same pace as demand. A review of the linguistic and cultural backgrounds of today's U.S. population will assist SLPs in understanding the experiences of students/clients who need speech and language services. Awareness of the clients' background will enable clinicians to select the most appropriate procedures for assessing their clients' linguistic skills. (It is appropriate, for example, to avoid the use of certain tests which may be biased, and to collaborate with interpreters if there is need to assess the client in his or her primary language.)

This chapter will provide information on various facts and figures related to CLD student/client populations—including those populations that have been identified as having various speech, language, and communication impairments. Refer to the chapter outline for topics discussed in this chapter.

DEFINING CULTURALLY AND LINGUISTICALLY DIVERSE (CLD) POPULATIONS

Several terms have been used to designate those individuals who differ from the Anglo-European mainstream. Terms include "minority groups," "minority language groups," and "culturally and linguistically diverse (CLD) populations." Also, terms such as "race" and "ethnicity" are used to differentiate those groups.

Nieto (2004) defines culture as "values, traditions, social and political relationships, and a world created, shared, and transformed by a group of people bound together by a common history, geographic location and language, social class, religion or other shared identity" (p. 146). As noted, the word "culture" includes aspects of a group's identity that comprise some observable patterns—such as traditions and social relationships—as well as characteristics that are translated into the group's values, beliefs, and religion (Trumbull et al., 2001). Additionally, "language" is embedded in the definition as a way to translate the group's history and ideas. However, "language" does not capture all the possible variants (noted in any combinations of phonology,

grammar, vocabulary, and pragmatics, including nonverbal communication) that may exist in that language. Some of the expressive language variations are referred to as dialects. For example, the Spanish spoken in Spain and Mexico share the same grammar, but there are phonological and semantic variations across the two languages. Similarly, the English spoken in England or Australia is very different from the English spoken in parts of Africa or the United States. Furthermore, the English spoken in the South of the United States is different from the English spoken in the Northeast. In all cases, the Spanish or English variations spoken in each region or country are marked primarily by differences in pronunciation, vocabulary and/or grammatical usage, but the speakers of each language group can understand one another despite these differences. Cantonese and Mandarin, on the other hand, are referred to as "dialects of Chinese"; but although they are understandable in written form, they are mutually unintelligible in their spoken form.

Two speakers of the same language may communicate verbally and nonverbally in a different way depending on social class, formal education, gender, age, or any combination of these variables. For example, in the Hispanic culture it is not unusual to address someone who is experienced and older as "maestro" or "maestra" (master-teacher) in order to acknowledge their expertise—regardless of their profession and level of formal education. It is also not unusual to use the more formal "usted" instead of "tú" (Condon, 1986). In contrast, different forms of "I" and "you" are used in Vietnamese depending on the age and status of interlocutors who are speaking in Vietnamese. In Japanese there are more than 100 words for "I," whereas in Chinese there are 10 words for that same pronoun (Cheng, 1991).

While verbal communication may be easier to describe, because the various components can be broken down into words and sentences, nonverbal communication is more difficult to interpret because it depends on the backgrounds and cultures of the persons who are interacting with each other. Several researchers have indicated that nonverbal communication conveys a greater proportion of meaning than verbal communication (30%) (Birdwhistell, 1970; Mehrabian, 1972). Nonverbal communication includes several aspects: kinesis (movement of the body and face); proxemics (how space is used between individuals while they communicate); and paralanguage (use of intonation) (Chen & Starosta, 1998; Lustig & Koester, 1999). Even though most emotions such as fear, surprise, anger, and disgust are displayed similarly across cultures, there are some differences in the interpretation of smiles. A smile can signal embarrassment, friendliness, or tension. Generally speaking, Middle Eastern and Latin American cultures express their emotions more readily than North Europeans or North Americans. In several Asian cultures, the use of eye contact is a taboo. Within these nonverbal communication patterns, there are variations in how conversations and conversation topics are initiated within a given group.

The variations will be discussed in greater depth in Chapter 4.

The concept of culture is not static. Instead, it evolves with time—especially when members of a given group interact or intermarry with members of the mainstream culture. Interacting with and becoming part of the American culture was more prevalent in the past as immigrants believed that learning English was an essential asset for assimilating into the mainstream culture. The use of English by the younger members of the family continues to be the norm. At times, these individuals may continue to interact in the family's language with parents and older relatives, but this is not always the norm. However, the older family members of past and more recent immigrants have more often continued to speak their native language at home with consistency. Thus, Veltman (1988) found that a language may "survive" for three generations but that variations may exist from case to case. By the time Hispanic immigrants have lived in the United States for 15 years, about 75% of them speak English on a regular basis. Furthermore, 7 out of 10 children of Hispanic immigrant parents become English speakers for all practical purposes. Nevertheless, "losing" the primary language does not necessarily mean that the group "feels" part of the mainstream American society represented in Figure 1-1.

In his theory of assimilation (also referred to as acculturation), which means adaptation and/or feeling part of the major culture (in our case, we would call this "Americanization"), Sandberg (1986) suggested that ethnic identity decreases with time. Assimilation and ethnic identity can be represented along vertical and horizontal lines that intersect, resulting in four quadrants. Each quadrant represents one of four types of individuals. Figure 1-1 illustrates the continuum of assimilation, ethnic identity,

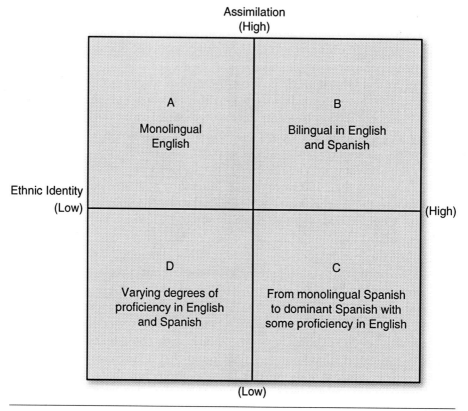

FIGURE 1-1 *Relationship of Assimilation, Ethnic Identity, and Proficiency in L1 and L2. Assimilation.* (Adapted from Pedersen, 1989.)

and language use (L1—native language, L2—English), according to Kitano's (1989) model.

Type A individuals are high in assimilation and low in ethnic identity: these individuals are "Americanized" (i.e., have assimilated into mainstream culture). They may continue to associate with members from the same ethnic group, however. Type B individuals are high in assimilation and high in ethnic identity and, essentially, bicultural. Individuals whose occupation and/or personal ties enhance opportunities to visit their country of origin and who continue to use their native language with native speakers of that language are part of this group. Type C individuals are high in ethnicity and low in assimilation. Recently arrived immigrants and

older persons who have spent most of their lives in ethnic communities within the dominant culture fit this category. Finally, Type D individuals are low in assimilation and low in ethnic identity. They not only have difficulty accepting and adjusting to the mainstream culture—they have difficulty accepting their own ethnic background, as well. No individual fits "neatly" into any of these categories, and there may be differences from generation to generation. Although Kitano (1989) does not address directly the role played by the native or acquired languages, it is possible to hypothesize that their roles vary from category to category. Type A persons seem likely to be essentially monolingual in English. Type C and D persons may have varying proficiencies in each language, but Type C persons are likely to use their native language primarily. Type B persons are probably bilingual, with equivalent proficiency in both languages. The examples provided in Figure 1-1 are for English and Spanish—but in fact the examples apply to any combination of two languages in which one is the majority language and the other is the first language of the client.

In addition to culture and language, "race" and "ethnicity" are terms that are frequently used interchangeably to mark distinctions between various groups. "Race" is used to make differentiations based primarily on physical characteristics, such as skin color and facial features, whereas the term "ethnicity" adds on the idea of customs, values, ancestry, tradition, religion, and history (Trumbull & Farr, 2005).

In the process of assessing the speech, language, and communication skills of an individual, consideration of the individual's race, ethnicity, culture, and language must be taken into account. In addition, the impact of the individual's age, gender, experiences, contact with individuals from the mainstream, formal education, economic opportunities, personality, and motivation should be considered. These variables will be further discussed in the next chapters.

While dividing 300 million people into categories based on race/cultural and ethnic differences is convenient, it does not do justice to the diversity within diversity, as each individual within any one grouping is just as unique as anyone's fingerprint.

CLD POPULATIONS: FACTS AND FIGURES

Hispanics, Asian-Americans and Pacific Islanders, blacks (African-Americans), and Native Americans and Alaskan Natives are often referred to as "minority group popula-

tions." However, the term "minority" is not applicable in all parts of the U.S. For example, these "minority groups" represent more than one-half of the population 18 years and older in states such as Arizona, California, Hawaii, New Mexico, and Texas. In turn, each of the major groups, such as Hispanics, or Asian-Americans and Pacific Islanders, include a large variety of different groups. The groups mentioned above will be reviewed in greater detail because they are the most prevalent groups currently living in the U.S. The classification is used as a convenience for studying similarities and differences among different groups. However, the delineation of each group is distinct—because an individual has parents who come from two different groups. This phenomenon of an individual coming from two different backgrounds surfaced while gathering data during the 2000 Census.

Hispanics

As previously discussed, Hispanics will become the largest minority population living in the United States within the next few years. Although considered as a distinct group, the background of Hispanics is as diverse as their countries of origin, which may be situated in Latin America (Central and South America, and the Caribbean). Hispanics have also been referred to as Latino. However, the word Latino also includes those who live in Brazil, where Portuguese is spoken. Therefore, the term Hispanic is more accurate when describing those who have Hispanic ancestry.

Latin America includes seven countries, three major islands of the Caribbean, Cuba, Puerto Rico, and the Dominican Republic in addition to most of South America with the exception of Brazil and the Guyanas. Details about each country of the Hispanic world, including historical backgrounds and geographical as well as population characteristics (culture and languages), can be found at the Department of State Web site: http://www.state.gov/.

1. Hispanics are descendants of Native Americans who settled in the Americas long before the Spanish conquest. The Mayans, for example, lived in what is today Guatemala, Mexico, Honduras, and El Salvador. The Aztecs settled primarily in Mexico, and the Incas in Perú, southern Colombia, Ecuador, Bolivia, and northern Chile. Some Hispanics are direct descendants of Spanish and European settlers, but the great majority is Mestizo, having both Indian and European heritage. Still other Hispanics have African-American ancestors, and a few have Asian ancestry as well. Those who are primarily of blended African-American and white heritage are referred to as mulattoes. Many of these are referred to as Creoles, which denotes those mulattoes born on the American continent whose direct ancestors are of European or Spanish descent. Discrimination based on racial heritage may occur among the different subgroups and even within a given subgroup.

2. The Hispanic group includes five subgroups: 66% are Mexican; 15% are Central or South American; 14% are Cuban; 9% are Puerto Rican; and 2% are originally from Spain (U.S. Census Bureau, 2004). Although all subgroups speak Spanish, there are phonological and lexical variations in the Spanish spoken in their countries of origin; a diversity of Indian and European languages may be spoken as well. Each country has its own history, celebrates different patriotic holidays, and has its own music and food specialties. In addition to Spanish, as many as 62 Indian languages are spoken in Mexico alone. Of particular interest is that currently more and more immigrants from Mexico may not speak Spanish as their first language. For example, a growing immigration from Oaxaca where natives speak Mixteco and Zapotec has been identified in California.

The majority of Hispanics are Roman Catholic, but religious symbols such as the Virgin Mary are represented differently based on the specific ethnicity of the particular populations. Important statistics on age, income, education, healthcare accessibility, and other characteristics is provided by Ramírez (2004).

Blacks (African-Americans)

As noted earlier, blacks (also referred to as African-Americans in much of the literature on various diverse cultures and languages) have been accounted for in Census data. Because Hispanics and Latinos may be of any race, the races of those populations may overlap. According to McKinnon (2003), the overlap is only 3.7%. But no matter how small such an overlap is, it is important to remember that members of a given group represent a diverse group, and this also applies to the group referred to as "black." For example, there are differences among Africans from different African countries, among black persons from the West Indies, or among black Hispanics.

Following the original Spanish settlements that began in the first part of the sixteenth century (in primarily the central and southern parts of the American continent), a wave of immigrants from various European countries such as France, Great Britain, and the Netherlands began to infiltrate the mainland of the United States. At the same time, the slave trade, which had begun in the 1600s in order to supply a workforce for a growing agricultural and industrial culture, continued well into the middle of the eighteenth century. As many as 10 million Africans, primarily from West Africa, were brought to America within a span of 200 years. Even though these immigrants originated from nearby regions of Africa, they spoke a variety of languages.

For more information on the early history of African-Americans, the reader is referred to Kolchin (1995) and Thomas (1998). African-Americans represent a diverse community that includes long-time residents of the U.S., first-generation refugees from Africa, and immigrants from the West Indies and the Caribbean.

The largest majority of blacks reside in the South, and more black than non-Hispanic populations live in metropolitan areas (51.1% as compared with only 21.1%). The black population is generally younger and there are fewer 65-year-old females and males as compared with the non-Hispanic group. Fewer black families consist of married couples (33.2%)—as compared with non-Hispanic white families (47%). There are educational discrepancies as well. More black females than males complete bachelor's degrees, but in total, there are fewer blacks with bachelor's degrees than non-Hispanic whites (17.5% vs. 27.3%). In general, blacks account for about one-quarter of the U.S. population living in poverty (McKinnon, 2003).

Asian-Americans and Pacific Islanders

The members of this group constitute an even more diverse population than the Hispanics. Some early records indicate that the Chinese have been emigrating to the United States for the past two centuries. During that period, several Asian groups, including Chinese, Japanese, Filipinos, and Koreans settled in Hawaii first. In the last 30 years, countless Southeast Asian refugees have moved to the United States. Cheng (1993) reports that the earlier Chinese, Japanese, and Filipino immigrants have assimilated more easily into the American culture and language than have more recent immigrants originating from Indochina, Hong Kong, China, and other Pacific Rim countries.

Cheng (1991, 1993), in her review of major Asian-American and Pacific Islander groups, provides information on each group's cultural and linguistic characteristics, including religious and philosophical beliefs, that are essential to understand when working with these populations. Table 1-2 lists the backgrounds of the various Asian-American and Pacific Islander groups, including the major languages spoken and religions practiced. Note that as many as 1,200 indigenous languages are spoken throughout Asia and the Pacific Islands and include languages such as Chamorro, Marshaleese, Carolinian, Samoan, Hawaiian, Fijian, and Tahitian, among others.

There are language representatives from various other language families. For example, Tagalog and Illocano, spoken in the Philippines, belong to the Malayo-Polynesian family. Tai, Yao, Mandarin, and Cantonese belong to the Sino-Tibetan family, whereas Vietnamese, and Khmer belong to the Austro-Asiatic family. For more details about the origin and some characteristics of various languages, the reader is referred to Baker and Prys Jones (1998), Campbell (1995), and Katzner (2002). The countries comprising the various regions of Asia and the Pacific Islands, as well as the languages and major religions practiced in those regions, are listed in Table 1-2. As noted, different languages are spoken and different religions practiced in each country—even if all the countries are included within the same continent. The religions represented include Hinduism, Buddhism, Confucianism, Taoism, Shintoism, Animism, Protestant Christianity or Catholicism, and Islam (Cheng, 1993).

TABLE 1-2 Major Languages and Religions in Asia and the Pacific Islands

Geographic Location	Country/Region	Major Languages	Major Religions
East Asia	China	Chinese and dialects such as Mandarin, Wo, Min, Yue, and Hakka, including Hmong*	Buddhism and Taoism
	Taiwan	Taiwanese (variety of Min dialect), Mandarin Chinese	Buddhism, Confucianism, and Taoism
	Hong Kong	English and Cantonese	Buddhism, Confucianism, and Taoism
	Japan	Japanese	Shintoism and Buddhism
	Korea	Korean	Buddhism and Confucianism
Southeast Asia	Philippines	Bisayo, Tagalog, Illocano, and another 80 languages	Christianity
	Vietnam	Vietnamese and another 50 other languages	Confucianism
	Cambodia	Khmer	Buddhism
	Laos	Lao and about 90 other languages, including Hmong*	Buddhism
	Malaysia	Bahasa Melayu (plus many varieties of Chinese)	Buddhism and Taoism
	Singapore	Chinese, Tamil, Malay, and English	Buddhism and Islam
	Indonesia	Bahasa Indonesia and 600 other languages	Islam (Majority)
	Thailand	Thai, Chinese, English, and Hmong	Buddhism
South Asia	India	Hindi and English (and another 15 languages that include Panjabi, Urdu, Gujarati, Sanskrit, Tamil, Kannada, etc.)	Hinduism
	Pakistan	Panjabi, Pashto, Urdu (official language), and many other languages	Islam
	Bangladesh	Bengali and English	Islam
Pacific Islands	Hawaii	Hawaiian and English	Protestant Christianity, variety of languages
	Guam	English, Chamorro, and Tagalog	Catholicism
	American Samoa	English and Samoan	Congregationalist, Roman Catholicism
	Tonga	English and Tongan	Christian
	Fiji	Fijian and Hindi	Christian and Hindu
	Micronesian Islands (includes Palau, Yap, Kosrae, and Truk)	English and a variety of other languages, including Kosraen, Pohnpelan, Chuukese, and Yapese	Various religions

*Hmong is highlighted because a large number of immigrants live in certain areas of the U.S., including Wisconsin, Minnesota, and California.
Source: Compiled from Cheng, 1991, and Katzner, 2002.

Native American and Alaskan Populations

These two groups are the least numerous; only 2.5 million people responded to the 2000 Census by stating that they were Native American or Native Alaskan—and this number represents only approximately 0.9% of the total American population. Additionally, 1.6 million indicated they were biracial—that they were Native American or Alaskan Native and have "another race." "The other race" included "Native American, Alaskan Native, and White" (66%), followed by "Native American, Alaskan Native, White, and Black or African-American" (11%). The rest of the respondents listed a different race. Responses came from 4.1 million people, representing 1.5% of the total American population (Ogunwole, 2002). It is estimated that today only 150 Native American languages are alive; several Native American languages are spoken by only a few older persons; and just a few are spoken by 10,000 persons or more (Francis & Reyhner, 2002).

Four out of 10 Native Americans live in the West, Southwest, or Midwest with some also living in New York and North Carolina. These individuals reside in states that include California, Oklahoma, Arizona, Texas, and New Mexico, with the largest numbers living in California and New York. The 10 largest Native American tribes include Cherokee, Navajo, Latin American Indian, Choctaw, Sioux, Chippewa, Apache, Blackfeet, Iroquois, and Pueblo.

LINGUISTIC GROUPS: FACTS AND FIGURES

This section includes data on both the general U.S. population's use of other languages than English and this population's proficiency in English. Another part of this section reports various data related to English-Language Learners (ELL). The term "ELL" refers to students who have not mastered the English language enough to be able to follow the academic curriculum in English without added instructional support.

General Population

In 2003, 18%, or 47 million people, reported that they spoke a language other than English (U.S. Census Bureau, 2003). Table 1-3 lists the 10 most frequently spoken languages.

In the U.S., the most widely spoken language other than English is Spanish, followed by Chinese. However, there is a wide gap between the number of Spanish speakers (28 million) and Chinese speakers (only 2 million). Other languages include a variety of Asian languages and a few European languages, such as German (spoken by 1.4 million people),

TABLE 1-3 Ten Languages Other Than English Most Frequently Spoken at Home

Language	Number of Speakers
Spanish	28.1 million
Chinese	2.0 million
French	1.6 million
German	1.4 million
Tagalog	1.2 million
Vietnamese and Italian	1.0 million each
Korean	0.9 million
Russian and Polish	0.7 million each
Arabic	0.6 million

Source: Adapted from Shin and Bruno, 2003.

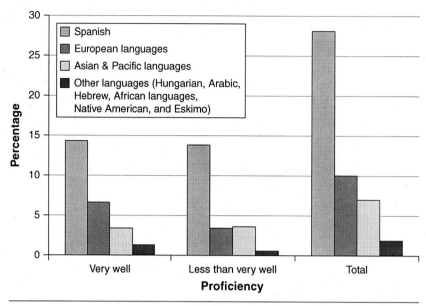

FIGURE 1-2 *English Proficiency of Various Linguistic Groups.* (Adapted from Shin and Bruno, 2003.)

French (spoken by 1.6 million people), and Russian and Polish (spoken by only about 700,000 people) (Shin & Bruno, 2003). Since 1990, the number of Vietnamese speakers has doubled from half a million to one million speakers, while the number of Russian speakers has tripled from 242,000 to 706,000, and the number of French Creole (Haitian Creole) speakers has doubled from 188,000 to 453,000 (Shin & Bruno, 2003). Figure 1-2 lists the various linguistic groups' proficiency in English.

Approximately 50% of the total number of Census respondents who speak Spanish or a variety of Asian and Pacific languages reported that they speak English "very well"—as compared with 66% of respondents whose native language is in the European or "other languages" group. However, the data need to be interpreted with care because "not being able to speak English very well" does not mean that the individual cannot read or write the language. Also, the data do not take into account the level of the respondents' linguistic ability or level of literacy in their own language.

School-Age Population

Within the last decade, the number of English-language learners (ELL) who are in the process of acquiring English as their second language has grown to almost 5 million nationwide, representing approximately 10% of the K–12 school population. Several names and acronyms have been used for these students over the last 30 years. In the 1970s a distinction was made between "Non-English-Speaking (NES)" and "Non-English-Proficient (NEP)" students, followed later by the term "Limited English Proficient (LEP)" students, a designation used for most of the 1980s and the beginning of the 1990s. The students who fit into these categories are currently referred to as ELL or English-language learners.

TABLE 1-4 States with the Largest Number of ELL Students

State	Number of ELL Students	Percentage of the Total Number of Students
California	1.6 million	26.6%
Texas	570,000	14.1%
New York	239,000	10.7%
Florida	254,000	9.3%
Arizona	135,000	15.7%

Source: Adapted from National Clearinghouse for Language Acquisition and Language Instruction Educational Programs, 2002.

TABLE 1-5 Ten Languages Most Frequently Spoken by ELL Students Nationwide

Language	Percentage
Spanish	76.9%
Vietnamese	2.4%
Hmong	1.8%
Korean	1.2%
Arabic	1.2%
Haitian Creole	1.1%
Cantonese	1.0%
Russian	0.9%
Tagalog	0.9%
Navajo	0.9%

Source: Adapted from Hopstock and Stephenson, 2003.

The states with the largest numbers of ELL students are listed in Table 1-4.

California, with 1.6 million, is the state with the largest number of ELL students (representing one-third of the total number of identified ELL students nationally), followed by Texas, New York, Florida, and Arizona.

In some districts, ELL students whose primary language is something other than English represent 400 different languages. Since 1990, the regular school population has increased about 19% as compared with 110% for the ELL student population (National Clearinghouse for English Language Acquisition and Language Instruction Educational Programs, 2003).

The top 10 languages most frequently spoken by ELL students are listed in Table 1-5. As noted, Spanish is the first most frequently spoken language, and there is a large discrepancy between the percentage of students who speak Spanish as their first language and the percentage of students who speak all the other languages listed. From a high of almost 80% for Spanish, the percentage decreases to only 2% for Vietnamese; all the remaining languages are below that level. Linguistic characteristics as well as the cultural characteristics of many of the principal languages spoken by English Language learners can be found in sources such as Campbell (1995), Roseberry-McKibbin (2002), and Swan and Smith (2004). For details about the top five languages spoken by ELL students by state, the reader is referred to Kindler (2002).

School-Age Children with Communicative Disorders

It is important to have information on the percentage of the CLD populations that are currently enrolled in special education and to identify those students who have more medical problems as compared with the normally developing CLD populations. Having this information helps avoid the over- or under-identification of CLD populations in the designated categories for special education services. Individuals who have learning difficulties and are eligible to receive additional assistance from special education are identified as qualifying for services based on a number of possible diagnoses, such as speech and language impairment (SLI), mental retardation (MR), Autism, and many others. Figures 1-3 A through G list percentages of students from various minority groups who are classified as being eligible for the various categories of special education programs. This comparison shows that there are more Hispanic and Native American students than white students labeled under Specific Learning Disability (SLD) (60.3%), and more Asian-American students than white students diagnosed with speech and language impairments (25.2%). Also, more African-American students have been identified as mentally retarded (18.9%) and relatively more Asian-American students have been labeled as autistic (3.4%) as compared with the white populations. This data certainly merit further investigation. However, more white students than students in any other category have been identified as having hearing impairments (5.9%). It is possible that more families of white children have access to health care or may be more aware of children's ear infections and the risk of decreased hearing. To avoid making incorrect diagnoses, these factors need to be considered when working with individual CLD students.

SLPs working with CLD students should be aware of information related to the identified health issues of various groups as these issues may impact hearing and speech/language development. Table 1-6 lists some health statistics that are helpful in working with CLD students and may explain the incidence of certain conditions that have ramifications for speech and language development.

The data reported in Table 1-6 indicate that there is a greater incidence of cleft lip/palate among Native Americans/Alaskan Natives as compared with any other group. Fetal alcohol syndrome is more prevalent among African-Americans, Hispanics, and Native Americans/Alaskan Natives than in the total population. For more references on various speech, language, and hearing impairments among CLD populations, the reader is referred to an excellent overview compiled by Castrogiovanni for the American Speech-Language-Hearing Association in 2004 (ASHA, 2005b). However, as noted by Castrogiovanni,

> There are few reliable data on the general incidence or prevalence of communication disorders among culturally and linguistically diverse populations in the United States. Estimates are based on projections from data founded on the mainstream population.... [Moreover,] there may not be adequate data on certain categories or illnesses such as otitis media among Hispanics. Further research into the Centers for Disease Control Web site have not yielded additional results" (A. Castrogiovanni, personal communication, August 11, 2005).

CURRENT SERVICES AVAILABLE TO CLD POPULATIONS WITH SPEECH AND LANGUAGE IMPAIRMENTS

The information presented in the previous sections indicates that SLPs can no longer rely on a "one-size-fits-all paradigm" that is based on one type of population, but must adjust to a variety of populations with different primary languages and cultures. In addition, SLPs must comply with new federal laws such as the Americans with Disabilities Act (ADA, 1990) and PL-94-1942 (which was enacted in

Specific Learning Disability (SLD)

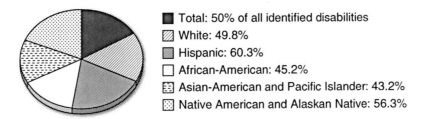

■ Total: 50% of all identified disabilities
▨ White: 49.8%
▦ Hispanic: 60.3%
☐ African-American: 45.2%
▣ Asian-American and Pacific Islander: 43.2%
▨ Native American and Alaskan Native: 56.3%

Note: The largest percentage is for the Hispanic and Native American–Alaskan Native groups. Percentages do not add up because they are related to the total number of students classified as White, Hispanic, or any given category.

A

Specific Language Impairment (SLI)

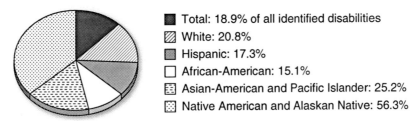

■ Total: 18.9% of all identified disabilities
▨ White: 20.8%
▦ Hispanic: 17.3%
☐ African-American: 15.1%
▣ Asian-American and Pacific Islander: 25.2%
▨ Native American and Alaskan Native: 56.3%

Note: The largest percentage is for the Native American and Alaskan Native group. Percentages do not add up because they are related to the total number of students classified as White, Hispanic, or any given category.

B

Mental Retardation (MR)

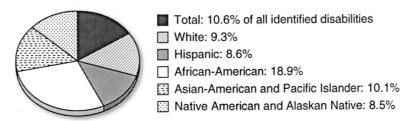

■ Total: 10.6% of all identified disabilities
▨ White: 9.3%
▦ Hispanic: 8.6%
☐ African-American: 18.9%
▣ Asian-American and Pacific Islander: 10.1%
▨ Native American and Alaskan Native: 8.5%

Note: The largest percentage is for the African-American group. Percentages do not add up because they are related to the total number of students classified as White, Hispanic, or any given category.

C

FIGURE 1-3 *A. Percentage of CLD Students Classified under Specific Learning Disability (SLD). B. Percentage of CLD Students Classified under Specific Language Impairment (SLI). C. Percentage of CLD Students Classified under Mental Retardation (MR). (Continues)*

Emotional Disturbance (ED)

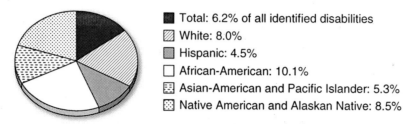

Total: 6.2% of all identified disabilities
White: 8.0%
Hispanic: 4.5%
African-American: 10.1%
Asian-American and Pacific Islander: 5.3%
Native American and Alaskan Native: 8.5%

Note: The largest percentage is for the African-American group. Percentages do not add up because they are related to the total number of students classified as White, Hispanic, or any given category.

D

Autism

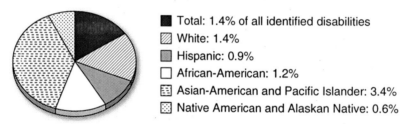

Total: 1.4% of all identified disabilities
White: 1.4%
Hispanic: 0.9%
African-American: 1.2%
Asian-American and Pacific Islander: 3.4%
Native American and Alaskan Native: 0.6%

Note: The largest percentage is for the Asian-American and Pacific Islander group. Percentages do not add up because they are related to the total number of students classified as White, Hispanic, or any given category.

E

Hearing Impairment (HI)

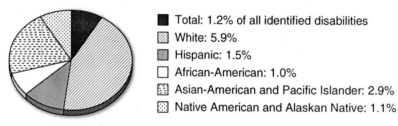

Total: 1.2% of all identified disabilities
White: 5.9%
Hispanic: 1.5%
African-American: 1.0%
Asian-American and Pacific Islander: 2.9%
Native American and Alaskan Native: 1.1%

Note: The largest percentage is for the White group. Percentages do not add up because they are related to the total number of students classified as White, Hispanic, or any given category.

F

FIGURE 1-3 *D. Percentage of CLD Students Classified under Emotional Disturbance (ED). E. Percentage of CLD Students Classified under Autism. F. Percentage of CLD Students Classified under Hearing Impairment (HI). (Continues)*

Traumatic Brain Injury (TBI)

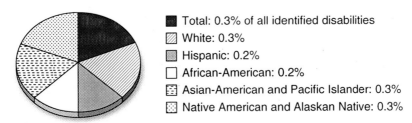

Total: 0.3% of all identified disabilities

White: 0.3%

Hispanic: 0.2%

African-American: 0.2%

Asian-American and Pacific Islander: 0.3%

Native American and Alaskan Native: 0.3%

Note: Percentages are equal among most groups. Percentages do not add up because they are related to the total number of students classified as White, Hispanic, or any given category.

G

FIGURE 1-3 *G. Percentage of CLD Students Classified under Traumatic Brain Injury (TBI).* (Adapted from U.S. Department of Education, 2001.)

TABLE 1-6 Health-Related Data for CLD Students

Health Issues	Total	White	Hispanic	African-American	Asian-American/ Pacific Islander	Native American/ Alaskan Native
Cleft Lip/Palate	1‰ births	N/A	N/A	1/2500 births	1.7‰ births	3.6‰ births
Fetal Alcohol	0.6‰ births	N/A	5.21‰ births	5.41‰ births	N/A	5.2/‰ births
Otitis Media	25.2%	26.2%	N/A	22.2%	N/A	N/A
Sickle Cell Anemia	N/A	N/A	1/‰ births	1/500 births	N/A	N/A

Source: Adapted from American Speech-Language-Hearing Association (ASHA), 2005b.

1975 and reauthorized in 1997 as the Individuals with Disabilities Education Act—IDEA.) The IDEA was revised in 2004 and reiterates what had been stated in previous legislation: that "assessment must be provided and administered in the language and form most likely to yield accurate information on what the child knows and can do academically, developmentally, and functionally" (IDEA, 2004, Sec. 614b). For a summary of main amendments to the IDEA 2004, the reader is referred to Mandlawitz (2006).

A survey of public school clinicians' comments on delivery of services to English-language learners (ELL) that was conducted in 2001 compared results with data from an earlier survey carried out in 1994. The responses indicated that clinicians from the West and Southwest of the U.S. had received more coursework in the area of assessment and intervention for multicultural/multilingual populations as compared with clinicians from other areas of the country. These same clinicians had more ELL students in their caseloads than clinicians from other regions did. The authors of the study, Roseberry-McKibbin, Brice, and O'Hanlon (2005), conclude that not only are there more ELL students attending public schools in the West and Southwest, but those clinicians who had taken coursework were more aware of communication disorders among ELL students. Seventy-three percent of a total of 1,145 participants had taken a university course in the area of nonbiased assessment; this is in contrast with only 23% who had taken such a course in the earlier (1994) study. Those clinicians who had taken courses were more aware of the complexities involved in assessing ELL students than were those who had not taken any coursework. The main challenges faced by clinicians were similar in both the 1994 and 2001 surveys, and included (in order of importance) the following: (1) "clinicians don't speak the language of the student"; (2) "there is a lack of appropriate, less-biased assessment instruments"; (3) "there is a lack of availability of other professionals who speak the students' language"; and (4) "there is a lack of developmental norms in the student's primary language." In both surveys, participants wished to have more continuing education in "assessment procedures and materials," and wished to know more about the "effects of bilingualism on language learning." However, the researchers did not report their findings about the tools the survey participants used to assess ELL students, and questions related to the process of collaborating with an interpreter/translator were not fully answered (Roseberry-McKibbin et al., 2005).

Another survey conducted by ASHA (2003) of clinicians working in various settings indicated that only 5% of 115,000 ASHA members (approximately 7,000 people) provide services in a language other than English (V. Deal, personal communication, fall, 2004). This number includes approximately 50% who reported using manual communication. The definition of "bilingual clinician" is based on a self-nomination process and includes no validation of the clinician's command of a language or ability to treat all aspects of the client's speech, language, and communication abilities (ASHA, 1988). This definition appears in Box 1-1. Only 3,500 members, or approximately 3% of the total membership, stated that they could offer bilingual services to their clients in a language other than English.

As noted earlier, assessment, intervention, and interaction with the student/client and contact with the student/client's family all constitute different contexts and demand different levels of linguistic proficiency. The communication interactions and skills needed to take a developmental history are different from assessing a child's phonological and linguistic development, which necessitates transcribing and analyzing a language sample. In the first case, the speaker may not need to know or listen to linguistic nuances as carefully, whereas in the second case, familiarity with patterns of speech and phonology and syntax errors is fundamental to an accurate analysis. Furthermore, the bilingual SLP must be familiar with patterns of normal monolingual and bilingual language development, as well as with the interferences that occur between two languages—the particular language and English.

The definition of the bilingual SLP is very ambitious because knowledge of monolingual language development in most languages other than English (with the exception of Spanish and a few other languages) is only emerging. Furthermore, studies on bilingual language development in English and other languages (primarily Spanish), although spanning decades, are still incomplete. This issue is discussed in greater detail in Chapter 2. Therefore, spoken

---

BOX 1-1

Bilingual Speech-Language Pathologists and Audiologists: Definition

This ASHA 1989 document that defines the roles and responsibilities of bilingual speech-language pathologists or audiologists who present themselves as bilingual for the purposes of providing clinical services. According to the definition, such professionals must be able to speak their primary language and to speak (or sign) at least one other language with native or near-native proficiency in lexicon (vocabulary), semantics (meaning), phonology (pronunciation), morphology/syntax (grammar), and pragmatics (use) during clinical management. The bilingual clinician who provides bilingual assessments and remediation services in the client's language must have several of the competencies that are listed below:

1. The ability to describe the process of normal speech and language acquisition for both bilingual and monolingual individuals and how these processes are manifested in oral (or manually coded) and written language

2. The ability to administer and interpret formal and informal assessment procedures to distinguish between communication differences and communicative disorders in oral (or manually coded) and written language

3. The ability to apply intervention strategies for treatment of communication disorders in the client's language, and provide language pathology and audiology services to the client's language community

4. The ability to recognize cultural factors which affect the delivery of speech-language pathology and audiology services to the client's language community

Source: Adapted from "Bilingual Speech-Language Pathologist and Audiologist Definition," by the American Speech-Language-Hearing Association (ASHA), 1988, *Asha, 31*, p. 64.

---

and written proficiency skills in another language are not sufficient parameters for ensuring adequate clinical services in speech-language pathology in that language. An individual clinician may be very proficient or even be a native speaker of a given language, but nevertheless lack practice in using the language in the context of clinical-service delivery. In addition, incomplete knowledge of a particular language's development—and of bilingual language development in that language and English—makes clinical-service delivery very difficult.

Therefore, knowing a language does not necessarily mean that one is proficient in using the language in all possible contexts. This concept is also important in the selection of interpreters/translators, because the person available might know the languages well enough to translate meaning in certain contexts but not in others. Knowledge of procedures and specific terminology are necessary (Langdon & Cheng, 2002). In addition, the likelihood that a clinician's language will match that of the client is often minimal. A clinician who speaks Spanish may need to work with someone who speaks only a certain dialect of Arabic. Bilingual and monolingual clinicians therefore face similar challenges. An ASHA omnibus survey (2003) indicated that of 1,871 respondents, only 37.7% understand well and can apply information based on knowledge of

PERSONAL STORIES

Bilingual SLP: A Personal Story

I am a native speaker of Spanish, who was trained in the field of speech and language pathology in English. Because I spoke Spanish, I was hired to provide bilingual Spanish-English services in a major children's hospital in the Boston area, working primarily with children from Puerto Rican Spanish-speaking backgrounds. Even though I was a native speaker of Spanish and I had both native command of the oral and written language, I needed to learn to use Spanish in a specific way, which I had never done before. It was like learning a new role using that language. I had to learn to use the language to interview a parent, to translate terms that I had never used in Spanish such as "language disorder," "articulation skills," "auditory association," "receptive and expressive language," and many other professional terms. I had to learn to scaffold my language to maximize my clients' Spanish-language comprehension and expression. In addition, I had to modify some of the words I used because I speak the Mexican dialect. I had to learn to name a bird "pichón" and not "pájaro"; name a bus "guagua" and not "camión"; and name a banana "guineo" and not "plátano." This process took some time.

normal stages of second-language acquisition; only 15.9% understand the impact of simultaneous vs. sequential bilingual-language development, and only 22.4% comprehend the role of code-switching (which is defined as using two different languages within a phrase or sentence). Only 29.9% of respondents reported understanding the impact of second-language acquisition on academic success, and 27.4% understood how the role of social and environmental factors affects second-language acquisition. Overall, slightly higher numbers of respondents, who understood and could apply their knowledge in the areas mentioned above, provided services to CLD populations in school as opposed to hospital settings. Compared with participants in the survey who worked in hospital settings, participants who worked in school settings demonstrated a greater understanding of the skills just mentioned, and were more suc-

cessful in applying their knowledge when working with CLD populations.

Therefore, the 2003 ASHA survey, as well as the recent findings by Roseberry-McKibbin et al. (2005), clearly show that there is a need to assist both students-in-training as well as practicing clinicians in developing the competence to work with linguistically and culturally diverse clients.

SUMMARY

This chapter provided the reader with some facts and figures related to the current diversity of populations residing in the United States. The groups that were primarily discussed included Hispanics, African-Americans (although the term "blacks" was often used because it figures in statistical data), Asian-Americans and Pacific Islanders, and Native

OUR CLIENTS

Eric, Ana, Jack, Grace, and Leonardo

Throughout the book we will follow five cases of individuals of various ages, linguistic backgrounds, and experiences. Our first three clients are school-age children, the other two are adults.

1. Eric is a 4-year-old preschool child whose parents speak primarily Vietnamese to him and who is referred to the SLP because of low expressive skills in both Vietnamese and English.

2. Ana is a 9-year-old enrolled in fourth grade; she emigrated from Mexico at the age of 5 and is having difficulty reading in English.

3. Jack is a 14-year-old of African-American descent; he has difficulty with subjects such as social studies, English, and writing.

4. Grace is a 60-year-old Mandarin-speaking former business woman who sustained a stroke while visiting the United States.

5. Leonardo is a 45-year-old fieldworker from Guatemala who suffered a traumatic brain injury following a dispute with a neighbor.

Americans and Alaskan Natives. These groups were discussed at greater length than others were because there is much more statistical information available for these groups regarding population numbers, education, health, and occupation—as compared with the many other groups from the Middle East, or from Eastern Europe. It was noted in this chapter, as well as in this book's Preface, that the language most frequently spoken in the home is Spanish (spoken by as many as 28 million people), followed by Chinese (spoken by only 2 million). Other languages are cited in Table P-1 in the Preface, and include German, Italian, Arabic, and Russian. These languages are spoken by only 1 million or fewer people, respectively.

Although Spanish is the most prevalent second language spoken in the United States, various other populations currently living in the nation use 400 other languages. Not only does this result in a significant number of language variations, but the experiences and cultures of the individuals who speak those languages also vary a great deal. These variations depend on factors such as the number of years of U.S. residency, education, issues of assimilation and acculturation, and last (but not least), individual differences. Therefore, no two persons from a given group are the same; each individual must be treated as unique. Working effectively with CLD populations means understanding their unique backgrounds in order to best assess and treat their communication disorders.

FURTHER READINGS

Baker, C., & Prys Jones (1998). *Encyclopedia of bilingual education and bilingualism*. Clevedon, UK: Multilingual Matters.

Edwards, V. (2004). *Multilingualism in the English-speaking world*. Malden, MA: Blackwell Publishing.

Nieto, S. (2004). *Affirming diversity: The sociopolitical context of multicultural education* (4th ed.). Boston: Pearson.

C H A P T E R 2

SECOND-LANGUAGE DEVELOPMENT AND DUAL LANGUAGE PROCESSES

"Human beings have the brain capacity to learn and retain several languages. In many countries it is not just the advantaged 'elite' who are multilingual, but the majority of the population, of all social classes" (Baker & Prys Jones, 1998, p. 19).

C H A P T E R O U T L I N E

INTRODUCTION

The above quotation serves to remind us that as human beings, we can learn and use two or more languages. However, the term bilingual *may have different meanings to different people. For some, it may mean the ability to communicate orally and in writing in more than one language, while for others, it may mean being able to understand, speak, read, or write in more than one language. However, these definitions do not include the individual's level of proficiency in, or preference for, one language or the other, nor does it include the individual's language performance in specific contexts. For example, one may be more proficient in speaking about certain topics in one language, but feel more proficient in writing in the other language. In very few cases do bilinguals have a balanced competence in all of their languages, or possess this competence at the level that a monolingual speaker of either language does (Baker, 2006; Baker & Prys Jones, 1998; Bialystok, 2001).*

This chapter will discuss issues related to dual-language development, including the use of and interaction between two languages. Having prior knowledge of these issues is vital for speech-language practitioners if they are to avoid under- or overdiagnosing a communication disorder in multilingual culturally and linguistically diverse (CLD) populations. The information presented in this chapter is important for the speech-language pathologist (SLP) because it can help the SLP: (1) avoid confusing a possible language disorder with the normal process of bilingual language acquisition; (2) keep in mind common phenomena that occur when two languages are developing either simultaneously or sequentially, and (3) understand factors that may accelerate or deter bilingual language development.

BILINGUAL LANGUAGE DEVELOPMENT

The available literature of the last 30 to 40 years has shed light into many aspects of first- and second-language acquisition and development. However, the field is still relatively in its "infancy" with regard to providing data about the language development of monolingual speakers of languages other than English. Some exceptions include information on the development of Spanish, African-American English, French (North America), Korean, and Inuktitut (Inuktitut is described in a volume edited by Taylor and Leonard, 1999).

Research on Spanish, French, and Korean bilingual children is now emerging, but continues to be fragmentary (Goldstein, 2004a). For example, there is more information about the bilingual phonological, semantic, and morphological development of bilingual Spanish/English-speaking children than there is about bilingual French/English- or Korean/English-speaking children (Choi, 1999; Fortin & Crago, 1999; Goldstein, 2004a).

The studies that have been conducted report the development of linguistic structures during various stages of language development, but it is difficult to compare the studies, because of differences in the focus of each study. One study may refer to the use of certain grammatical forms in a given language, while a study of another language may focus on different grammatical forms. (Refer to Romaine, 1995, for a discussion of some studies of simultaneous bilingual language development.) Also, the research is less systematic because most of the studies in other language combinations are cross-sectional rather than longitudinal, and only selected linguistic aspects have been analyzed. This is not unusual given that such studies are difficult to design and very costly to carry out. With the exception of studies on Spanish and French, there are no systematic studies that I know of that have followed bilinguals in most of the languages that are represented in the demographics of the United States. Examples of such bilingual language combinations include Vietnamese-English, Hmong-English, and Chinese-English. Furthermore, the majority of the longitudinal studies on bilingual children are case studies conducted by linguists in additive bilingual environments. In referring to those studies, Bialystok (2001) comments, "The majority of these accounts, however, reflect a single reality: an educated middle-class family that has made a conscious decision to raise the children with two languages. Although this does not undermine the reliability of the descriptions produced by these studies, it does leave open a question about their generalizability to other social contexts" (p. 10).

Simultaneous vs. Sequential Bilingualism

In his Acquisition-Learning Hypothesis, Krashen (1981, 1982) proposes two ways to explain the process of bilingual language development. The first is the spontaneous "acquisition" of a language, which is a subconscious process occurring in both children and adults. The other is the "learning" of a language, which is attained through formal education. In the next section, when relevant, I will refer to my personal experiences with the four languages I speak as a way to illustrate certain points. Chapter 3 will discuss in greater depth the issues inherent in the process of "learning" another language.

"Acquired" bilingualism can occur principally within three different scenarios: (1) parents speak a different language to the child than the one spoken by the community; (2) each parent speaks a different language; or (3) the child is exposed to a second language through daycare or playgroup activities. For example, each parent in a family may speak a different language and the community a third language, or the child may speak one language at home, another in the community, and a third language at school (where the third language is the language of instruction) (Baker, 2000, 2006; Genesee, Paradis, & Crago, 2004).

When children acquire two languages simultaneously prior to age 3, they are considered to be simultaneous bilingual learners, and when they acquire a second language after the first has developed, they are referred to as sequential language learners. There is, however, disagreement among researchers about the specific linguistic stages (one vs. more words at a time) involved in establishing the simultaneous-sequential bilingualism dichotomy (Bialystok, 2001; Hammer, Miccio, & Rodríguez, 2004). We can, nonetheless, describe typical characteristics of bilingual children's language skills—whether they are simultaneous or sequential learners. The following characteristics can be described: (1) the different timelines for the development of vocabulary and language skills, (2) the learner's awareness of two languages, (3) the issue of code-switching, and (4) the cognitive implications of learning two or more languages.

Different Timelines for the Development of Vocabulary and Language Skills

Unless two languages are used under identical conditions, the differences between those languages with regard to vocabulary, syntax, and grammar will be noted. Efficiency in the processing or production of oral language in particular contexts will vary as well. For example, a child might have a larger vocabulary for household items in one language, or use more detail in telling a story in one language as compared with the other. Thus, it is important to assess the individual's competence in both languages and to document the particular contexts in which each language is used. The collaboration of a trained interpreter/translator (I/T) will therefore be essential when the SLP and the client do not speak the same language. Langdon and Cheng (2002) outline steps to follow when collaborating with an interpreter to assess individuals. This topic is further discussed in Chapter 5.

A timeline for the child's acquisition of each language (obtained from the parent or main caregiver), and a description of contexts in which each language is used, is helpful for understanding differences in bilingual language performance.

Awareness of Two Languages

Bilingual children have the ability to perceive that the two languages they are exposed to are different, as evidenced by comments such as, "I speak like Mommy" and "I speak like Daddy"— or by the fact that the children respond in the language in which the interaction is taking place. Ronjat (1913) (French-German) and Leopold (1970) (German-English) are some of the pioneer linguists who documented their bilingual children's ability to differentiate between two languages from as early as 18 months of age. Other studies on young children speaking combinations of various languages report the same phenomenon (Langdon & Merino, 1992). More recently, experiments described in Genesee (2003) and Genesee, Nicoladis, and Paradis (1995) that were conducted with young 2-year-old English-French bilinguals document this important concept. The researchers report how young bilingual children were observed to use more English when they spoke with the parent who addressed them in English, and more French with the other parent. Furthermore, when monolingual strangers addressed the children in their respective languages, the children were observed to use more of the language in which the stranger communicated with them. Some aspects of each language develop autonomously, while others are more dependent on the other language. For example, phonology may develop more autonomously, while syntax may depend more on the combination of the two languages. If children code-switch from one language to the other within one sentence, they seem to do it according to the accepted patterns of code-switching that would be found in their adult model (for a review of this subject, refer to Genesee, 2003). A possible language disorder manifests itself when the child is unaware of which language he/she speaks, or does not respond in the language of interaction at the same level of competence as do other children in the community.

Issues of Code-Switching

Bilingual children typically mix the two languages; they insert a word from one language while conversing in the other (Genesee et al., 2004; Nicoladis & Secco, 2000). Children

PERSONAL STORIES

A Personal Note

I was a simultaneous bilingual in Polish and Spanish. My parents and grandparents spoke to me in Polish and I acquired Spanish as a result of living in Mexico since infancy. I became a sequential bilingual in French at the age of 5 when I entered first grade in an immersion French school in Mexico City. I learned English more formally at the age of 12. While a preschooler, I remember communicating in each of the two languages, Polish and Spanish, with ease. My mother reports the following incident when I was 3 years old. While riding my 2-year-old brother on the stand of my tricycle, my brother said, "Teta [my nickname], jéchame más" [a combination of the prefix of the Polish "jechac," which means "give me a ride," and the Spanish "más," which means "more"]. To this I replied, "ya te jeché bastante," using once again the prefix of the Polish "jechac" and adding the "é" for past tense in Spanish: "I have given you enough rides." This is an example of code-switching.

For most of my childhood, I navigated effortlessly between Polish, Spanish, and French. Each language "meant something different" in my daily life and different people interacted with me in each of those languages. However, neither my oral nor my written proficiency in Polish, Spanish, French, or English is equivalent. Today, because I work with primarily Spanish-speaking children and adults, and I read and write the two languages on a daily basis, I am equally proficient in most language areas in both Spanish and English. My oral and written proficiencies are not as complete in French due to lack of practice. I can discuss both abstract and everyday topics in Polish but I cannot read or write the language as fluently as I speak it due to a lack of explicit instruction in that language.

may also make up a new word utilizing the prefix of the word in one language and inserting the suffix in the other language. Nevertheless, the child can be understood and progresses in each language as long as the environment provides opportunities for further development, and as long as comprehension in each language (which often is not discussed in the literature) is normal as reported by parents and caretakers. As will be further discussed in this chapter, it is not unusual in bilingual communities for bilingual speakers to alternate languages (code-switch). Therefore, this phenomenon should not be viewed as a sign of disability.

Cognitive Implications of Learning Two or More Languages

The simultaneous exposure to and use of more than one language does not cause harm or constitute a too-demanding cognitive task for the child—if the language-learning occurs in an environment where there is support for the development of two languages (Genesee, 2003). In other words, whether a child is harmed or disadvantaged in some way by simultaneous language exposure depends on how and when the languages are "nurtured." Children who have learned a variety of combinations of two languages show no difference in their performance of specific phonological, syntactical, or lexicon-related tasks as compared with monolingual or bilingual children. Studies on this topic have examined language combinations such as Spanish and Catalan (Bosh & Sebastián-Gallés, 2001), French and English (Goodz, Legarré, & Bilodeau, 1990; Paradis, 2001; Paradis & Genesee 1996), and Spanish and English (Pearson, Fernández, & Oller, 1993; Umbel & Oller, 1994).

A bilingual child may have different abilities in each one of the two languages depending on the child's exposure to the language. For example, the child may have a large vocabulary for home- and food-related items in one language and a large vocabulary for animals in the other language. The child may respond with longer and more complex sentences in one language but not in the other—because of having had greater practice in expressing ideas in one and not the other. Thus, assessing only what may be considered the "dominant" language is not desirable, because it does not provide sufficient information about the individual's true language proficiency as manifested across both languages. Instead, both languages should be assessed.

Factors Affecting Bilingual Language Development

Several factors influence the rate of and success in acquiring two languages: (1) socioeconomic status (SES), (2) attitude of the community toward bilingualism, (3) the learner's age, and (4) personal factors such as motivation and aptitude. Second-language pedagogy and bilingual programs, which can influence success in learning another language, will be discussed in greater detail in Chapter 3.

Socioeconomic Status (SES)

A family's high socioeconomic status is a factor that can contribute to the acceleration of a learner's acquisition of language skills. Socioeconomic status can also play a role in arresting the process of language loss (Anderson, 2004; Hammer et al., 2004; Oller & Eilers, 2002; Wei & Milroy, 2003). Poverty negatively affects a child's language and cognitive development because of fewer opportunities to be exposed to diverse experiences and literacy-based events such as joint reading. One of the disadvantages of poverty is that students may take more time to arrive at comparable levels of competence in relation to their more socioeconomically advantaged peers.

However, the type of bilingual programs in which the student is enrolled also plays a role in the student's ultimate linguistic and academic achievement. Oller and Eilers (2002) compared the performance of over 950 bilingual children (Spanish-English) from two different socioeconomic groups (SES) in Miami at three different grade levels using various tasks such as narrative production and knowledge of grammar. In the earlier grades the higher SES students performed better in English while the lower SES students performed better in Spanish. The two groups scored comparably in English by the fifth grade. Comparison of two-way programs, where both English and Spanish were used in instruction, showed a slight advantage over English immersion programs. Thus, the students instructed in both English and Spanish performed better as compared with those students who attended English immersion programs exclusively. Therefore, SES might not have played as big a role in the children's language acquisition as did the amount of English exposure they received and the appropriate instructional program that was adapted.

Attitude of the Community toward Bilingualism

In extensive, pioneering studies of language immersion programs in Canada, Peal and Lambert (1962) addressed the importance of the community's attitude toward the learning and maintenance of the learner's native language. Additive bilingualism occurs when the community's attitude toward bilingualism is positive. This is contrasted with subtractive bilingualism, where maintenance of the speaker's native language does not occur. A positive attitude toward the learner's native language, which infers acceptance of the culture, will facilitate the acquisition of a second language and have positive effects on cognitive skills (discussed later in this chapter) (Bialystock, 2001; Cummins, 2000). However, the "survival" of the native language is often the result of families' efforts to maintain the native language at home in spite of a neutral or negative attitude from the community toward it. This phenomenon is quite common in the United States and, for that matter, around the globe—where children lose their native language due to the mainstream culture's lack of exposure to and appreciation for the language and its heritage.

The Learner's Age

The influence of age on language acquisition has been discussed widely in the literature, which has suggested that there may or may not be critical periods for acquiring certain language features such as phonology, syntax, or pragmatics. However, the outcomes of the research studies have varied depending on the methodology used (for a review of this subject, see Bialystok, 2001). There is no simple answer to the question of which age is best for acquiring a certain language, because there are other intervening factors such as the learner's personality, motivation, and first-language level of proficiency. Other variables include the similarity and differences between the two languages being learned, the learner's aptitude, and last but not least, the learning context and type of instruction. It is often believed that younger students learn faster and better and that older students have more difficulty, but in fact it is difficult to draw specific conclusions. Although many features of a language may be acquired later in life, accent (pronunciation) seems to be the most liable. Therefore, the length of time necessary for children, adolescents, or adults to master a second language depends on the linguistic area considered. For example, adolescents and adults may initially acquire morphological and syntactical skills in the second language rapidly. However, those who begin learning a second language at a younger age will attain higher levels of performance in the language. There may be critical times when certain language features, such as accent, are acquired with greater facility, but the acquisition of other language components may not be as time-sensitive. As an example, Flege, Frieda, and Nozawa (1997) studied the accent of various second-language learners of different ages and found that a native-like pronunciation (i.e., native to the second language) was perceptible for those sounds that were either most similar to or different from the learner's native language. Those sounds that "fell in between" were the ones in which the speaker's native accent (i.e., native to the first language) was most perceptible; these were also the sounds most difficult to learn past the age of 7. These findings contradict somewhat some researchers' earlier claims that foreign accent is most perceptible when the learner is older than age 12 (Singleton, 1989).

Some conclusions from an extensive research study conducted 20 years ago still

PERSONAL STORIES

The History behind the Four Languages I Speak

I learned Spanish and English simultaneously from birth. When I speak Spanish, my accent is reflective of the Mexican native accent (i.e., the accent used in Mexico City) and it becomes refined when I visit Mexico.

On the other hand, despite my fluency in Polish, one can detect that I do not speak Polish as a native, even though Polish is my "native" language. Nevertheless, because I have spoken Polish since I first began to speak, natives have been impressed by my fluency in the language despite my "nonnative" accent. The noticeable "foreign accent" heard when I speak Polish may be due to the fact that I interacted in the language with adults only (i.e., with my parents and grandparents but not with peers).

I spoke my first sentences in French when I was 5 ½ years old, and had opportunities to hear and interact with native French speakers of all ages for the duration of my primary and secondary education. When I am in France or when I meet native speakers of French, they are impressed by my genuine French pronunciation.

This is not the case with English. Even though I have spent most of my adult life in the United States, the minute I speak, others can detect a nonnative accent. I attribute the "foreign" accent heard when I speak English to the fact that I learned English from bilingual speakers of French and English, whose accents were distinct. My first introduction to English occurred at a crucial time (between the ages of 12 and 14) (Lenneberg, E. 1967). However, the opportunities to interact with English-speaking peers were almost nonexistent at the time. Factors like these need to be considered when judging the language and speech patterns of a person interacting in more than one language.

have implications regarding the best time to learn another language. Collier (1987) studied 1,500 students who were learning English on a "pull-out basis" (pulling a student out of their regular classroom to receive more individual assistance in a small group), in addition to being immersed in all English classrooms. The students came from middle-class backgrounds and performed at grade level in their native languages (Spanish, Vietnamese, Korean). Controlling for the students' length of residency, Collier found that 8- to 11-year-olds were the fastest achievers; they required two to five years for reaching 50% in the National

Curve Equivalents (NCEs), which are national norms for all academic areas. Those in the 5- to 7-year-old age group were one to three years behind the 8- to 11-year-olds. Adolescents who were 12 to 15 years old experienced the most difficulty, requiring as much as six to eight years for attaining grade-level norms.

The results of this study indicate that age alone is not a factor in predicting success in learning another language. However, it is true that the facility with which a second language—or for that matter, any learning—is acquired may decline with age. This difficulty is related to decreasing skill levels in certain prerequisites necessary for successful language learning—such as auditory perception and working memory. This is true especially for populations who are 65 and older, a fact which has the greatest implications for those SLPs who work with older clients. For a review of the various aspects of language ability and learning in older populations, the reader is referred to de Bot and Makoni (2005).

Personal Factors

Personal factors such as the motivation and aptitude for learning a second language are important to consider. Genesee et al. (2004) reported that motivation might be a stronger factor for adults than for children. Gardner (1985) distinguishes between two types of motivation: instrumental and integrative. Learning or preserving a language may take place because of instrumental/personal reasons, such as being able to obtain a better job or being able to communicate with desirable persons. Integrative motivation means that the person will preserve or learn another or other languages to "be like or identify with members of a particular language community" (Baker & Prys Jones, 1998, p. 651). There are communities all over the world where adults may never have to use the majority language, because there are neither instrumental nor integrative motivations to learn it. Their daily lives do not depend on communication in the other language.

Differences in motivation for learning a language emerge early. Wong-Fillmore (1983) observed the behaviors of 48 kindergarten children whose native language was either Cantonese or Spanish and who were enrolled in an English classroom. The children who learned English with the greatest ease were either very social (they approached other children to interact with them) or very shy—but shyly attentive to the learning environ-

ment. Observing students in a learning environment assists in identifying the unique strategies they use to acquire skills in the new language. In my practice I have witnessed cases of children who clearly stated that "they did not like speaking English." At the time it was difficult to determine whether this statement was something the child had thought of on his or her own or if it was something that was repeated from what a parent may have said.

Some persons may learn another language more easily than others. Aptitude may be considered to be a special skill or ability. However, aptitude for language learning should not be compared to general intelligence. Aptitude is more like "the ability to rapidly and accurately decode unfamiliar speech into phonetic (sound) units and parts of speech (e.g., nouns, verbs, adjectives) and it is considered to be an intrinsic, not a learned skill" (Genesee et al., 2004, p. 139).

Second-Language Pedagogy and Bilingual Programs

A significant shift in attitude toward offering "bilingual" education (a misnomer, because the reference primarily applies to Spanish-English programs) in the United States has taken place in the last 10 years. Even in the mid-1980s about 23% of English-language learners (ELL) received some form of bilingual education. By contrast, in California, after the passage in 1998 of Proposition 227, the percentage of students receiving some form of bilingual education dropped from 29% to 11% in only one year (Rumberger, 2000).

In summary, when attempting to determine whether or not a student/client may have a language learning disability, it is important to consider all the variables that have been discussed so far in this chapter: the context in which two languages were acquired, the age of the learner, the amount of formal and informal exposure to both languages, and the type of second-language instruction provided. For example, one cannot expect a student to read in the first language (L1) unless the student has been taught how to read in that language. A student who began schooling at age 6 in the second language (L2) may not have all the vocabulary necessary to read at grade level in L2. In addition, it is important to analyze the client's language patterns in both languages to decide whether they (1) signal a possible language difficulty, (2) reflect the process of acquiring the second language, or (3) are simply indicative of the language patterns that occur when two languages come into contact. There is no simple answer to these questions. One must take into account the variables mentioned previously and explore the processes we will describe next.

Oral vs. Written Language Skills

Historically, more research has been conducted to study the oral, rather than the written, development of language and bilingualism. This is because oral language is considered a natural process while written language reflects the influence of formal education and is not as universal (Crystal, 1997). Just as languages have different sounds and sound combinations, written alphabets vary a great deal in number and shape as well as in script direction—for example, Arabic and Hebrew (right to left) or Japanese (top to bottom) (Campbell 1995, 1998; Cook & Bassetti, 2005; Katzner, 2002). There are also languages with no written alphabetical representation, but which may consist of symbols that have not yet been deciphered. Interest in written language forms has increased for languages of which there are very few remaining speakers, and this interest has resulted in

the creation of written forms that use the Roman alphabet instead of the original written or symbolic representations. The various scripts that may impact the ability of CLD populations to acquire written language skills in English will be discussed at greater length in Chapter 6. One helpful resource is a book edited by Cook and Bassetti (2005). A list of the languages most frequently spoken by English-language learners (ELL) and the languages' script types appear in Table 2-1. As noted, there are great variations in script from language to language, as well as variations in word order.

It is important to keep the dichotomy between oral and written language in mind for three main reasons: (1) to determine if the student/client has oral and written language skills in each language; (2) to assist in preparing a more comprehensive assessment of the student/client's language abilities; and (3) to assist in developing writing goals and objectives that will better facilitate the student/client's progress with further acquisition of academic or job skills.

Bilingual Language Proficiency and Dominance Issues

Proficiency and dominance are two terms that are commonly used to quantify and qualify the level of mastery of two or more languages. *Proficiency* refers to the degree of mastery of the individual's linguistic ability within the various components of language (listening/understanding/speaking/reading/writing), whereas *dominance* indicates which language is mastered with greater competency. However, the influence of context needs to be taken into account in evaluating both proficiency and dominance. Additionally, primary or dominant may not refer to the language of greater competency, but the language that is most

TABLE 2-1 Scripts of Languages Most Frequently Spoken by ELL Students

Language[*]	Frequency[*]	Script[**]	Word Order[**]
Spanish	76.9%	Roman alphabet	SVO-VSO
Vietnamese	2.4%	Roman alphabet and diacritics to mark vowels	SVO-OSV Tonal language
Hmong	1.8%	Recently developed Roman alphabet	SVO-OSV Tonal language
Korean	1.2%	Mixed script (Indigenous and Chinese)	SOV
Arabic	1.2%	Naskhi script—reading right to left	VSO
Haitian-Creole	1.1%	Roman alphabet	SVO
Cantonese	1%	Logographs—12,000 characters—reading may have been reformatted left to right instead of up-down	SVO-SOV
Russian	0.9%	Cyrillic	SVO-SOV
Tagalog	0.9%	Roman alphabet	Variations
Navajo	0.9%	Roman alphabet and marks for specific pronunciation	S, V, O free

Source: [*]Adapted from Zehler, Fleischman, Hopstock, Pendzick, and Stephenson, 2003.[**]Adapted from Campbell, 1995 and 1998.

often spoken. (The term *dominant language* is often used interchangeably with *first language* and *native language*.) For example, greater dominance in reading or writing a certain language may not signify greater proficiency in performing those tasks in general. Specifically, a person may be more proficient in writing about concrete topics in one language, but may be able to express more abstract ideas in the other. Unless two or more languages are acquired and used in exactly the same contexts, the level of competence of each language will vary depending on the given situation. For example, a student/client might know one word in one language, but not in the other due to lack of exposure. For example, bilingual students may have labels for certain items in one language but not in the other. If L1 is used at home to label objects such as furniture, kitchen items, or gadgets, it is more likely that the individual may have those labels in L1 but not necessarily L2. The student/client may be more at ease speaking about certain topics in

one language as compared with another. Finally, a student/client's reading and writing skills may vary across languages depending on a number of additional factors, such as need and exposure. Thus, expecting equivalent knowledge of vocabulary or competence across two languages may not be realistic when working with bilingual individuals.

Therefore, exposure and use are important variables to consider when assessing language competence in multilingual populations. No single test or series of tests can capture all the elements of the concept of proficiency and dominance. A comprehensive assessment of the student/client in the various aspects of spoken and written language in both languages should be paired with observations in various settings such as home, school, and/or work. As suggested by some researchers (Gutiérrez-Clellen & Kreiter, 2003; Langdon, 1992a; Restrepo, 1998; Roseberry-McKibbin, 2002), these observations should be provided by families, teachers, and persons who know the

PERSONAL STORIES

A Personal Note Regarding Proficiency and Dominance

Polish and Spanish are my native languages; however, Polish is not my dominant or more proficient language. Yet, Spanish is a dominant language for me, as is English, although I consider English to be my most proficient language at this time. French, on the other hand, is somewhere "in between." I am proficient in French, but not at the same level and in as many contexts as I am in Spanish or English. Even though I am able to discuss in French various topics related to history, geography, and literature—both orally and in writing— because of my elementary and secondary schooling in a French Lycée, I did not have everyday French words such as the equivalents of "pacifier," "diaper," and "crib" when I decided to raise my daughter bilingually in French and English. Today, I can lecture in both English and Spanish on topics related to speech-language pathology. I can conduct and discuss reports in English, Spanish, and French, but I still prefer to write in English on all of the above topics.

individual best. It is important to compare the student/client's responses to a particular task with the expected responses—but the efficiency and ease with which those responses are provided should also be noted. This topic is further elaborated in the section of this chapter that discusses language processing in bilinguals.

Cummins (1981, 1984) proposed a framework of communicative proficiency that incorporates a developmental perspective, takes into account differences between the language demands of the classroom and those of nonacademic settings, and captures the relationship between proficiency in the first language and proficiency in the second language. With these factors in mind, he proposed a model in which two continua intersect. One continuum represents the degree of cognitive demand involved in the communication task, and the other represents the extent to which context contributes to expressing and receiving meaning. Thus, all communication tasks can

be placed in one of four quadrants. This is presented in Figure 2-1. Even though the model was proposed 25 years ago it is still referred to in the literature and in academic discussions about categories of language proficiency.

Quadrant A tasks are the least cognitively demanding, while those in Quadrant D are the most demanding. In addition, the model differentiates two types of language proficiency: (1) the language proficiency noted in a context-embedded face-to face situation, which is referred to as Basic Interpersonal Communicative Skills (BICS), and (2) the language proficiency acquired in a context-reduced (academic) situation, which is referred to as Cognitive Academic Language Proficiency (CALP).

Second-language learners usually acquire the first type of language proficiency (BICS) within two years of contact with the second language, whereas they may require five to seven years of exposure before the second type

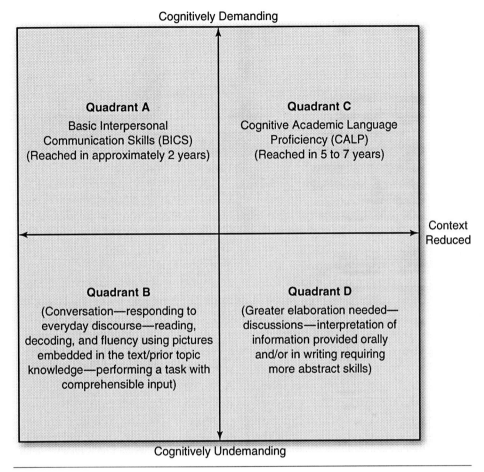

Cognitively Demanding

Quadrant A
Basic Interpersonal
Communication Skills (BICS)
(Reached in approximately 2 years)

Quadrant C
Cognitive Academic Language
Proficiency (CALP)
(Reached in 5 to 7 years)

Context
Reduced

Quadrant B
(Conversation—responding to
everyday discourse—reading,
decoding, and fluency using pictures
embedded in the text/prior topic
knowledge—performing a task with
comprehensible input)

Quadrant D
(Greater elaboration needed—
discussions—interpretation of
information provided orally
and/or in writing requiring
more abstract skills)

Cognitively Undemanding

FIGURE 2-1 *The Relationship of BICS and CALP.* (Adapted from Cummins, 1981.)

of language proficiency (CALP) is comparable to that of a native speaker. As mastery is developed, the degree of difficulty that an individual can manage moves from bottom to top in the proficiency model along the vertical continuum. For example, producing sounds in certain words may be difficult for a 3-year-old at first; therefore, the task would be placed in Quadrant B. As the child becomes more proficient in the language, the task would be placed in Quadrant A. Similarly, the task of mastering basic sentence structure may begin in Quadrant B for second-language learners, but move to Quadrant A as the learner

progresses in acquiring the language. As another example, school-based tasks that are context-reduced are often "cognitively demanding" to the student. With the use of appropriate instructional strategies, the material should eventually become "cognitively undemanding" and its difficulty level would move from Quadrant D to Quadrant C.

It is rare to find individuals who have completely mastered all components of two languages with the same degree of skill. Generally, bilinguals show greater dominance in one language component than another. For example, although bilingual persons may be able to carry on a conversation on many topics with the same degree of ease in two languages, they may prefer to read or write about certain topics in one of the two languages. The variations of each bilingual individual's exposure and proficiency in each language add to the complexity of assessing the language proficiencies of bilinguals who may have a language disorder. Therefore, to accurately assess results of tests that determine levels of proficiency in a given language, the SLP should be familiar with the construction of the proficiency test used and consider the student/client's learning experiences and educational history.

The focus of this chapter only allows for a summary of language proficiency tests. Most of these assess one or several linguistic areas. As an example, the Bilingual Syntax Measure (BSM-I and -II) (Burt, Dulay, & Hernández-Chávez, 1975, 1980) assesses students' level of syntax and grammar by asking them to respond to questions based on cartoon-like pictures. Proficiency levels in each language (Spanish and English) are established based on the number and type of responses given in each language. The Bilingual Verbal Abilities (BVAT), (Muñoz-Sandoval, Cummins, Alvarado, & Ruef, 1998) measures language proficiency by assessing children's and adults' abilities to name pictures of different objects or concepts, to provide synonyms and antonyms, and to make analogies in English and in any one of 14 other languages. Other tests such as the Language Assessment Scales (LAS) (De Avila & Duncan, 1978, 1991, 2005) assess a wider range of language skills in school-age children that include listening, speaking, reading, and writing. In all cases, the purpose of each test is to classify the English-language learner's language proficiency skills into levels of ability using 5 levels, which range from "nonspeaker" to "fluent speaker." The objec-

tive is to provide more "adequate" language instruction and teaching techniques. Unfortunately, many students who score in the "fluent" category may not be ready to learn in English-only language classrooms, and may need additional instructional modifications to benefit from instruction.

Most current proficiency tests are designed to assess the student/client in English and in Spanish only, one exception being the BVAT. More recent tests, created by various states, are only available in English. For example, the California English Language Development Test (CELDT), first implemented in 2001, assesses English listening, speaking, reading, and writing abilities and was created to determine the proficiency of ELL students in each of the four language areas. Specific standards are listed for each curriculum area and at five levels of proficiency: Beginning, Early Intermediate, Intermediate, Early Advanced, and Advanced. Exit criteria for each level are also delineated for each one of the language areas (listening, speaking, reading, and writing). The reader can refer to the California Department of Education (http://www.cde.ca.gov/) under ELD (English-Language Development). Many of the proficiency tests were developed to provide "quick" measures of these students' proficiency. This tends to sacrifice the accuracy of the results, and therefore the outcomes may only be available as guides for placement; they do not offer practical suggestions for the teacher. Kuhlman (2005) comments: "In other words, teachers typically aren't given a consistent and formal way of either diagnosing exactly what students know and can do, based on their state's ELD/ESL standards, or of monitoring students' language growth and development. What teachers need to supplement these statewide language tests is a performance-based instrument that they can use on a regular basis to document their students' growth and development in English and that will inform their teaching" (Kuhlman, 2005, p. 3).

Knowing about the general language proficiency of the student/client in both English and his or her native language provides the SLP with a profile of the student/client's bilingual language skills. However, the SLP must be familiar with the particular tests used to interpret and evaluate the significance of the results. Thus, if a student/client is dominant in one language, it does not mean that he/she has no proficiency in the other language. It is therefore important to provide assessment of both languages spoken. More information on this topic will be discussed in Chapter 5.

In summary, the various components of the term "bilingual" must be analyzed. The SLP who plans to assess a bilingual individual needs to consider the type of bilingualism (oral, written) and the proficiency/dominance dichotomy as well as the contexts in which the languages have been used.

USE OF AND INTERACTION BETWEEN TWO LANGUAGES

This section discusses four different phenomena that occur when a bilingual speaker uses two languages. These phenomena include code-switching, language transference and interference, language loss, and the influence of bilingualism on language processing and cognitive development.

Code-Switching

Code-switching, code-mixing, and code-borrowing are terms that have been used interchangeably to describe when a speaker uses a word, phrase, or sentence from one language while communicating in the other language. Code-switching is a common occurrence in bilingual communities both in the United States and around the globe. Code-switching may be enhanced when the conversation occurs in a "bilingual mode" or at the same "level of activation of two languages, one of which is the base language" (Grosjean, 2001, p. 4). The frequency of code-switching depends on variables such as proficiency in each language, language mixing habits, socioeconomic status, and the type of the message being conveyed and the context in which it is being conveyed. Code-switching is very common to a young child's process of acquiring two languages and has been observed in studies analyzing various combinations of languages. In most cases, the patterns are systematic and follow the grammatical constraints of the two languages (Genesee et al., 2004). For example, adjective order is often switched by individuals from Spanish or French backgrounds who are learning English; in Spanish and French, the adjective is usually placed after the noun. Code-switching between two languages has some negative connotations—for example, derogatory references to Spanglish, Tex-Mex, Franglais, and Hindish are common. Examples of some code-switching patterns occurring at word and sentence levels are listed in Table 2-2.

Code-switching serves social and pragmatic purposes when a speaker is communicating in two languages or two dialects (for details on the nature of code-switching between Standard American English and African-American English, see Seymour and Roeper, 1999). Grosjean (1982) identified nine situations that are conducive to code-switching: (1) filling a linguistic need for a lexical item, phrase, or stretch of discourse, (2) quoting someone, (3) marketing and emphasizing the group identity, (4) conveying confidentiality, (5) excluding someone

---

TABLE 2-2 Examples of Code-Switching at the Word and Sentence Levels

Word level	"Voy a necesitar un bandaid" [I am going to need a bandaid]. (No available vocabulary word for the term/ curita) (Spanish-English)
	"Carlos would never talk to his abuelita this way." (Spanish-English)
	"Ja nie znam jego backgroundu" [I don't know his background]. (No available comparable term for "background"—note that the word has a morphological ending denoting the "object" case) (Polish-English)
	"Ella se anda parqueando" (estacionando) [She is parking]. (Spanish-English)
Sentence level	"Yo me limpio la cara, mi mamá me pone shampoo and she makes it clean." (A four-year-old bilingual Spanish/English-speaking child)
	"My brother went there et puis il a decidé de ne plus revenir." (French-English)
	"Avant d'entrer dans la chambre, ona pomiszlala ze muszi zadzwonic do matki" [Before she entered the room she thought she had to call her mother]. (English-Polish)

---

from conversation, (6) changing the role of the speaker (i.e., raising the speaker's status), (7) adding authority, (8) showing expertise, and (9) using a word or phrase that may not have an equivalent in the other language.

Code-switching follows some strict rules. First, a switch may not violate the syntactic rule in either language. In English the order is article-adjective-noun whereas in Spanish for the most part it is article-noun-adjective. For example, one may say "Me compró a red car" (he bought me a red car), but not "Me compró un red carro." Second, as in the following French-English example, there cannot be a switch between a pronoun and a verb as in "I joue the piano" (instead of "Je joue the piano") or "Nous do the dishes in the evening" (instead of "Nous lavons the dishes in the evening") (Myers-Scotton, 1992). Poplack (1979) found that there seemed to be strict rules with regard to code-switching across the languages he studied (English and French). Myers-Scotton (2002) further confirms this observation by stating that the main language, which she refers to as the "matrix language" (ML), is the base for the grammatical frame or rules for grammar. A preliminary study comparing the code-switching patterns of children with and without speech and language impairments and who had varying degrees of bilingual ability found no difference between the two groups in the code-switches the children made. Furthermore, the bilingual students who had a speech-language impairment (SLI) did not violate the rules of code-switching (Gutiérrez-Clellen & Erickson, 2003). The researchers' observations were different from Restrepo (2003), who found differences in the code-switching of one of the two children they studied. Restrepo and Gutiérrez-Clellen (2004) attribute these differences to the environment in which the students were learning English. In the Restrepo (2003) study, the students were learning English in a subtractive environment (an environment where knowing a second language is not regarded as an asset), whereas the subjects studied by Gutiérrez-Clellen and Erickson (2003) were developing their English skills in an additive environment (one where knowing a second language is regarded as an asset). Even though the researchers do not mention this possibility, it could be that the two subjects studied by Restrepo (2003) were unique. Conclusions are difficult to draw, because the number of subjects studied in the Gutiérrez-Clellen and

Erickson study was not mentioned. However, the authors accurately indicate that more research is needed to determine the environmental conditions that enhance or reduce code-switching in bilingual individuals.

Language Transfer and Language Interference

In a previous section (page 26), it was reported that many grammatical features in two different languages develop in a similar fashion in each language, regardless of the nature of the two languages. In the 1950s and 1960s, contrastive analysis (the pointing out of phonological and grammatical differences between first and second languages) prevailed in second-language curricula. It was believed that awareness of those differences would in-crease proficiency in the second language. This strategy soon fell into disfavor, however, when second-language acquisition studies seemed to indicate that there were common strategies for second-language acquisition, independent of the native language. In fact, Dulay and Burt (1973, 1974) concluded that, in acquiring English, most errors made by second-language learners resemble those of first-language learners. They indicated that only 5% of errors were due to native language interference. Thus, the type of error may not be as important as the quantity of those errors. In my research (Langdon, 1977, 1983), I found that a group of 6- to 8-year-old students whose L1 was Spanish and who had been identified as language-disordered made very many of the same types of errors in English that a matched group of normally developing students of the same L1 backgrounds did. Similar errors were noted in both groups' use of various grammatical forms (plural agreement and use/omission of prepositions in prepositional phrases in English). However, there were differences in the quantity of errors. A recent study conducted by Paradis (2005) of children who spoke a variety of languages (such as Korean, Mandarin, Romanian, Japanese, Arabic, Farsi, Ukrainian, and Dari) as their first language and who were learning English, indicated that the children made errors that were similar to those made by a group of language-impaired native-speakers of English. The types of errors analyzed consisted of various grammatical forms such as present tense, third-person singular, regular and irregular past tense, auxiliaries and the copula "do," prepositions, plurals, and determiners. The kinds of errors made were similar in all groups, when the children were tested and compared with others who were experiencing difficulties in English and were of monolingual backgrounds. Therefore, analysis of morphology alone is not helpful in differentiating a second-language learner who might have a language impairment from a child who is a native speaker of English and who might have a language impairment. This study confirms earlier findings and suggests that more sensitive measures should be used to detect language impairments in second-language learners. Nonetheless, predicting some common transfer errors from one language to the other can be very helpful. Obtaining other measures, such as by comparing the second-language learner to a child with a similar language background is suggested. It is also important to obtain a careful history of the child's first language development if assessment in that language is not possible due to lack of appropriate measures, or lack of personnel fluent in the student/client's first language.

Most frequently, the "interference" of one language with the other is more prominent at the phonological level than at any other level. Therefore, the use of correct phonology may be important to the process of following certain syntactic rules, such as correctly using plurals, past tense, and other morphological endings.

TABLE 2-3 Examples of Contrasts between English and Other Languages

Phonological Contrast	Language	English Rendition
No final /b/	Spanish	[ca] for [cab]
No /tʃ/	Vietnamese	[sue] for [shoe]
No /Ø/	Hmong	[sum] for [thumb]
Different /r/ (like French)	Haitian Creole	[red] for [red]
No final /l/	Cantonese	[ba] for [ball]
Omission of final cluster	AAE	[rus] for [rust]—[des] for [desk]
Grammatical Contrast	**Language**	**English Rendition**
Use of negative	Spanish	[No help him]
Omission of article ([a] and [the])	Asian Languages	[I have key to car]
Omission of copula	AAE	[She pretty girl]

Source: Adapted from Campbell, 1995, and Swan and Smith, 2004.

The work of Swan and Smith (2004) is a helpful resource; the editors outline areas that are difficult for second-language learners of English who speak one of many different languages as their primary language (examples include Arabic, Farsi, Spanish, Italian, and several others). Being aware of the sound system of a given language, as well as any possible "interference" of a given language with English, is important for avoiding a misdiagnosis. It also assists in making the learner aware of language differences; such awareness will assist both oral and written communication. Some examples of differences between English and other languages are listed in Table 2-3.

"Transfer," or its more pejorative synonym "interference," is a common phenomenon for individuals who are learning other languages. The various components of language—phonology, grammar, syntax, reading, and writing—are not necessarily relearned with the addition of a new language. Having two languages does not mean using "two different language systems." The concept of transfer is related to the hypothesis developed by Cummins (1981, 1984) that there is an underlying proficiency common to two languages. For example, while learning to read in Spanish, the student not only develops skills in Spanish, but also acquires a deeper conceptual and linguistic proficiency that influences the development of English literacy and general academic skills. (This topic will be discussed in greater detail in Chapter 6). The metaphor of the "dual iceberg" illustrates this concept (Cummins, 1984, p. 143). (See Figure 2-2.)

Two different languages express similar functions, such as sharing information, requesting, denying, predicting, or hypothesizing. Both languages may also share the concepts of liberty, honesty, freedom, sadness, and happiness even though there might not be exact verbal equivalents. The similarity in concepts can be included as the common underlying proficiency illustrated in Figure 2-2 in the shaded area "underneath the iceberg" (central operating system). In that area we may also find the cognitive basis of language processing that includes perception, attention, working memory, and emotion (Kohnert & Derr, 2004). The surface features, or relationships between morphemes, include the

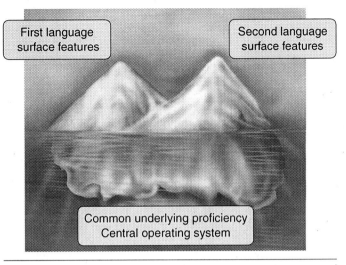

FIGURE 2-2 *The Iceberg Analogy.* (Adapted from Baker and Prys Jones, 1998.)

lexicon, syntax, grammar, and phonology that differ from language to language. As a matter of fact, the "surface structure" of one language, in the form of vocabulary words, does not transfer from one language to the other; however, the underlying concepts do. For example, earlier I gave the example of how I knew certain words in one language but not in the other: I knew the word "pacifier" in Spanish, English, and Polish, but not in French. I knew the label, because I was exposed to the term in all three languages, but I didn't know the label in French despite having a high proficiency in the French language—because I hadn't been exposed to the term in French. I did, however, understand the *concept* underlying the label.

The concept of underlying proficiency assists in understanding why skills gained in one language can be transferred to another language, benefiting the overall bilingual linguistic performance of the individual. Therefore, if a student learns, for example, the concept of quantity in one language, this skill will transfer to a new language, if there is an opportunity to learn words that denote quan-

tity (i.e., "number," "more," "less," "greater," etc.). Some recent studies confirm the hypothesis that skills learned in one language will transfer to the other language (Dopke, 2000; Gutiérrez-Clellen, 1999). This concept has implications for treatment planning. (The issue of transference across languages for purposes of clinical intervention will be discussed in Chapter 7.)

Language Loss

It is common for second-language learners to lose their first language if its use is discontinued. Anderson (2004) differentiates "language loss" from "language attrition," both of which are symptomatic of "language shift." Language "loss" is a more rapid phenomenon, whereas language "attrition" is generally considered to be a slower process of the arrest or decline of the first language over time.

Language loss has been observed as a shift in proficiency in both additive and subtractive environments. However, language loss in a subtractive environment may erroneously be considered symptomatic of a language disability. Often, in both additive and subtractive situations, the individual (child or adult) may be proficient in social situations in the first language, but have more difficulty performing decontextualized language tasks, such as comprehending written text. This phenomenon is even more pronounced if the individual has not been exposed to more academically based tasks in the primary language. It may also occur with adults who have only rare opportunities to interact and read in their first language. When evaluating the primary language of a student/client, clinicians should always consider the possibility of language loss. Finding out the extent to which each language is used and the environment in which it is used is very important. Anderson (2004) lists reasons for language loss in bilingual Spanish-English communities and these reasons may be generalized to other bilingual communities. These reasons are reported in Figure 2-3.

In addition to the phenomena listed in Figure 2-3, there is another important factor to consider: aging. Aging does have an impact on the language skills of a bilingual individual. The term "aging" is used to denote different ages in different cultures. For example, Giles and Makoni (2005) found that the perception of aging was different in North America than in South Africa and Ghana. Students in North America considered that being elderly begins at age 60, whereas students in South Africa and Ghana considered that it begins at only 50. To ensure an accurate assessment, a language history for the older patient, who may have sustained a stroke or brain injury, or may be suspected of having dementia, should be collected. For more information on aging and communication in multilingual contexts, the reader is referred to De Bot and Makoni (2005). Chapter 8, which addresses adult CLD populations, provides further discussion about the currently known general patterns of language recovery in bilinguals following trauma and stroke.

Influences on Language Processing and Cognitive Development

The relationship between cognitive development and bilingualism has been measured with a variety of procedures. Some researchers have

1. Females tend to experience more language loss than males (more common in rural communities where higher proficiency in English is rewarded).
2. Role of sibling—older sibling(s) may act as interpreters/translators for their families, thus maintaining their proficiency in L2.
3. Early preschool programs are often available in the majority language only.
4. The low status of L1 accelerates loss; there are more vocational and educational opportunities in L2.
5. There is a lack of opportunity to interact with peers in L1.
6. Siblings interact in the majority language (a common phenomenon in bilingual environments).
7. Parents are bilingual and will speak L2 more frequently.
8. There may be lower education levels attained by the family in L1.
9. The family has a belief that L1 preservation is important despite all odds.
10. L1 loss is a consequence of the aging process.
11. There is a lack of opportunity to visit the country where L1 is spoken.

FIGURE 2-3 *Eleven Factors Accelerating L1 Loss.* (Adapted from Anderson, 2004.)

analyzed subjects' performance on traditional intelligence tests that measure linguistic and general intellectual skills, while others have focused on tests that measure divergent thinking, academic performance, and metalinguistic awareness (Bialystok, 1991, 2001; Swain & Cummins, 1982). As a result, the outcome of two similar studies may vary as a result of the nature of the tasks analyzed. Sources that date from almost the beginning of the century illustrate researchers' evolution of thought on the effects of bilingualism on cognitive development, a controversial topic that has ramifications for education and politics. Early studies on the relationship between cognitive skills and bilingualism concluded that bilingualism had a negative effect on general intelligence. Positive effects are documented following some of the pioneering work done with bilingual French-English children (Peal & Lambert, 1962).

Negative Outcomes

Studies carried out in the 1920s and 1930s that examined a variety of language combinations (Saer, 1924; Smith, 1923, 1931, 1939; Yoshioka, 1929) concluded that bilingualism had a negative impact on intellectual ability. For example, Goodenough (1926) concluded that children's intelligence was affected by their amount of exposure to another language. Negative outcomes were obtained because several of the studies were based on inappropriate methodology, partly because testing intellectual ability was a relative new construct at that time, but also because control of variables was not carried out appropriately. For example, subjects were tested in only their second language, which was their weaker language. Also, the researchers did not control for variables such as the subjects' attitudes, experience with testing, and other cultural variables. In summary, research studies were not designed carefully to determine the

impact of bilingualism on different measures of cognitive ability. To demonstrate that bilingualism does indeed have a positive impact on intellectual ability, the subject must have reached a certain "threshold of performance in both languages, in order to avoid cognitive deficits and allow the potentially beneficial aspects of becoming bilingual to influence cognitive growth" (Cummins, 1984, p. 107). This is illustrated in Figure 2-4.

Longitudinal studies conducted by Hakuta and Díaz (1985), Galambos and Hakuta (1988), and Yelland, Pollard, and Mercuri (1993), found positive correlations between degree of bilingualism and the subjects' performance on metalinguistic tasks that required detecting ambiguities in words. Outcomes of the studies confirmed the "threshold hypothesis": subjects performed best when their proficiency in at least one language was sufficiently high to enable them to respond to the task at hand. As mentioned by Bialystok (2001), "the important point is that children have not been found to suffer any disadvantages from learning and using two languages, even in academic settings, providing that one of their languages is established at a level appropriate for children their age" (p. 227).

Positive Outcomes

The Canadian studies reported by Peal and Lambert (1962) were among the first to demonstrate that bilingualism has a positive effect on different measures of cognitive development. Even when studies indicate that bilingualism has a positive impact on cognitive and intellectual functioning, the subjects' proficiency in two languages is not necessarily the only variable to consider. Other factors such as attitude, motivation to learn the language, and the community's attitude toward bilingualism are also important.

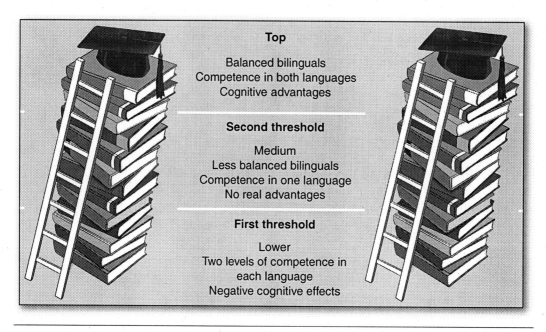

Top

Balanced bilinguals
Competence in both languages
Cognitive advantages

Second threshold

Medium
Less balanced bilinguals
Competence in one language
No real advantages

First threshold

Lower
Two levels of competence in
each language
Negative cognitive effects

FIGURE 2-4   *Illustration of the Threshold Hypothesis.* (Adapted from Baker and Prys Jones, 1998.)

Research on the benefits of bilingualism have focused on various linguistic and cognitive tasks: (1) the use of more complex sentence structures (Barik & Swain, 1978; Ekstrand, 1978); (2) metalinguistic awareness, including the ability to detect ambiguity in sentences or detect the different meanings of words (Ben-Zeev, 1977; Galambos & Hakuta, 1988); and (3) metapragmatic ability, such as the ability to efficiently explain rules to listeners who are blindfolded (which therefore forces the speakers to use language alone to convey meaning, instead of relying on expressive gestures and facial expressions) (Genesee, Tucker, & Lambert, 1976), or identify facial expressions with greater accuracy (Bain & Yu, 1978). For example, the significance of a smile tends to vary from culture to culture (Russell J. 1994).

More recently, studies have focused on bilinguals' ability to sustain attention in the presence of competing/misleading information. Research has begun to explore the role of the right and left hemispheres of the brain; that is, how the brain functions in the process of becoming bilingual. Research is beginning to uncover the overall organization of the "bilingual brain." For a review of various studies related to the topics mentioned above, the reader is directed to Bialystok (2001).

In summary, it appears that research on the relationship between bilingualism and different aspects of cognitive development have begun to yield more positive results because of more careful research design procedures.

Language Processing in Bilinguals

Successful language development involves acquiring both the ability to comprehend and express more complex linguistic structures and the ability to perform tasks that require the processing of specific information. In the last 10 to 15 years, studies conducted with monolingual speakers who may have a language impairment have documented the effectiveness (speed and accuracy) with which the participants process various linguistic structures; these studies have also measured language competence. *Information processing* refers to the psychological components involved in attention, perception, memory, concept formation, problem solving, and information management (Snyder, Dabasinskas, & O'Connor, 2002). Two basic levels of processing (LOP) have been identified: "bottom" and "top" (Gromme, 1999). The "bottom" levels make fewer cognitive demands on the individual and consist of a perceptual analysis of input. More cognitive demands are made of individuals when they use "top" levels of processing. Tasks demanding bottom-level processing (such as understanding the phonetic aspects of a given word) are recalled with less success than tasks requiring top levels of processing (such as associating new information with what is already known). In the first example, the task requires learning new information, whereas in the second task, the information can be more easily learned because it can be associated with something that is already known. (Hamman & Squire, 1996, 1997).

The implications of this for clinical assessment are multiple. It is important to analyze the nature of language-related tasks at hand and the processing demands made on the individual. For example, it may be easier for an individual to select a picture that illustrates a given word or concept than it is for the individual to define the word. It is also important to differentiate knowledge from efficiency. For example, recalling numbers, words, or sentences constitutes a different task than does formulating sentences (Snyder et al., 2002). Immediate recall of information is generally easier than making up a sentence using a specific word or concept. In addition, even if an individual can perform well on both tasks, it is important to observe the speed and accuracy with which the tasks are performed. This is referred to as "a processing model"—as opposed to a "knowledge-based" model which is considered to be more static and abstract. Weismer and Evans (2002) report studies in which processing-dependent measures (such as repetitions of nonsense words) and verbal working memory tasks (such as asking the subjects to answer yes/no questions while simultaneously recalling the last word in each set of sentences) were more effective in differentiating the subjects' level of English proficiency than were the traditional knowledge-based tests. On the other hand, the exclusive use of "processing-based" tasks may result in bias because such tasks may be "stripped away from their 'linguistic code' and primarily evaluate executive function or language-neutral ability such as attention and memory that are common to all human processing of linguistic material" (Weismer & Evans, 2002, p. 24). However, the researchers conclude that using a combination of both types of tasks might indeed be important for evaluating and differentiating language disorders in normally developing monolingual or bilingual individuals.

In a series of experiments reported in Kohnert (2004), the author and her colleagues analyzed the ability of bilingual Spanish-speaking individuals aged 5 to 22 (who had a specific number of years of experience with English) to perform on various tasks that assessed their comprehension and expression skills in each language, Spanish and English. These tasks focused on speed and accuracy of performance. In the comprehension portion of the experiment, the subjects had to pay attention to competing

OUR CLIENTS

Eric, Ana, Jack, Grace, and Leonardo

A description of each client's specific linguistic background is provided below. At the end of each description is a list of conclusions that might be drawn from the information presented in the description and from the concepts discussed in this chapter.

Eric

Eric is a 4-year-old preschool child whose parents speak primarily Vietnamese to him and who is referred to the speech-language pathologist (SLP) because of low expressive skills in both English and Vietnamese. Eric was born in the United States; his parents immigrated to the United States from Vietnam when they were teenagers. He is the youngest of three children; his siblings are 8 and 10 years old. Eric's parents speak English but, even after their years in the U.S., they still feel more at ease speaking in Vietnamese, which is the language spoken in their home. Eric's siblings speak English to him and among each other, but they communicate with no difficulty in Vietnamese with their parents and family members. Eric's mother completed high school and works in retail, whereas his father completed two years of college and owns a restaurant. Eric's speech development proceeded at a slower pace than that of his siblings. At first, his parents were not alarmed; they felt that because he was spoiled and everyone in the family treated him as the "baby," his speech was understandably slower in developing. However, now that he is in preschool he is behind other children in acquiring English. He prefers to play by himself. He has difficulty concentrating for more than a few minutes at a time unless he is watching his favorite cartoons or videos. His health has been good and there are no concerns about his hearing.

Based on this information about Eric, it is possible to draw the following conclusions:

- His parents compared Eric's language development to that of to his siblings but made excuses for his delays.

- Eric has had input in English because his siblings speak English to him.

- Preschool interaction revealed a tendency for Eric to isolate himself from peers.

- His choice of activities revealed that Eric has difficulties with sustaining attention, which is unrelated to bilingualism.

- Visual stimulations such as cartoons or videos seem to help focus his attention.

It will be important to assess Eric in both Vietnamese and English to obtain a more accurate picture of his overall language skills.

Ana

Ana is a 9-year-old enrolled in fourth grade; she emigrated from Mexico at the age of 5 and is having difficulty reading in English. Ana lives with her parents and two younger siblings (aged 5 and 3). Her parents are originally from Michoacán, a state neighboring Mexico City. She was raised by her maternal grandparents beginning at the age of 6 months; after five years she was reunited with her parents. Ana attended kindergarten in Arizona but moved in the middle of that year when her parents found better jobs in California. Her mother works in her school's cafeteria. Ana has learned English quite well but her teachers have said she is behind in reading. All of her schooling has been in English. She speaks Spanish to her parents and to some relatives who live nearby, but she talks to her siblings in both English and Spanish. Her parents insist that only Spanish should be spoken at home.

Based on this information about Ana, it is possible to draw the following conclusions:

- Ana is a sequential bilingual whose language proficiency seems appropriate at the conversational level in English (BICS), but not for academically related tasks (CALP).

- We do not yet have sufficient information about the particular reading instruction methodology that Ana has been exposed to.

- We have no information about how Ana feels about her school experience or about what accommodations may have been made to assist her.

It is possible that Ana may need more time in acquiring reading skills; the comments we have from her teachers seem general because we don't know whether she is weak in reading fluency, or comprehension, or both. Therefore, collecting more information will be necessary.

Jack

Jack is a 14-year-old of African-American descent who has difficulty with subjects such as social studies, English, and writing. Mrs. G., Jack's paternal grandmother, adopted him when he was 2 years old because his single mother could not raise him. Jack was born and raised in Louisiana, and he has been living with his grandmother in California for the past four years. Prior to entering School District A (summer 2002), Jack attended a private school for two years. Mrs. G. is a nurse in the surgical ward in one of the hospitals. When she is not home a neighbor supervises Jack's whereabouts.

Jack had to remain in the ICU for about seven days after birth due to respiratory distress. His developmental milestones occurred within a normal timeframe, except for his speech, which was delayed: Jack did not put words together until he was about 3 years old. His latest vision and hearing screenings (fall, 2002) were unremarkable. Mrs. G. reports that Jack is on daily medication for anger, anxiety, and agitation. He is receiving counseling to address his emotional issues. A previous school assessment report written by the SLP and the psychologist indicated some learning difficulties, but their severity did not warrant intervention from special education. Because the results of this assessment were not satisfactory to Mrs. G., she sought an outside assessment by a neuropsychologist. Results indicated that Jack has difficulty with working memory and sequencing skills. Mrs. G. states that Jack has difficulty synthesizing oral and written information. Writing is difficult for him: Jack does not respect rules of grammar and punctuation. She is requesting a second evaluation from the school assessment team.

Based on this information about Jack, it is possible to draw the following conclusions:

- Jack has a significant health history.

- His grandmother is aware of his problems and has already sought some evaluations.

- There is no information about whether Jack speaks African-American Vernacular English (AAVE).

Jack's learning difficulties have not been recognized by the school assessment team, which may mean that school expectations are low and/or that Jack has been able to compensate for his disabilities. A more in-depth language assessment is warranted.

Grace

Grace is a 60-year-old Mandarin-speaking former businesswoman who sustained a stroke while visiting the United States. She is originally from Shanghai. She speaks Mandarin, Cantonese, English, and French. She completed her business degree in China, but spent five years in the United States when she was first developing her business. The languages she speaks most frequently are Mandarin and English. She communicates in Cantonese with her relatives and speaks French when she visits Canada

(Continues)

(Continued)

and France for business transactions. Prior to her stroke she could converse on several topics in all the languages she knew. However, she felt most at ease reading and writing in Chinese and English. Before the stroke she was very proficient in reading and writing English but her strongest area was business English.

Based on this information about Grace, it is possible to draw the following conclusions:

- Grace is a simultaneous learner of Mandarin and Cantonese and a sequential learner of French and English.

- Her proficiency in each of the languages is different—but her English skills are comparable to Mandarin in at least one domain, business, because she transacts business in both China and the United States.

- Grace is well educated so she has reading and writing skills in all languages, although we can suspect that these skills are stronger in Chinese and English than they are in French.

- Grace's French skills may not be as strong because she uses the language less frequently than the others.

As in the case of Eric who has been exposed to another language, it will be important to assess Grace's linguistic skills in all of the languages that she spoke prior to her injury to determine her overall language skills. Assessing only one or two languages may not render a fair portrayal of her language performance.

Leonardo

Leonardo is a 45-year-old fieldworker from Guatemala who suffered a traumatic brain injury following a dispute with a neighbor. Leonardo is an illegal immigrant who has been traveling back and forth between the U.S. and Guatemala for more than 20 years. He works as a crop picker in several states including Washington, Ohio, Michigan, California, and Oregon. He completed seven grades in Guatemala but was able to get his GED in the U.S. after attending night classes. His family lives in Cobán, Guatemala, and he has some friends that he has met over time. He is able to speak in English, but given a choice, he prefers to interact in Spanish because he feels more at ease expressing his thoughts in that language. Prior to his accident he could read newspapers in both English and Spanish but concentrated primarily on sports and local news. His family and relatives depend on the money he sends them every month. During a recent party he got into a fight with someone over money that he had borrowed but had not returned on time. Two heavier persons attacked him and hit his head with a baseball bat. He remained unconscious in the hospital for more than a week. At this time, he can walk but he cannot easily remember what is said to him. He is disoriented, he cannot keep track of time, and he forgets daily routines. After spending two weeks in a rehabilitation center he was dismissed and he is currently living with some friends.

Based on this information about Leonardo, it is possible to draw the following conclusions:

- Leonardo has similar language skills in both Spanish and English although he prefers reading in Spanish and is particularly interested in sports and the news.

- His work demands physical fitness and effort.

- Leonardo is in this country without his family, and is living with friends.

- He is illegal and most likely avoids medical establishments due to the fact that he has no proof of citizenship and no medical insurance.

As in the previous case (Grace), obtaining background information on the client's preferences and language abilities in each language prior to the injury are important for accurately assessing the current oral and written language skills of the client. This information will also be important for intervention.

Grace and Leonardo's assessments will be fully described in Chapter 8, which discusses assessment and intervention issues for adult ELL clients.

visual and auditory messages and press a "happy face" if the picture was correctly named, and a "sad face" if it was incorrect. This task was performed using one language at a time. A subsequent task consisted of presenting the pictures and stimuli using either Spanish or English randomly. The expressive portion of the experiment required the subjects to name pictures in either Spanish or English—or in a mixed mode (some words had to be named in Spanish and others in English). Results indicated that the older the individual, the faster the responses were made. After one year, the greatest gains in proficiency were noted for the mixed-mode task across all individuals. However, there were variations across participants and for individual participants, depending on the participant's age; some performed faster and with greater accuracy in English, whereas others performed better in Spanish. Over time, however, the overall performance was greater in English because this was the language to which the individuals had had more exposure (i.e., in school).

The implications of this research is that assessments of CLD students who have possible speech and language impairments should focus on the speed and accuracy of performance in each language, because this may be a viable way to determine the difference between a language acquisition problem and a language disorder. By assessing the learner using various tasks that require different levels of cognitive processing, one may have a clearer picture of students' progress in improving linguistic performance. More on this topic will be discussed in Chapters 5 and 6, which focus on assessment issues.

SUMMARY

Several important aspects of bilingualism were reviewed in this chapter. First, the definition of bilingualism was discussed and found to be a complex concept because it includes many developmental, social, and personal variables. Two languages can be acquired simultaneously or sequentially, and variables such as age and social status, as well as personal characteristics such as motivation and aptitude, must be considered. Second, this chapter discussed various phenomena that occur when individuals learn a second language: code-switching, language transfer, and language loss. Finally, the chapter examined research on how bilingualism relates to cognitive development and language processing.

In conclusion, the SLP who works with CLD populations needs to be aware of a multitude of variables in order to avoid misdiagnosing a communication disorder in a bilingual individual.

FURTHER READINGS

Baker, C., & Prys Jones, S. (2001). *Encyclopedia of bilingual education and bilingualism.* Clevendon, UK: Multilingual Matters.

Bialystok, E. (2001). *Bilingualism in development: Language, literacy and cognition.* New York: Cambridge University Press.

Genesee, F., Paradis, J., & Crago, M. (2004). *Dual-language development and disorders: A handbook on bilingualism and second-language learning.* Baltimore: Brookes.

C H A P T E R 3

OPTIMAL SECOND-LANGUAGE LEARNING FOR CLD POPULATIONS

"The learning 'disabilities' of many students are pedagogically induced rather than a reflection of some intrinsic processing deficit" (Cummins, 1984, p. 223).

CHAPTER OUTLINE

INTRODUCTION

*C*hapter 2 included a discussion of factors that play a role in the development of a second language. Examples of such factors are an individual's age, motivation, attitude, aptitude, school, and support from the community. There are two additional variables that merit more discussion. The first is the process of acquiring a second language in a classroom environment, referred to by Krashen (1981, 1982) as "conscious acquisition of language." The second is the students' and their families' learning experiences in their own country of origin. Understanding the students' and families' experiences with formal education and the types of programs attended by the student assists SLPs and other professionals in connecting those experiences with educational expectations and preferred teaching strategies.

Several models of bilingual education instruct students in reading in one or the other language, depending on their grade. Consequently, a student's reading skills may not be at grade level in either Spanish or English, for example, because of insufficient or inadequate instruction. Knowing about the recommended practices for instructing CLD students assists SLPs and other professionals in differentiating a language disorder from language difficulties that are due to inadequate pedagogical practices. As an example, a student may not be able to process the teacher's instructions because the teacher's rate of speech is too fast. This situation can be easily remedied by teacher awareness.

Seeking further information about the students' and the families' previous schooling can assist in planning a more appropriate course of action, assessment, and, if needed, treatment. For example, parents who may have had limited formal education in their own country may not be as familiar with grade-level expectations. Additionally, students may not be on an academic par with peers because they missed certain levels of instruction in the past, or transferred between schools too frequently.

BILINGUAL EDUCATION IN THE UNITED STATES: A HISTORICAL OVERVIEW

CLD students are often referred for assessment because of language difficulties that do not necessarily stem from a basic language disorder. Implementation of inappropriate, or unfamiliar instructional strategies may be the primary cause of the student's lack of progress, as noted in Cummins' comment at the beginning of this chapter. This comment applies not only to students for whom English is their second language, but also to those children living in the U.S. who speak African-American Vernacular English (AAVE), also referred to as Ebonics, Black Vernacular, or Black English Vernacular. In 1996, the board of the Oakland Public Schools in California passed a resolution to outline the best way to educate these children. As noted by Perry (1998), circumstances were somewhat similar to those in an Ann Arbor case, which took place 20 years earlier. Perry states, "Sixty-six percent of the plaintiff children in the Ann Arbor case had been classified as special needs. In this liberal, affluent college town, African-Americans were also overrepresented in the number of suspensions and underrepresented in honors classes. In the predominantly white school district of Ann Arbor and in the minority/majority district of Oakland, the caste positionality of African-Americans was the same. So much for the promise of multiculturalism" (p. 4). The past and current political climates have shaped the implementation of educational programs available for CLD students as well as for all students, including those who have various language and learning disabilities.

With the 2004 Individuals with Disabilities Education Act (IDEA) signed into law, students who have difficulty in academics are identified for eventual special education instruction based on their progress as a result of intervention. This progress is also referred to as Responsiveness to Intervention (RtI), and this model of identifying students needing services from special education programs will eventually be favored over the more traditional discrepancy model. In the discrepancy model, the student is placed in a special education program if there is a significant discrepancy between the student's academic performance and his or her potential to learn— which is based on results from intellectual and cognitive testing. Therefore, SLPs need to collaborate more regularly with teachers and other specialists as well as with families; intervention should come from all quarters. "Now more than ever, students with disabilities are viewed as the responsibility of the entire school community, including general education" (Ehren & Whitmire, 2005, p. 169).

As mentioned in Chapter 1, approximately 47 million, or 18% of the population in the United States, speak a language other than English (U.S. Census Bureau, 2003). Of those, 21 million (children and adults) reported that they do not speak English very well. Of those, 5 million are students (English-language learners or ELL) who are enrolled in the nation's public schools. This number has doubled within the last 10 years (National Clearinghouse for English Language Acquisition and Language Instruction, 2003). The states with the largest number of ELL students are California, Texas, Florida, New York, and Arizona.

There is also great diversity among this group of ELL students because many speak various dialects of English. The amount that an individual speaks of each variety of English depends on a number of variables such as socioeconomic status, context (whether the communication is informal or formal), and the particular geographical region in which the individual lives. African-Americans who live in the same community may use AAVE and even a number of its variations. Spanish- or Chinese-speaking individuals may also use a variety of dialects of their own language.

Hispanic and African-American students have the greatest challenges with regard to completing their education. Greene and Forster (2003) report that only 70% of all students in public high schools graduate and only 32% attain a college degree. College graduation rates in the sampled class of 2001 are 72% for white students, 79% for Asian-American students, 51% for African-American students, 52% for Hispanic students, and 54% for Native American students. The conclusion of the report states that "This suggests that the main reason that these groups are underrepresented in college admissions is that these students are not acquiring college-ready skills in the K–12 system—rather than inadequate financial and or affirmative action policies" (Greene & Forster, 2003, p. 2).

Thus, the students' lack of proficiency in English, coupled with instruction inadequate for preparing them to succeed in achieving curricular demands are the main causes for the high dropout rates among various racial and ethnic groups (Crawford, 2004). The solution to this problem is expressed by Crawford in the following quote: "One way is to stress things that can be accomplished in the classroom, such as offering state-of-the art programs to address limited English proficiency and provide trained personnel and adequate resources. Another way is to support goals that help students adjust to American life both inside and outside of school. One of these goals is heritage language development" (Crawford, 2004, p. 21). Another researcher, commenting on African-American students' failure to complete their studies, echoes Crawford: "I'll be the first to agree with those who say this problem is not just about Ebonics. It's about inadequate facilities and lack of supplies. It's about pay for teachers, particularly for those who work in districts with larger numbers of black speakers, who are not paid as much as teachers in other districts" (Professor John Rickford, as quoted in Perry & Delpit, 1998a. p. 63).

Therefore, CLD students are often overrepresented in special education for two principal reasons. The first is that lack of academic attainment is directly related to the students' inadequate English language proficiency. The second reason is that teachers are insufficiently prepared to implement adequate teaching practices for CLD students due to lack of training and resources. The following section presents a historical perspective on strategies that have been used in the past to address the educational needs of CLD students. This information can assist SLPs in gaining a perspective on the intricacies of research and practice.

Bilingual Education: Dependent on Cycles of Tolerance and Restrictiveness

Bilingual education in the United States is not new. The degree of tolerance and levels of support for other languages and multiculturalism in this country have fluctuated from the time of the Continental Congress in 1774 to the present. Four different historical periods in bilingual education can be identified and outlined (Ovando, 2003). Table 3-1 summarizes those different periods.

The period from 1774 to the end of the nineteenth century is referred to as the "permissive period." A strong sense of self-identity

TABLE 3-1 Attitudes Toward Bilingualism: Four Historical Periods

Name	Period	Ramification
Permissive	1774 to 19th century	Preserving the first language
Restrictive	End of 19th century through World War I until 1950s	Sense of nationalism
Opportunist	1960–1980	Implementation of bilingual programs. Promotion of dual language proficiency.
Dismissive	1980 to present	Accelerated movement toward diminishing the availability of bilingual programs: Negative feelings about bilingualism reflected in banned bilingual programs

among immigrants permitted them to "hold onto their languages" while also acquiring English and the new country's culture. A "restrictive period" beginning toward the end of the nineteenth century and reinforced by World War I, enhanced a sense of nationalism, and during that time, "It was expected that immigrants would learn English, forget their native language and integrate into the "'American ways' of life" (Ambert & Meléndez, 1985, p. 5). Attitudes changed again after political events of the late 1950s at home and abroad. Examples include the launching of the Sputnik satellite by the Soviet Union, previously considered a technologically less advanced nation; Fidel Castro's assumption of power in Cuba, which resulted in a flood of middle- and upper-class Cuban immigrants to the United States; and the civil rights movement of the 1960s. The feeling that the United States needed to increase its contact with other nations by encouraging instruction in other languages and providing non-English students with the right to receive an appropriate education led to the passage of the Bilingual Education Act of 1968 (U.S. Code Title 20, 1968). Thus began the "opportunist period" commencing in the 1960s and lasting for the next 20 years.

The Bilingual Education Act had two main objectives: (1) to develop programs that utilized two languages as an instructional medium and, (2) to maintain the foreign language resources of the United States. However, the Bilingual Education Act contained no clear guidelines for ways to implement bilingual programs; this resulted in a great deal of confusion. Many different programs have been called "bilingual programs," but they have varied a great deal as to philosophy, implementation, and ultimate effectiveness in preparing CLD students to achieve success in the mainstream. This incon-

sistency is one of the main reasons why bilingual programs have not received complete support from society at large. The lack of agreement about what would be the best program, and what would be the best way to best allocate monies for educating ELLs and students in general, began to be a source of debate beginning the early 1980s. This debate led to the "dismissive period" that characterizes bilingual education today. Although the Bilingual Education Act was reauthorized in 1974, it was short-lived following studies that were conducted by the American Institute of Research (AIR) and published by Dunoff, Coles, McLaughlin, and Reynolds (1977, 1978). These studies concluded that bilingual education as implemented in its "maintenance" form (i.e., education that seeks to maintain the home language) was not effective in promoting language minority students' acquisition of English or their ability to develop academically. Consequently, federal support for bilingual programs decreased, resulting over time in further legislation that declared English as the official language in various states, beginning with California in 1986. The debates of the merits of bilingual education continued for almost 10 years until, through the efforts of millionaire Ron Unz, the program was banned completely in California. The result of this is that Proposition 227 was successfully passed in 1998.

A review of the history of bilingual education reveals that the various programs were established to assist students in gaining English language proficiency. Yet, although temporarily nurturing and enhancing the development of the native language, that language was "dropped" once the student appeared to have sufficient skills in the second language to follow the regular English-only academic curriculum. Ramos (2005) reports that prior to Proposition 227, only 29% of teachers worked in bilingual programs. This percentage decreased to 14% in 1999 and was only 6.3% during the 2002–2003 academic year. Similar propositions were passed in Arizona in 2000, and in Colorado and Massachusetts in 2002. Despite all the prior research evidence that has supported bilingual education, and teachers' difficulties in meeting frustrating new criteria that demands parent waivers be obtained before even short-term bilingual instruction is permitted, most public schools in the states mentioned above continue to offer mostly English-only classroom instruction to ELL students.

The controversy over the effectiveness of bilingual programs began when the AIR studies were released and followed by the reports of Baker and De Kanter (1983). These two documents claimed that bilingual education had a negative impact on the academic achievement of Hispanic ELL students. A careful analysis of the reports revealed that their conclusions were based on a heterogeneous group of programs, which included 38 programs and more than 7,000 students in 150 schools. The reading and mathematics scores of elementary school-aged children enrolled in bilingual programs were compared with the scores of others of the same backgrounds who did not attend bilingual programs. Baker and de Kanter reviewed 300 studies, half of which were primary evaluations of actual programs. The programs varied in many aspects, from their philosophy toward bilingual education to actual instructional methodology. One principal conclusion of these studies and reports was that there was insufficient evidence to recommend a maintenance approach, and that because students were isolated from the mainstream during maintenance teaching, a transitional method was preferable. In addition, the researchers advocated more local control by the school districts. These sugges-

tions matched the political trends of the late 1970s and early 1980s, which emphasized more local government control.

On the basis of a meta-analysis, Willig (1985) challenged the conclusions of the earlier reports. The meta-analysis accounted for 183 variables that the previous studies had not considered, such as student and teacher characteristics, methods of instruction, and the language of the achievement tests. Willig found small to moderate differences among the students' achievements that actually favored bilingual instruction. Furthermore, she found that in the AIR studies, as many as two-thirds of the students who were in the monolingual classrooms (comparison groups) had previously been in bilingual programs. Thus, in fact, the students in monolingual classrooms had received instruction in Spanish and were outperforming their counterparts whose exposure to English was still minimal. Subsequently, the statistical methodology of Willig's study was criticized. For example, Willig had used averaging techniques by which mean effect sizes or differences between programs that were too small to be statistically significant were combined. The effects of the bilingual programs were based more on how the various researchers had decided to analyze the outcomes of the various studies than on the true characteristics of those programs.

This research debate highlights the importance of defining terms more precisely and choosing appropriate research designs to confirm or reject any given hypothesis. There is evidence that bilingual programs, if implemented appropriately, can be beneficial in increasing CLD students' academic achievement in both the native language and in English, a point to be discussed in the next section of this chapter. One of the positive outcomes of the debates was that the various research studies indicated the need for consistency in the definition and implementation of bilingual education programs. For a history of the legal underpinnings of bilingual education and their ramifications for education in states like California, the latest edition of Crawford's book, entitled *Educating English Learners: Language Diversity in the Classroom* (2004), is a good resource.

There is no question that English is the official language used for legislation, treaties, federal court rulings, and all official/government-regulated business. However, there are some states and territories that are still bilingual— including, for example, Louisiana (English and French), New Mexico (English and Spanish), Puerto Rico (English and Spanish), Guam (Chamorro and English), and the Northern Mariana Islands (English, Chamorro, and Carolinian).

Throughout its existence, the United States has attempted to accommodate the communication needs of new immigrants. This accommodation has fluctuated, however, due to historical events such as the outcomes of the two world wars and the events of 9/11/2001. Accepting open tolerance for other languages and dialects might have been a sign of fear of losing power. Despite the current negative feelings about immigration, the standard census questionnaires distributed in 2000 were printed in English, Spanish, Korean, Mandarin, Vietnamese, and Tagalog, indicating an acceptance of linguistic diversity on at least a federal level.

MODELS OF BILINGUAL EDUCATION

The term "bilingual education," like the term "bilingualism," is difficult to define, as both terms encompass many variables. The lack of a common philosophy about language use and curriculum guidelines has been one of the reasons for the contradictory data about the effectiveness of using bilingual programs to educate CLD students. When defining the nature of a bilingual program, it is necessary to consider how the two languages are used during the day and in the curriculum, and to take into account the background of the students attending the program.

Baker and Prys Jones (1998, p. 464) propose that program planners consider six questions when designing bilingual instructional programs: (1) Are both languages used in the classroom? (2) For how long during the day are the languages being used? (3) Are the two languages used by all or only some of the students? (4) Are the two languages used by the teachers or just by the students? (5) Is the aim to teach a second language or to teach *through* a second language? and (6) Is the aim to support the home language or to move to an alternative majority language?

Crawford (2004), Herrera and Murry (2005), and Ovando (2003) describe in greater detail the various types of bilingual programs traditionally implemented in the United States. In most cases, the aim of the programs has been to eventually move to English-only instruction—at which point the home language is no longer maintained. (An exception is the Maintenance Program, also called the Developmental Bilingual Program or Two-Way Bilingual Program). Unfortunately, not all programs are explicit about which language of instruction should be used for specific subjects. The Case Studies project (Crawford, 2004), in which the California State Department set out to improve school practices, rather than attempting to demonstrate the effectiveness of bilingual education, is an exception. The instructional model in this project was based on information from second-language acquisition research and included five principles: (1) the concurrent development of both the native and English language should have a positive impact on academic achievement; (2) language proficiency needs should be reflected in both Basic Interpersonal Communication Skills (BICS) and Cognitive Academic Language Proficiency (CALP); (3) improvement of the native language should have positive effects on the acquisition of oral as well as written skills in the second language (i.e., teachers should avoid mixing English and the native language during instruction); (4) sufficient comprehensible input should be offered in English, and (5) attention should be given to the students' language proficiency in each one of their languages and their interaction with teachers and other students. Specific subjects taught in either Spanish or English were also specified for each grade level (for details and further discussion refer to Crawford, 2004).

Brisk (2005) indicates that the lack of survival of bilingual programs and bilingualism is due to the fact that bilingualism has been associated with "remediation." Bilingual education in the United States has implied an alternative method for educating children whose home language is not English. Elsewhere in the world, however, it refers to education in two valued languages. Another challenge faced by bilingual education is that in the United States, the term "bilingual programs" is thought of as almost synonymous with bilingual programs for Spanish and English. Very few other bilingual programs have been developed other than for Chinese, Vietnamese, and some Native American languages. That this is a moot point is often argued by families of children who speak any of the other 100 or more languages that may be represented within one single school district.

Methodologies for Teaching English as a Second Language (ESL)

Methodologies for teaching English as a second language (ESL) vary significantly. Instruction in English may range from the submersion, or sink-or–swim, model (no specific language support) to other models where the use of language in the classroom is tailored to enable ELL students to benefit from instruction.

Three of the methodologies most frequently discussed in the literature include (1) the Cognitive Academic Language Learning Approach (CALLA) (Chamot & O'Malley, 1994); (2) Specially Designed Academic Instruction in English (SDAIE), and (3) Sheltered Instruction Observation Protocol (SIOP) (Echevarría, Vogt, & Short, 2004). Use of the language is carefully tailored to ensure that students are learning the content of the instruction. Strategies such as checking for comprehension, enabling more interaction between teacher and students and students and other students, and implementing activities to apply the content learned are applied. Only short descriptions of each program are provided here. More comprehensive reviews can be found in the references at the end of this book. See, for example, Herrera and Murry (2005) or Trumbull and Farr (2005).

The CALLA approach employs various learning strategies in three areas: metacognitive, cognitive, and social affective. For example, graphic organizers, charts, and self-monitoring are tools used in the metacognitive area. Reference to the students' background knowledge on a given topic of instruction, and the enhancement of skills for predicting and making inferences are targeted. The social affective strategies include questioning for clarification, and cooperative learning in the metacognitive area. The SDAIE and SIOP models share commonalities such as hands-on activities, cooperative learning, teacher's control of language in the classroom (slower rate of speech, simplified vocabulary, and avoidance of idioms) as well as use of visual aids such as graphic organizers, charts, diagrams, and tables. Although the SIOP model is similar to the SDAIE, it has been expanded to include lesson outlines with carefully written objectives and materials. The SIOP model also includes descriptions of the best strategies for implementing those lessons. In addition, Echevarria et al. (2004) emphasize the importance of frequent language interaction between students and teacher.

The teaching strategies described above can be implemented in any classroom where there might be students with various linguistic and cultural differences, including African-American students who speak a variety of dialects. In reference to those students, Delpit (1998) indicates that "educators need to understand that the linguistic form a student brings to school is intimately connected with loves ones, community, and personal identity.... On the other hand, it is equally important to understand that students who do not have access to the politically popular dialect form in the country are less likely to succeed economically than their peers who do" (p. 19).

Several strategies for working effectively with African-American students include creating situations where students are engaged, instruction is paired with visual aids, and drama, music, and movement are utilized. To improve the academic performance of some African-American students, specific schools have been created to respond to their unique needs. For example, African-American-centered programs emphasize literacy and critical thinking; the teaching of African and African-American history, heritage, and culture; and the development of students'

Submersion
Structured Immersion
Transitional Programs
Maintenance or Developmental Bilingual Programs
Two-Way Bilingual Programs

FIGURE 3-1 *Types of Bilingual Program Models.*

self-concept, self-expression, and self-confidence. For more details on these programs readers can refer to Gay (2000), Lipman (1998), and Riley (1995). The following section describes specific bilingual programs that are delivered in one or two languages at various phases of the student's education.

Bilingual Education Programs

Figure 3-1 lists five different bilingual education program models. For further details about each of the programs, the reader is referred to Brisk (2005), Crawford (2004), Herrera and Murry (2005), Lessow-Hurley (2005), and Nieto (2004). Highlights of each program are described in the next sections.

Submersion

In this program, the native language is not used during instruction, but students may attend ESL classes (which, however, might vary in duration and quality of instruction). Minimal or no support at all in English or the primary language is available, and these submersion programs have been referred to as "sink-or-swim " programs.

Structured Immersion

This program has been referred to as sheltered English, content-based ESL. The language of instruction is English and the programs are available to students for one to three years. The teaching approaches are similar to the submersion model except that instruction in the student's native language is offered about one hour daily.

Transitional Programs

Instruction is provided in both English and the student's native language. There are many more of these programs for Spanish than for any other language. The student is exited into the mainstream English programs when "ready"; at that point, instruction in the native language ceases. Early-exit transitional programs last for two or three years, whereas late-exit programs last five to six years. The first language is used for reading instruction.

Maintenance or Developmental Bilingual Programs

These are intensive programs that prepare students to be bilingual and biliterate; they continue instruction in the native language even after the students have sufficient mastery of English.

Two-Way Bilingual Programs

The structure of the two-way bilingual programs is to place speakers of both languages in bilingual programs to learn each other's language. These programs are also referred to as dual immersion, or dual language, two-way immersion. Native speakers of English and native speakers of other languages learn together. As a result, the students become fully bilingual and biliterate.

Other Ways of Promoting Bilingualism

Bilingual education programs proliferated in the late 1960s until the late 1980s. However, there were also situations in which no provisions were made for instruction in the children's first language and the children needed to adapt to a learning environment conducted in the majority language only. This model is increasingly more frequent throughout the United States, and more and more immigrant children attend nursery and preschool programs where English is used exclusively. If parents wish their children to continue speaking the family's language at home, the language needs to be reinforced at home by interaction in that language on a consistent basis. This can be accomplished by arranging playgroups with other families who speak the language and hiring caretakers who speak the language, as well (Baker, 2000). The latter demands a great deal of effort on the part of the family.

Maintaining the language of the home is particularly difficult in countries such as the United States, because English is so highly valued throughout the world. Maintaining the home language may be easier to carry out in other countries where other languages are spoken, or where the status of the majority language does not have such a global importance. For example, my parents and grandparents communicated in Polish with me and my brother, instilling a sense of pride in the language. This did not deter us children from learning Spanish, the majority language of Mexico where my family resided at the time. Maintaining Polish was easier in Mexico, where the majority language doesn't have quite the "status" that English does in a global context.

There are still Head Start programs where the majority of the instruction is conducted in Spanish, but the use of Spanish and English varies from program to program depending on the availability of bilingual staff and their ease in using their first language. The advantage of conducting preschool programs in the children's primary language enables further development of that language. The home language gains status and respect and the communication between parents and teachers can be reinforced (Baker & Prys Jones, 1998). Baker and Prys Jones indicate that the success of bilingual nursery and preschool programs depends on three factors: (1) whether the second language is used at the expense of the first language (both the majority and minority languages should be assigned equal status); (2) whether bilingual instruction is continued and nurtured beyond this early period of education and, (3) whether parents who send their child to a bilingual preschool are disappointed if the child's acquisition of the second language is not on a par with that of other children who are native speakers of the second language. As discussed in Chapter 2, it takes time to learn and have a command of a second language.

In order to rule out the impact that an inconsistent or inadequate education might have on ELL students who may not be progressing sufficiently in their acquisition of English (and often in reading and academics), it is important to have information on the type of program or programs these students have attended. It is possible that the student may not be progressing because of an interrupted education caused by moving from one district to another or one state to another. There may have been a period when the family returned to their country of origin. Interrupted education can happen to students of all ages, including those children who attend nursery or preschool programs.

Efficacy Studies

Results of studies on the effectiveness of various programs that are designated as "bilingual" is important for identifying the best teaching strategies. Krashen and Biber (1988) analyzed the effectiveness of seven bilingual programs in California that met the following three criteria: (1) translation was not used when the curriculum was taught in the students' first language, (2) the development of literacy in the first language was enhanced, and (3) there was ample opportunity for comprehensible input in English. (The term "comprehensible input" refers to one of Krashen's five hypotheses of second language acquisition. This hypothesis states that best learning occurs when students are exposed to material they can understand, but which also offers some challenges.) Although the results of the research must be evaluated with care because the studies were not longitudinal, the researchers demonstrated that the ELL students in these programs outperformed other ELL students who were not enrolled in the bilingual programs.

On average, it took the students in the bilingual programs at least three years to attain reading skills in English at the 50th percentile level relative to the English-speaking monolingual group. It was concluded that "children who participate in properly designed bilingual programs acquire English rapidly. They typically achieve at grade level norms for English and math after three to five years. Furthermore, bilingual education in fact may be the best English program we have" (Krashen & Biber, 1988, p. 63).

A comparison between Canadian and American bilingual programs is described in Table 3-2.

Table 3-2 is an outline of aspects of the Canadian immersion programs and the more recent types of programs implemented in the United States, such as the Case Studies project and the two-way bilingual programs. The latest U.S. programs are versions of transitional programs, but have six additional features: (1) the program lasts four to six years; (2) instruction is adjusted to the students'

TABLE 3-2 Bilingual Programs in Canada and the United States

Program	Government Policy	Parent's Status and Views	Teachers	Curriculum
Immersion in Canada	Enhancement of bilingualism and multiculturalism Promotion of international economic advantage	Additive—Middle class—Parents initiate and support the program. Students' skills in both languages are valued.	All teachers are bilingual. Have the support from the community and administrators. Are offered a uniform preparation.	Students are expected to use both languages. All students begin at the same level of L2. Literacy in both languages is emphasized. Both languages have the same value. No real transition in programs.
Transitional programs	No clear policy Bilingualism is not viewed as an advantage	Programs are viewed as remedial in nature. Generally, bilingualism may be considered as an advantage but is difficult to maintain.	Only some teachers are bilingual. May have community and administrators' support. Training institutions offer great variation in preparation. Requires large numbers of bilingual teachers. Many rely on teacher aides.	Use of L1 until L2 is mastered. Students need to catch up to function in an all-English curriculum. Transition to English is often made when surface language skills (BICS) are judged adequate. Some other programs may transition students when sufficient (CALP) skills are acquired.
Other models in the U.S.	Flexiblity at the local level Bilingualism is viewed as an advantage	Socioeconomic status is generally low. Parents' participation is generally promoted but in actuality parents have little to say. *There may be exceptions, however.*	Only some teachers are bilingual. May have community and administrators' support. Training institutions offer great variation in preparation. Requires fewer bilingual teachers. Use of language grouping. More emphasis on teacher cooperation.	Use of L1 and L2 is acquired. L1 is valued. Provision is made for uniformity in language instruction. Transition to English is done only when student has higher language skills in L1 (CALP).

level; (3) oral language development is implemented in conjunction with academic subjects; (4) languages are separated during instruction; (5) students have opportunities to interact with native speakers; and (6) there is home-school collaboration to reinforce the native language and enhance the potential for success in academic subjects (Crawford, 1989, p. 167).

Such programs were in operation in California, New York, and Massachusetts until the various propositions to declare English as the official language were passed. One fundamental factor differentiating the U.S. programs from the immersion programs in Canada is that the latter have the support of community at large.

Recent studies by Thomas and Collier (1997, 2002) compared various models of bilingual instruction over a period of four to eight years. These studies indicated that the most effective programs had four main characteristics in common: (1) the status of each language was equal; (2) parents were involved; (3) instructional approaches included strategies that emphasized whole language, language scaffolding for content areas, and cooperative activities; and (4) the programs lasted for six years at least. Best outcomes were reached when students had been schooled in their own language for at least two or three years. These students required five to seven years to reach the 50th percentile for performance on standardized tests in English. Students who had not been schooled in their native language required 7 to 10 years to attain the same 50th percentile performance level. The least successful program was the traditional "pull-out" program and the most successful was the two-way developmental bilingual program.

Since 2001 and the passage of the No Child Left Behind Act (2001), more attention has been given to results of national testing to determine the effectiveness of a given school program. No public school in the country is exempt from the process. All ELL students need to take a yearly language proficiency test to document their progress in gaining language and academic skills. When students exit the category of being ELL, they are treated like any other mainstream students. A few accommodations, however, are made for these former ELL students—they don't have to take the state tests during the first year of their enrollment as mainstream students in a U.S. school, and they are permitted to take the tests in their native language for three to five years. States are not required to develop those tests, however, and even if the ELL students take

the tests in their native language, they must take the test in English after three years.

OPTIMAL TEACHING/ LEARNING STRATEGIES FOR CLD POPULATIONS

In their extensive review of bilingual programs, August and Hakuta (1998) offer suggestions for optimal teaching and learning strategies for CLD students. These suggestions are divided into two major areas: (1) the climate of the school and the classroom, which includes the teacher's expectations and philosophy; and (2) the "research-based" teaching techniques required for both ELL and special education students. Helpful sources for the topics discussed in this section include Díaz-Rico and Weed (2005), Echevarria, Vogt, and Short (2004), Herrell (2000), and Trumbull and Farr (2005).

Climate of the School and District

In their analysis of 33 studies, August and Hakuta (1998) found that successful ELL programs included a supportive school-wide climate that encouraged an explicit respect for the students' linguistic and cultural backgrounds while maintaining high expectations for student performance (Berman, McLaughlin, McLeod, Minicussi, Nelson, & Woodsworth, 1995; Moll, 1988). ELL students' performance increased when there was communication between the school and the family (this will be discussed in greater detail in Chapter 4), as well as the inclusion of the students' experiences in the curriculum.

School leadership (principals or other personnel who may have the role of coordinators or facilitators) is another important variable for securing the success of ELL students (Carter & Chatfield 1986; Goldenberg & Sullivan, 1994). Coordination among teachers within a school and district is another important consideration, especially because each school may have some programs that others do not—such as after-school programs, cross-age and parent tutoring, specialized instructional personnel who teach specific subjects, and teachers who collaborate by sharing their classes for certain subjects. Careful monitoring of the students' progress and transition to the next language development level is another variable to consider (Berman et al., 1995; Moll, 1988; Short, 1994).

The Curriculum

Grade-level expectations specify the material that students need to learn. With No Child Left Behind, teachers may feel more restricted in their ability to implement their preferred teaching techniques because they have to adhere to a script. Furthermore, there might be less time for additional activities that could reinforce academic content because of pressure to prepare students for state-mandated tests. As expected, there may be variations within schools, districts, counties, and states because of interpretations of the law.

In the absence of "bilingual programs," CLD students can achieve academically if and when they learn through effective teaching strategies. The role of the SLP is to observe whether the CLD student who may be experiencing language and learning difficulties has been included in a learning environment that promotes such strategies. The following sections discuss this subject in more detail. (For further information on the strategies discussed in the following sections, please refer to Crawford (2004), Díaz-Rico and Weed (2005), Herrera and Murry (2005), and Trumbull and Farr (2005). Another useful resource is a video produced by Silver (1995), entitled *Profile of Effective Teaching in a Multilingual Classroom: Featuring Robin Liten-Tejada.*

The following teaching strategies are divided into teacher's responsibilities and students' responses. Many of the strategies are based on Cummins' (1989) "interactive/interactionist" model, as well as on the "contextualized/interactionist" models created by Tharp and Gallimore (1988), which will be discussed again in Chapter 7.

The Role of the Teacher

Researchers who have studied the best teaching strategies for students who are learning English as a second language or speak a distinct dialect (such as AAVE) share a number of conclusions. The seven strategies listed below are those most frequently mentioned by researchers as being the most useful for instructing CLD students.

The following sections discuss each of these strategies in detail; each section is followed by references to research studies.

- Use of thematic approach
- Explicit teaching of learning strategies
- Utilization of media
- Incorporation of the student's experience in the learning process
- Vocabulary building
- Teacher discourse
- Scaffolding

Use of a Thematic Approach

In this approach, the same theme is used to reinforce a topic throughout the curriculum (to enable growth in overall oral and written language skills). If a goal of the curriculum is to examine the formation of clouds and rain, the topic can be applied by having students read about the topic in an appropriate book that describes the process. Beaumont (1992) lists some activities that can embrace various areas of the curriculum. For example, before students begin reading about the formation of clouds and rain, words that are connected to the topic can be listed on the board by the teacher. A definition of each word can follow. In social studies, students may apply the concepts by interpreting a weather map, or by following the weather patterns occurring in other cities. "Conceptual learning is promoted because students repeatedly encounter a set of interrelated meanings, and language learning is enhanced because students are reading, writing, listening, and speaking to general meaning related to the theme at hand" (Kucer & Silva, 1989, p. 18). More recently, Farr and Quintanar-Sarellana (2005) have indicated that "thematic instruction can increase motivation, engagement, and a sense of purpose. Working together on projects, students use language to ask questions, solve problems, negotiate, and interact with and report to their peers" (p. 260). This same approach can be used in intervention strategies for CLD clients with various language and learning disabilities. These strategies will be discussed in greater detail in Chapter 7.

Explicit Teaching of Learning Strategies

In this model, specific instruction about the material to be learned is provided; that is, the "why and how" of what is going to occur in the classroom. For example, prior to initiating a unit, a discussion about what the students already know takes place and the points that are going to be covered are written on the board. Before reading a textbook, chapter headings and subheadings, diagrams, and pictures are presented and a discussion about the text's content is carried out. Also, students are assisted in thinking about their own learning. This process taps metacognitive and cognitive understanding that is achieved through awareness, reflection, and interaction. Further information about explicit teaching of learning strategies can be found in Duffy (2002), McLaughlin and Allen (2002), and Echevarría et al. (2004).

Utilization of Media

Robin Liten-Tejada, featured in the video *Profile of Effective Teaching in a Multilingual Classroom* (Silver [producer], 1995) reminds viewers that filling out blanks on a page is a very specific but minimal way to demonstrate one's knowledge. In her classroom, teacher Liten-Tejada enhances the students' ability to use and demonstrate their knowledge through sociodramatic play and other media such as art. One connection between symbolic play and literacy lies in organizational schema between play episodes and narratives. Sociodramatic play is also helpful for school-aged children who need practice in the pragmatic aspects of language, such as making requests, using an appropriate level of verbal specificity, and repairing communication breakdowns. When Ruiz (1988) studied sociodramatic play used with bilingual special education students, she noted a significant improvement in their oral language skills over their performance in more structured classroom academic tasks. As children discussed key elements of their play, such as scene, actors, and props, their ability to negotiate meaning improved. The negotiation process may require the use of particular language structures, turn-taking, convention, and message repair (Beaumont, 1992). Similar strategies have been followed by teachers of children who use an African-American dialect. Role-play and puppet shows are used to make students aware of the differences between AAVE and Standard English: "Role-playing eliminates the possibility of implying that the child's language is inadequate—and suggests, instead, that different language forms are appropriate in different contexts" (Delpit, 1998, p. 20). The author cites other techniques that include drama—such as having students produce a news show every day. The students take on the role of famous newscasters and read their news reports. This type of activity would be appropriate for older elementary students and beyond.

Incorporation of the Student's Experience in the Learning Process

The goals of this approach can be reached through using recounts of the students' background culture and experiences when teaching new concepts, or previewing a reading selection. The focus is on assisting students in making a bridge between the academic content and their experiences and environment. Schools are a place to help students expand their minds and gain knowledge of other cultures. Not only cultural content but also culturally based modes of learning and communication ought to be tapped (Farr & Quintanar-Sarellana, 2005).

Beaumont (1992) provides a list of topics (based on suggestions from Brooks, 1986) that can enhance a dialogue between teacher and students. These topics compare and contrast various cultural viewpoints. Along with familiar topics, such as festivals and holidays, Brooks advises examining daily living patterns. Examples include questions such as: (1) How do Sunday activities different from weekly activities? (2) What are the most popular games that are played outdoors and indoors by children and adults? (3) What are typical errands that a young person is likely to be asked to do, either at home or in school? (4) What are the special characteristics of each meal, the food eaten, the seating arrangement, the method of serving dishes, the general conversation? and (5) What are some of the beliefs of the people of various countries? (For example, in the previously mentioned video, Liten-Tejada's students describe cultural superstitions, such as what people believe will happen when they see a black cat or an owl.) Using information gleaned from their interview with Oakland teacher Carrie Secret, Delpit and Perry describe in her words the following activity for students of African-American descent: "After the children have completed the page they have to go back and group at least four pictures together. Or they might group together four pictures that belong together and one that doesn't and tell why. I might also make a connection between the lesson and their lives. I will say, 'How would you connect the picture to your life, and why?'" (1998, p. 84).

Vocabulary Building

Vocabulary is an important component for improving the understanding and knowledge of content. Therefore, in order to assist students in expanding their vocabulary, the "weekly vocabulary list" should be linked to the content that will be taught. Echevarria et al. (2004) provide suggestions for increasing knowledge of vocabulary, such as providing a context for or alternatives to the different words that are discussed (for example, while reading a text, clarifying the meaning of a word by offering a synonym or cognate). In Liten-Tejada's video, she asks students to remember a word ("creek") that they learned the week before. They are then asked to connect it to a new, recently learned word ("stream"). Other techniques include making lists of vocabulary words and reviewing them either in small groups or with the entire class; creating dictionaries; and developing a "word wall" using the relevant vocabulary from a given lesson. Conceptual maps are also a helpful way to reinforce vocabulary. Delpit (1998) suggests that students create bilingual dictionaries with words from their own language and from Standard English. She recommends that teachers and students decide on the best possible translations of the various terms.

In a similar vein, exposing the students to the vocabulary and language of math is very important. Knowing numbers and solving computations is only part of the subject. Even though students might be able to solve a given mathematical problem using, for example, multiplication, it does not necessarily mean that they have the vocabulary for all numbers in tens, hundreds, or thousands—or for specific concepts such as "equal," "decimal," "place," "tens," and other terms. In Liten-Tejada's class, the students have a chance to practice the vocabulary by dictating math problems to one another. This incorporates the tasks of listening, speaking, reading, and writing. For example, students dictate to each other higher numbers such as "two-thousand and fifty-three" and then check to see if the numbers are correct. They also solve problems which require thinking about the particular computation necessary. Therefore, differentiating mathematical computation (adding, subtracting, multiplying, and dividing numbers) from mathematical problem solving (which requires applying concepts—such as realizing that "more" translates into addition, and that "sharing" translates into division) is important.

Teacher Discourse

At the heart of all instruction is the teacher's style of content delivery. Figure 3-2 lists some

- Speak more slowly.
- Use clearer articulation ("Do you want to?" instead of "D'ya wanna?")
- Emphasize intonation of important words and use body language when making a point.
- Use students' names instead of pronouns.
- Clarify the meaning of possibly unfamiliar words.
- Use visual aids (pictures, videos, real objects) to increase comprehension of ideas and concepts.
- Initially, do not "correct" students, but rather ocus on meaning.
- Allow for additional "wait time" to enable the student to process and formulate an answer.

FIGURE 3-2 *Suggested Teacher Discourse Strategies.*

teaching strategies that are suggested by Beaumont (1992). Note that the SLP who has ample knowledge of language development and intervention strategies can play a key role in outlining discourse and interaction strategies between teachers and students. The suggestions provided in Figure 3-2 are not listed in any particular order.

Scaffolding

Scaffolding is an instructional strategy that facilitates the students' acquisition of skills and is done in steps until the student can learn new material more independently. Consistent with the Zone of Proximal Development (ZPD) approach described by Vygotsky (1962), this approach is based on the assumption that students have a range of ability that is much wider than that revealed by a static picture of a particular developmental level. New learning does not await a given developmental level; rather, learning moves development forward. Furthermore, students' learning is expanded by interaction with more expert members of a society. Greenfield (1984) stated that scaffolding "does not involve simplifying the task during the period of learning. Instead, it

- Connecting the current task to something the student already knows.
- Using questioning techniques that lead the student to problem-solving strategies.
- Modeling mnemonics devices.
- Following the student's cues to decide when and how to intervene.
- Allowing for a balance of error and success that allows the child to use errors for growth without becoming discouraged by them.
- Verbal scaffolding—rephrasing what the student says in order to model the correct form.
- Rephrasing what the teacher says in order to obtain desired responses from the student.

FIGURE 3-3 *Scaffolding—Effective Strategies.* (Note These same strategies can be implemented during sessions with the SLP.)

holds the task constant while simplifying the learner's role through the graduated intervention of the teacher" (p. 11). Thus, instead of teaching discrete skills, the teacher identifies the larger context that the student needs in order to participate in authentic communication exchanges. Characteristics of effective scaffolding applied to an activity are listed in Figure 3-3 (Beaumont, 1992, p. 275). Naturally, the number of steps that a student needs to take to be at the independent level depends on the student's initial level of performance. These strategies can be reviewed in greater detail in Herrera and Murry (2005) and Trumbull and Farr (2005).

For example, for "connecting the current task to something the student already knows," the teacher can begin a discussion about a given topic by asking the students to share what they already know about that topic. If the topic is "the marine world," questions about the students' experience with visiting aquariums or seeing ocean animals can begin the discussion. In this fashion, each individual student can express what he or she already knows. The other students benefit by listening to peers' contributions. From that point,

everyone involved has a shared initial knowledge about the topic that will be expanded upon by the teacher.

The Students

Structuring the classroom to enable students to interact with each other and with the teacher is part of the curriculum. As Kagan (1986) noted: "In a relatively short time what appears to be a long-term minority student deficiency in basic language skills can be overcome by transforming the social organization of the classroom" (p. 246). Cooperative learning activities offer students the opportunity to use a variety of language skills in group interactions. In these situations, students listen, negotiate turn-taking rules, ask questions, clarify information, repair miscommunications, initiate and maintain topics, change roles, explain, persuade, record, summarize, and apply politeness conventions used when joining and taking leave of a group.

After working in their small groups, students conduct a debriefing session to evaluate both the product and the process followed. This debriefing assists them in developing functional communication skills and metalinguistic awareness. The group work provides experience in highly contextualized "here and now" activities that are more frequently associated with home cultures. It also enhances practice in school language skills, such as planning and reflecting.

In the video featuring Liten-Tejada's classroom, students had to plan how they would illustrate the lives of different Native Americans using various props. In a subsequent activity they were asked to work in groups of two and use a Venn diagram to list similarities and differences between two different versions of the same legend that was related to various Native American tribes. This activity enabled the students to engage in several of the reflective and metalinguistic activities that enhance learning. The value of cooperative learning has been summarized as follows: "The achievement gains in cooperative classrooms are particularly dramatic for minority students. Whereas nonminority and high-achieving students generally perform about as well as in traditional and cooperative classrooms, low-achieving and minority students appear to be considerably more motivated to learn in cooperative classrooms" (Cummins, 1989 p. 76).

The information presented thus far has outlined the best strategies suggested by researchers and teachers for teaching CLD students. However, it is important to consider the learners' (and their families') experiences with the teaching and learning process based on their own experiences in their home culture or country.

DESCRIPTIONS OF LEARNERS' PREVIOUS SCHOOLING

Recent immigrant children and adolescents who attend schools throughout the United States may come from many different countries and therefore various types of schools. Furthermore, their attendance in those schools may have been disrupted due to economic or political crises. In addition, they may have attended schools in rural (as opposed to urban) settings where resources may have been more scarce. Moreover, when teachers work with first-generation CLD students, it is helpful to understand the educational systems attended by the students' parents in order to be better able to facilitate involving the parents in the educational process. Also, having some information on higher-education facilities in those countries is helpful for understanding the

family's background experiences with regard to the educational process; such an understanding can assist in guiding parents through their children's transition from high school to college. This information is also useful for the SLP who is working with an older client who may have sustained a stroke or traumatic brain injury, or who may be suffering from dementia: inquiring about the client's previous schooling in his or her country of origin is helpful for planning assessment and intervention.

The scope of this book does not permit a review of all of the educational systems of the countries of immigrants who have recently settled in the United States. Therefore, the following sections describe selected educational systems. Keep in mind, however, that the best information comes from perspectives of the students and families themselves; thus, it is advisable to conduct a dialogue with the student/client and their families about their previous schooling and educational experiences. This information provides SLPs with strategies for planning an assessment and drafting a treatment plan. The questions listed in Figure 3-4 are helpful for determining the type and continuity of education received by the client/student and their families.

In the following sections, several school systems are described. They are representative of Mexico, Puerto Rico, Cuba, Vietnam, and China/Taiwan.

Mexico

Public schools in Mexico, free of charge, are usually attended by the low- to middle-class socioeconomic groups. Those same students who enroll in secondary schools may receive their tuition free but this is variable (Langdon, 1992a). Middle- and upper-class Mexicans, as well as many of the Europeans residing in the

Country of origin: _____ Primary Language:_____

STUDENT

- Number of years attended:_____
- Overall performance/grades:_____
- Disruptions in school attendance?   No   Yes
- Difficulty with learning?   No   Yes
- Repeated any grade?   No   Yes
- Did student need special education?   No   Yes

If (Yes) was an answer to any of the above questions, please comment:

_____

_____

MOTHER/FATHER/CLIENT

- Number of years attended:_____ Degree: _____
- Disruptions in school attendance?   No   Yes
- Difficulty with learning?   No   Yes
- Repeated any grade?   No   Yes

If (Yes) was an answer to any of the above questions, please comment:

_____

_____

Briefly describe the educational system of your country of origin (Elementary, Secondary, etc.)_____

_____

_____

- How many students in a class? _____
- What kind of tests are used? For example, written, oral, multiple-choice, etc. _____
- How did the interviewee perform on tests? _____

Further comments: _____

_____

FIGURE 3-4   *Obtaining Information about the Previous Schooling of Students/Clients and Their Families.*
*Note (Adapted from Langdon, 2002, pp. 33–34.)

country, send their children to parochial schools or to bilingual French, German, or American private schools.

In the early grades (1 and 2), the "global method" is followed; teachers integrate social and environmental studies. Foreign languages and art are part of the curriculum in the secondary schools. When completing the American equivalent of secondary school (secundaria), students select specific programs leading to a college, technical, or business career. Classrooms may have as many as 58 students; they are not grouped by ability. The teacher has no assistant and discipline as well as the teacher's authority is generally negatively impacted.

There can be broad differences between the kind of education available in urban areas and in more isolated or rural communities. It is very difficult to find a teacher in the more isolated communities and, once students complete elementary school, it is even more difficult to attend secondary school due to the distance students must travel to reach it. Furthermore, the expenses created by transportation, textbooks, and uniforms may be too costly for families. Some of the Native Mexican Indians, who live in the remote areas, do not speak Spanish, which constitutes an additional barrier for them as they seek access to education. The proportion of Indians to non-Indians is quite significant in countries such as Bolivia, Perú, Guatemala, Ecuador, and Mexico. Educating these children and adults poses immense challenges to their governments. As of 1984, bilingual textbooks in as many as 12 Indian languages and 26 dialects had been adopted in Mexico (Miller, 1984).

Higher education can be attained at several public and private colleges and universities located in major cities across the country. The University of Mexico, or Universidad Autónoma de Mexico, is the oldest university in Latin America and was founded in September of 1551. The Web site http://www.unam.mx/ is recommended for those who wish to learn about the University of Mexico's history and curriculum. For a helpful overview of education in Mexico the reader is referred to McLaughlin (2003).

Puerto Rico

The educational system in Puerto Rico is somewhat influenced by the U.S. system. Education is compulsory from age 6 to 17 just like on the mainland. The majority of schools in Puerto Rico are public, with only 20% of children attending private schools. Elementary education includes kindergarten through the 6th grade; junior high school is the 7th through the 9th grade; and high school is from the 10th through the 12th grade. Although Spanish was the main language of instruction until 1948, it was switched to English in that year. However, all schools, whether public or private, strive to be bilingual. At the college level, both Spanish and English may be used. Currently there are 51 private and 14 public institutions. The University of Puerto Rico was founded in 1903 and currently there are many branches on the island. Literacy has increased considerably—to 94.6% from only 67% in 1940. In addition, there are several technical and vocational institutions in Puerto Rico. For information on various aspects of educational and cultural aspects, the reader is referred to the website listed under Puerto Rico in the references "http://welcome.topuertorico.org/people.shtml.

There are, however, significant differences between the Puerto Ricans who live on the island and the mainland. For example, those who settle in large cities on the mainland, such as New York, frequently have limited resources. Some live in

PERSONAL STORIES

Attending a Mexican University

I attended the Universidad Autónoma Nacional de Mexico in the 1960s. Although it is old it is still considered one of the best universities/institutions in the region. The university does not have departments; instead it has "faculties" (facultades) because it is modeled after the European system where students begin their area of specialization beginning their freshman year. This system is similar to several European university systems even to this day. In my case, I attended the Faculty of Chemistry where I studied biology and chemistry. All students followed the same curriculum. At the end of four years I received the title of "Licenciatura" which is the equivalent of a bachelor's degree. All lectures and labs were conducted in Spanish. However, several textbooks were available in English only. Therefore, reading comprehension in English was a prerequisite for completing the course of studies successfully. After completing the degree, the course of studies was recognized by one major American university but I had to take and pass the Graduate Record Exam (GRE) and the Test of English as a Foreign Language (TOEFL).

Approximately 93% of students in Mexico attend elementary grade school; 86% attend secondary schools. Preschool enrollment is low (56%) as is upper secondary school/high school (51%). Out of an enrollment of 100 students who enter school, only 68% will complete the equivalent of junior high school. Thirty-five percent of those students graduate from high school, and only 8% of the population aged 18 and older in Mexico has a bachelor's degree (Saltibañez, Vernez, & Razquin, 2005). Students are graded on a scale of 0 to 10 and must have a 6 in exams to pass from grade to grade. When students do not achieve academically, they are asked to repeat the grade. Therefore, it is important for SLPs and teachers to learn whether a student has repeated a grade. It may signal that the student may have had some learning difficulties.

Access to special education services has increased since the 1990s following a series of international conferences in Spain in 1994 and Thailand in 1999 where the best strategies for offering services to students with special needs were discussed. Mexico voted only in 1994 on legislation that would provide services to students with special needs. These services would also include helping these students become integrated into the mainstream (Fletcher, Dejud, Klinger, & López-Mariscal, 2003). Until that time, students needing special education services attended separate programs and were not integrated into the regular classroom or curriculum environments, much like in the United States prior to the implementation of PL-94-142 (1976). Fletcher et al. (2003) indicated that even though a process had been implemented to integrate students with special needs, there were still many gaps in the ability of the process to successfully carry out this goal. Lack of teacher preparation for working with students with special educational needs, undefined roles and responsibilities of both regular and special education teachers, and lack of parent participation in the process seemed to be at the core of the problem. Change takes time; putting a great deal of effort into planning, coordinating the skills of professionals, and enlisting the participation of parents is necessary.

dilapidated, low-rent apartments called *caserias*. It is estimated that of all the Hispanic groups living in the U.S., Puerto Ricans have the highest proportion of persons living below the poverty level—26.1% as compared with 21.4% for the entire U.S. Hispanic population (U.S. Census Bureau, 2004).

Cuba

The Cuban revolution of 1959, although devastating to many of its citizens, increased educational opportunities for most of its population. The result is that, after 40 years, the literacy rate is very high: 96.9%. The beginning of the literacy campaign in the early 1960s was a daunting task, since most of the educated citizens had left the island. Some of the most striking curriculum changes consisted of a nationalized educational curriculum, a focus on arts in the curriculum, required texts that included political and moral messages, and the absence of school libraries or books for casual reading. Today, students' progress in each subject is evaluated each quarter and both students and teachers take a state-mandated exam at the end of the year. Teachers' salaries depend on teacher performance (Worthman & Kaplan, 2001).

Specific teaching strategies utilized in Cuba include reciprocal and collective discussions in the classroom (such strategies were previously mentioned in this text with regard to English teaching methodologies). Students demonstrate great respect for their teachers, who also visit their homes (Williams, 2002). Almost all children ages 6 to 11 attend school and complete primary school at least, then move onto secondary education. Regardless of where children live (urban, suburban, or rural areas) all Cuban children are guaranteed primary and secondary education. The crisis of 1990s, which coincided with the fall of the commu-

nism, resulted in many shortages of materials, resources, and teachers, which led to overcrowded classrooms. A great deal of effort has been put forth since then to train new teachers to take the vacancies left. At this time, a large proportion of teachers is very young—below age 25 (or approximately one-third of 38,000 teachers). However, every effort is made to offer support, including providing televisions, VCRs, and computers that can assist in instruction (Acosta, 2005). Special schools are available for students with mental and physical disabilities, as well as for those gifted in athletics and the arts.

Vietnam

For 11 centuries (the first century BC to the tenth century AD), Vietnam was ruled by the Chinese and therefore Chinese borrows many Vietnamese words. There was a large migration of Chinese people to Vietnam in the seventeenth and eighteenth centuries. However, many of the Chinese left after the reunification of Vietnam in 1976. The colonization of Vietnam by the French from 1880 to 1945 had a decided impact on the school system. Until 1945, French was the primary language of instruction and some French words are still used in the Vietnamese language.

Although there is an emphasis on education throughout the country today, funding comes from local sources, leaving poor areas with fewer resources. The overall structure of the schools and delivery of subject matter mirrors the French system, even though the French have not ruled the country since 1946. Primary school is compulsory, begins at age 6, and lasts five grades. There are preschool and kindergarten programs, but they are not compulsory. The focus at the primary school level is on mathematics and civics and the students take an exam at the end of the term. If they do not pass the exam, they can take it at the beginning of the following term, but if they fail their file is reviewed and the student may repeat the grade or be dropped. Upper secondary education lasts from the equivalent of Grade 6 to Grade 9 with a curriculum that is standardized and includes several subjects such as art, mathematics, chemistry, foreign language, and other subjects. The students are tested each term and at the end of Grade 9 they take an exam administered by the Ministry of Education. The students receive a Diploma of Completion of Lower Secondary Education, which is the minimum requirement for continuing in one of several tracks (vocational, technical, or academic) at the high school level. Upper secondary school lasts three years—from the equivalent of 10th to 12th grade—and students are streamed into one of four groups: natural science, social sciences, humanities, and technical studies. Upon successful completion of a comprehensive exam at the end of the upper secondary school education, the student can apply to a university program.

The student receives a certificate, the "Bang Tot Ngniep Pho Tong Trung Hoc," and is encouraged to enroll in a university program. Students who do so need to take an exam to enter the university; the exam tests a foreign language, philosophy, and a specialty. Depending on the specialty selected and number of years needed to complete it, the following degrees are awarded: associate bachelor's, bachelor's, engineering, medical, or law. A master's degree can be obtained after two years of postgraduate study, much like in the United States. A doctorate degree may be obtained following the award of a master's degree; a doctorate program may last from two to three years, and the student must complete a dissertation and defend it. Efforts are made to offer special education to students who need it in order to achieve their potential (Villa et al., 2003).

China/Taiwan

In general, students in China and Taiwan receive mandatory education for nine years. After the ninth year, students can choose to attend middle school for another three years, earning a high school diploma, or they can choose to attend vocational school for three years, earning a certificate for vocational training. In China, the students who have earned a high school diploma can participate in a national examination for higher education: they have to be qualified to enter the universities. In Taiwan, high school seniors apply for university admission and enter a university after receiving admission from the granting university.

Special education is available in China, and students with challenges are generally admitted to special schools. While there are schools for the deaf and blind, the needs of children with special challenges are often not met. Special education also exists in Taiwan and the government passed special education legislation in the 1980s that provided funding for the establishment of many special schools. Mainstreaming is also done. Box 3-1 describes an SLP's experience working in China with students needing special education.

SUMMARY

This chapter highlighted preferred teaching strategies for facilitating the second-language acquisition and learning of CLD students/clients in a classroom setting. Before engaging in an assessment, the SLP should review the type of programs attended by the student/client

BOX 3-1

An SLP's Experience Working in China

I lived in Xi'an for two weeks this summer and volunteered in a special education school that was started by a parent who could not find an appropriate education for her son, now about 10 years old. He appeared to me to be autistic. The student/staff ratio is superior (2:1) and there were about 40 students ranging in age from 3 to the early teens, most of whom were nonverbal and appeared to be on the autistic spectrum. Some appeared to have cerebral palsy and a couple appeared to have ADHD. None of the children actually had any kind of diagnosis and the staff asked for my input as to what was wrong with each child. The children had a regimen of physical exercise that took them through the day—the belief was that strengthening their [gross motor] muscles would facilitate speech. Some of the children did "homework" which consisted of drawing vertical and horizontal lines or actually doing workbook exercises. Behavioral management tended toward negative rather than positive reinforcement. As I had no advance notice about where I would be volunteering, I was not provided with appropriate materials for this population, but managed to create a reasonable facsimile of pictures so that I could begin using a picture communication system with one of the students. Staff and parents were impressed enough with the child's progress to invite me to do an in-service for the staff and to videotape me for training purposes. Although this was useful, I would still like to help set something up that will make a more lasting impact (L. R. Cheng, personal communication, December, 2005).

OUR CLIENTS

Eric, Ana, Jack, Grace, and Leonardo

Receiving an optimal education is paramount in the lives of all children, but it is particularly important that preferred teaching strategies be adapted when those children are learning in a different language. For each one of our clients we will outline how his or her individual situation impacts their progress in acquiring language. To remind the reader about each one of our clients, a synopsis of each case will be presented. (For more detail about each client's background, please refer to previous chapters.) At the end of each synopsis is a list of conclusions, suggestions, or questions that relate to each client's situation and that are based on both the information presented in this book about each client and the concepts discussed in each chapter.

Eric

Eric is a 4-year-old preschool child born in the United States. His parents are first-generation immigrants from Vietnam. Both Vietnamese and English are spoken in the home. His parents speak Vietnamese to him, whereas his two older siblings communicate in English with him. His parents are concerned because Eric's language skills in both languages are limited as compared with his siblings and other children who are growing up in similar bilingual backgrounds. Eric has been a healthy child. Eric's teacher has reported that he prefers playing by himself. His concentration is limited unless he watches cartoons or videos.

An evaluation of Eric should include a visit to the classroom attended by Eric in order to determine the opportunities he has for communicating with other children. The SLP should explore the following questions, which are based on the information presented in Chapter 3:

- Is the environment conducive to learning? Is there structure and a schedule?

- Does the teacher use some of the strategies outlined in this chapter? (Examples include evaluating Eric's rate of speech during instruction; using props; using a thematic approach; using various media; using vocabulary building tasks; and providing language modeling and expansion.)

- Because Eric wants to play by himself, do the teachers make an attempt to facilitate environments where he can interact with other children through the mediation of an adult?

Ana

Ana is a 9-year-old enrolled in fourth grade who emigrated from Mexico at the age of 5 and who is having difficulty reading in English. She is the oldest of three children. She was raised by her maternal grandparents beginning at the age of 6 months; after five years she was reunited with her parents.

Ana attended kindergarten in Arizona but moved in the middle of that year when her parents found better jobs in California. Ana has learned English quite well but she is behind in reading. All of her schooling has been in English. She speaks Spanish to her parents and to some relatives who live nearby, but she talks to her siblings in English and Spanish. Her parents insist that only Spanish should be spoken at home.

Based on the information discussed in Chapter 3, an evaluation of Ana should include:

- A review of Ana's cumulative school record. Notes from previous teachers can assist in determining if there were any concerns about her progress in learning English and acquiring reading skills.

- An interview with Ana's parents to see how they perceive the problem.

- A visit to Ana's classroom to determine if the instruction is conducted using the optimal strategies outlined in this chapter.

Jack

Jack is a 14-year-old of African-American descent who is has difficulty with subjects such as social studies, English, and writing. Mrs. G., Jack's paternal grandmother, adopted him when he was 2 years old because his single mother could not raise him. Prior to entering School District A (summer 2002), Jack attended a private school for two years. Even though both Mrs. G. and Jack have a Southern accent and speak AAVE, his use of a different syntax and vocabulary do not seem to interfere with his academic learning.

Jack had to remain in the ICU for about seven days after birth due to respiratory distress. His developmental milestones occurred within the normal accepted timeframe, except for his speech, which was delayed: Jack did not put words together until he was about 3 years old. His latest vision and hearing screenings were unremarkable (fall 2002). Mrs. G. reports that Jack is on daily medication for anger, anxiety, and agitation He is receiving counseling to address his emotional issues.

Mrs. G. reports that a previous school assessment report written by an SLP and the psychologist indicated some learning difficulties, but their severity did not warrant intervention from special education. Because the results of this assessment were not satisfactory to Mrs. G., she sought an outside assessment by a neuropsychologist. Results indicated that Jack has difficulty with working memory and sequencing skills. Mrs. G. states that Jack has difficulty synthesizing oral and written information. Writing is difficult for him: Jack does not respect rules of grammar and punctuation.

Points to consider based on the information discussed in Chapter 3:

- In Jack's case, there is no mention about his fluency in any English dialect such as AAVE. Reportedly, this not an issue that is related to his current academic difficulties.

- A visit to two or three of Jack's classes is warranted in order to determine which teaching strategies have been utilized by the various teachers. Preferably, this visit should be to a class where Jack is asked to work with others in collaborative groups, i.e., a lab as opposed to lecture-style classes.

(Continues)

(Continued)

- Observations should be made: Does Jack's behavior change depending on the teacher's teaching style? For example, does he take notes when he is supposed to? Does he participate during discussions? Does he ask for clarification?

Grace

Grace is a 60-year-old Mandarin-speaking former businesswoman who sustained a stroke in the right hemisphere of her brain while visiting the United States on a business trip.

Grace was a successful businesswoman prior to her accident. She speaks Mandarin, Cantonese, English, and French. She completed her business degree in China, but spent five years in the United States when she was first developing her business. The languages she speaks most frequently are Mandarin and English. Prior to her stroke she could converse on several topics in all the languages she knew. However, she felt most at ease reading and writing in Chinese and English. She was very proficient in reading and writing English but her strongest area was business English.

Points to consider based on the information discussed in Chapter 3:

- Grace has a command of four languages (oral language communication). She has learned the languages in various contexts. There is no information on how she first acquired English, but it is possible she attended a bilingual Chinese-English school or learned English through additional programs.

- Grace is very fluent in Chinese and English and we know she has spent five years in the United States conducting business. Her reading and writing skills in both of these two languages, which are very different, were, before the stroke, at sufficiently high levels to conduct business in either language.

- We do not have information on how she learned French, but can assume that it may have been as a foreign language in school.

Leonardo

Leonardo is a 45-year-old fieldworker from Guatemala who suffered a traumatic brain injury following a dispute with a neighbor. Leonardo is an illegal immigrant who has been traveling back and forth between the U.S. and Guatemala for more than 20 years. He works as a crop picker in several states including Washington, Ohio, Michigan, California, and Oregon. He completed seven grades in Guatemala but was able to get his GED in the U.S. after attending night classes.

He is able to communicate in English, but even after his years spent in the U.S., he is still much more fluent in Spanish than in English. Prior to his accident, he could read newspapers in both English and Spanish but concentrated primarily on sports and local news. At this time, he can walk but he cannot process what is said to him in either Spanish or English. He is disoriented, he cannot keep track of time, and he forgets daily routines. After spending two weeks in a rehabilitation center he was dismissed and he is currently living with some friends.

Points to consider based on the information discussed in Chapter 3:

- We do not have information on whether Leonardo attended bilingual programs. As was discussed in this chapter, the majority of bilingual programs are available at the elementary grade level. Therefore, most likely he learned English through one of the ESL programs described in this chapter (CALLA, SDAIE).

- He has been able to sustain his oral and written proficiency in Spanish by communicating in Spanish with friends and reading and watching the news in Spanish.

- Leonardo earned a high school diploma in the United States. He has a sufficient command of English to communicate in the language and read the newspaper.

in the past and visit the classroom to determine if the learning environment is optimal.

The review of the history of bilingual education in the United States presented at the beginning of the chapter will assist the SLP in gaining a broader perspective of the various political trends that have had a direct influence on public support of specific programs. An understanding of the various "bilingual" programs is important because the adjective "bilingual" is used to describe programs that are often very different from one another. In conducting a careful review of the student/client's past and current educational experiences, the SLP will be able to determine if the language or learning problem is most likely due to pedagogical issues or if, indeed, the client has a speech or language disorder. Finally, having an understanding of the student/client's educational experience in his or her country of origin will assist in gaining a more specific picture of the problem.

FURTHER READINGS

Brisk, M. (2005). *Bilingual Education: From compensatory to quality schooling* (2nd ed.). Mahwah, NJ: Lawrence Erlbaum Associates.

Crawford. J. (2004). *Educating English-language learners: Language diversity in the classroom.* Los Angeles: Bilingual Educational Services.

Echevarria, J., Vogt, M. E., & Short, D. J. (2004). *Making content comprehensive for English learners: The SIP Model.* Boston: Pearson.

Herrrera, S., & Murry, K. (2005). *Mainstreaming ESL and bilingual methods: Differentiated instruction for culturally and linguistically diverse (CLD) students.* Boston: Pearson.

C H A P T E R 4

CLD POPULATIONS' CONNECTIONS TO SCHOOLS, HEALTH CARE, AND OTHER AGENCIES IN THE COMMUNITY

"Communication goes beyond sharing the same language code. For educators and professionals working with CLD populations, it means providing them with tools and strategies for promoting their adaptation to new settings and situations while respecting their own methods of communication" (Author).

CHAPTER OUTLINE

INTRODUCTION

In most cultures, the family is one of the most important influential agents in the early development of children. In addition, schools and the community continue to have an impact on children's subsequent social and cognitive growth, as well. Although children spend only a portion of their day in school, this institution plays an important role in their lives. It is the place where they acquire new knowledge, and they must follow particular rules of discourse to be successful.

Speech-language pathologists (SLPs) who come in contact with culturally and linguistically diverse (CLD) students/clients and their families must consider these individuals' unique communication styles and their experiences with various educational, health care, and other community agencies. Understanding these differences has an impact on the successful identification and management of various handicaps that affect learning as well as the ability to function independently.

The topics outlined above will cover the characteristics and perspectives of Anglo-European, Hispanic, African-American, Asian-American and Pacific Islander, and Native American and Alaskan Native groups.

GENERAL GUIDELINES FOR UNDERSTANDING CROSS-CULTURAL DIFFERENCES

The importance, impact, and development of various types of communication styles that are related to specific contexts (also referred to as pragmatics or use of language) was not recognized until the mid-1970s by researchers such as Bates (1976), Dore (1975), Bloom and Lahey (1978), and Greenfield and Smith (1976). The study of intercultural communication began with the pioneering work of Hall in the 1960s and 1970s, followed by the work of Condon and Yousef (1975) in the 1970s and Samovar and Porter (1994) in the 1990s, and many others. For a historical review of intercultural communication the reader is referred

to works by Chen and Starosta (1998), and Lustig and Koester (1999).

Cross-cultural communication is complex because verbal and nonverbal cues such as eye contact, facial expressions, proximity, and touching vary from culture to culture. Several psychologists have provided models for interpreting the ways in which various cultures interact. For a review of this subject, please refer to Chen and Starosta (1998). We have selected one of the first models, described by Hall (1977). Although this viewpoint is 30 years old, it assists us in understanding how other cultures communicate and what they expect, and allows us to become more adept at interacting more effectively with those cultures.

In his book *Beyond Culture* (1977), Hall indicates that cultures can fit within a continuum of what he refers to as "high- and low-context" cultures. Certain cultures—for example, Asian-American, Native American, Latino, Arab-American, and African-American—are referred to as "high-context cultures." Communication in these cultures relies more on nonverbal cues and messages. Other cultures, referred to as "low-context cultures," rely more on verbal communication and less on nonverbal ways to communicate. Anglo-European cultures are an example of low-context cultures. However, there may be variations within any one type of culture depending on specific situations. For example, good friends, relatives, or spouses use fewer words when communicating and rely more on nonverbal cues. "A look, a word, or a gesture may convey the equivalent of paragraphs of spoken words" (Lynch, 2004, p. 61).

It is important to understand variations in discourse across various cultures and in specific situations. For example, the language used at home varies significantly from the language used in school. In this aspect, mainstream children have an advantage over their minority peers. Their parents are more familiar with school expectations, and they have greater access to different institutions and networks such as libraries and various educational events offered by the community (i.e., one-day programs that allow children to enjoy art, as well as music classes, camping trips, and various field trips). Recent immigrants must adjust to a new set of rules regarding schooling, employment, access to health care—all requiring a specific process that often varies significantly from that of their country of origin. Formal education or socioeconomic variables may not play a role in this case. For example, some elderly middle-class immigrants to the United States have difficulty accepting that doctors' house calls are uncommon. Medicare-based drug benefit programs for seniors are very confusing even for mainstream Americans. For example, in a 2005 *New York Times* article, a 73-year-old retired chemist from Wichita, Kansas, said, "I have a Ph.D., and it's too complicated to suit me"; and, after attending a seminar on the Medicare program, Pauline H. Olney, a retired nurse from Santa Rosa, California, commented, "The whole thing is hopelessly complicated" ("Confusion Is Rife about Drug Plan," 2005). These procedures are even more complex for recent immigrants.

Thus, many CLD students/clients and their families must cross two obstacles: overcoming the language barrier, and learning to adapt to a new set of discourse rules that vary from setting to setting. To be effective with these populations, SLPs, educators, health care and other professionals, and community agents must be attuned to their own set of beliefs and expectations. In addition, they should understand their clients' and their clients' families' experiences and expectations with regard to the specific topics that are the focus of this chapter. These topics include: (1) the rearing and communication patterns occurring within the families of students/clients; (2) the families' and children's experiences in attaining literacy and accessing formal education and various community agencies and health care establishments; (3) the way that students/clients and their families understand and react to various educational and medical disabilities; and (4) the best strategies for obtaining the information from CLD families that is needed in order to counsel and guide them in handling specific educational or medical issues. In summary: "All organizations have a culture or shared understanding of both explicit and implicit rules of thought and behavior. Also important to note is that these health-care cultures are influenced by the larger culture" (Threats, 2005, p. 4).

The four topics mentioned above could become the focus of an entire book. However, only relevant highlights will be discussed and the breath of information presented within each section will vary depending on the amount of research and information that is available concerning each cultural group being discussed. It is important to remember that no one can become an expert in all the cultural backgrounds of the diverse families that currently live in the United States. But, having some general background knowledge about important issues can assist the SLP in working with most populations. Bonder, Martin, and Miracle (2001); Gay (2000); Lynch and Hanson (2004); Luckmann, (2000); and Trumbull, Rothstein-Fisch, Greenfield, and Quiroz (2001) are helpful references. Suggestions for how to work effectively with CLD populations are provided at the end of this chapter.

REARING AND COMMUNICATION PATTERNS OCCURRING WITHIN FAMILIES

Childrearing and communication patterns within families are engrained early in the lives of family members. Such patterns vary from population to population because they are based on the cultural and communication characteristics of the group in question. In addition, there are differences that occur across generations and time. Understanding those patterns may explain the behavior and reactions of children and families to specific situations. In this chapter, some of these

characteristics and patterns are highlighted for various groups. However, the reader is cautioned to avoid generalizations. Parents and caregivers are the first "teachers" of their children, but there are cultural and individual differences across and within groups that need to be considered.

Vigil and Hwa-Froelich (2004) reviewed several areas of caregiver-parent-child interaction that should be considered when working with various CLD populations. For example, in North American–European families the caregiver adopts communication patterns that reflect a more "independent" style of interaction. These patterns include following the child's lead when responding to the child's exploration. This is opposed to a more "interdependent" style of childrearing where the child's attention is directed or redirected to join an ongoing activity. In comparing the childrearing styles of North American and European caregivers with those of other cultures, Vigil and Hwa-Froelich (2004) indicate that styles of communication may vary along the pragmatic continuum represented in Figure 4-1.

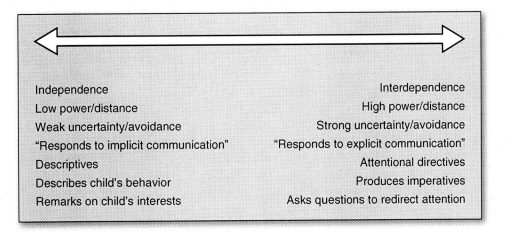

Independence	Interdependence
Low power/distance	High power/distance
Weak uncertainty/avoidance	Strong uncertainty/avoidance
"Responds to implicit communication"	"Responds to explicit communication"
Descriptives	Attentional directives
Describes child's behavior	Produces imperatives
Remarks on child's interests	Asks questions to redirect attention

FIGURE 4-1 *Characteristics of Caregivers' Pragmatic Input.* (Adapted from Vigil and Hwa-Froelich, 2004, p. 121.)

For example, caregivers who fall more into the "independence" group would be observed to use more "descriptives"; that is, they would describe the child's behavior and remark on the child's interests. On the other hand, the caregivers who belong to the "interdependence group" would use more "attentional directives"; that is, they would use more imperatives and ask questions in order to redirect attention. Keeping these differences in mind can assist SLPs, educators, and professionals in assessing children with greater accuracy, and can also assist in providing more relevant and realistic suggestions for intervention.

Anglo-European Perspectives

For many years, the "nuclear" family was defined as the mother, father, and children, where the mother was the "stay-at-home" parent and the father the sole breadwinner. Everyone knows this is not the case today, when a high percentage of women of young children work outside the home in addition to carrying out parenting and household duties. Up to 65% of mothers of children younger than 6 years old work outside the home (Children's Defense Fund, 2001). Families may be composed of single parents and their children, homosexual and heterosexual relationships, or parents who have remarried and who each have their own families.

Anglo-European families try to foster independence in their children from very early on. Children are reared to feed themselves as infants, to assist and dress themselves early, and to bathe with decreasing supervision. They are encouraged to take part in decisions such as selecting their clothes, and are assigned specific chores around the home. Many teenagers work while going to school and leave the home to pursue further education or take on a job. Elders in the family continue to live on their own or join senior citizens' homes, and they rarely live with their own children, although there may be exceptions. Even though the younger generation is encouraged to become independent, it is not uncommon for some children in their 20s and 30s to return home temporarily to save money in order to return to school or to have a down payment toward the purchase of an apartment or a home.

Depending on the level of formal education and personalities of the parents, children are addressed as if they were equal partners in the communication process, and are consulted about their feelings and opinions from very early on. Parents tend to expand on their children's utterances and encourage turn-taking between adult and child. I was "shocked" one day when I heard the mother of a 1-year-old tell her babysitter, "I hope you will have no difficulty with Adam today. He is not in a very good mood." Being a newcomer to the U.S. who grew up in an environment where adults were the ones in control in any situation regarding their children, this comment seemed out of the ordinary.

Research on how to best communicate with elderly populations in mainstream America and the world has received scarce attention. De Bot and Makoni (2005) found that language skills in older populations tend to decrease, but there is an imminent need to understand how to communicate more effectively with this population without undermining their cognitive skills, especially when they are in more vulnerable situations such as nursing homes or hospitals. For example, the researchers report a study by Hummert, Shaner, Garstka, and Henry (1998) in which persons interacting with older individuals who were hospitalized used more "patronizing language" than they did when interacting with a matched older population residing in the same community but who were not hospitalized.

Anglo-Europeans are generally driven by timelines, competition, and the fostering of individualism as well as privacy—yet there may also be informality in their ways of being. These characteristics have penetrated educational institutions such as schools and colleges and will be discussed further.

Hispanic Perspectives

Styles of interaction among Hispanic groups may be as varied as each group's specific Hispanic heritage, manner and level of assimilation into the mainstream culture, level of formal education, socioeconomic status, and personality. Differences exist among Hispanics who come from the various countries of Latin America and Spain but, generally speaking, some common patterns prevail. My personal experience of being raised in Mexico, along with comments and feedback from other persons who have lived or have grown up in the Hispanic world, support these conclusions.

It is not uncommon for young children of Hispanic backgrounds to lag behind in the performance of everyday skills such as knowing how to button jackets, tie shoes, or cut food—because parents, caretakers, and even older siblings have done it for them. This situation is even more prevalent for children with disabilities.

In many daily situations, parents and caregivers may not always comment on or make verbalizations about ongoing events. For example, while engaged in a daily activity such as cooking, shopping, or completing household chores, the parent may not necessarily pair the actions with words (e.g., "We are going shopping and first we need to get some tomatoes for the salad and beans to go on our tostadas"). Often parents and older siblings provide the directives for what the child should do. In turn, children's responses are rewarded with comments such as "good," "fine," "wrong," or "bad." Sometimes parents do not understand the value of playing with their child but, instead, consider that this activity is only appropriate among children and should not to take place in an educational setting (Delgado-Gaitán & Trueba, 1991). I remember how the parent of a young preschooler with language and developmental disabilities was unhappy with the program because she felt the child "was not learning anything; they play all day."

Hispanic children are taught to be respectful of adults and not interrupt conversations (Rodríguez & Olswang, 2003; Valdés, 1996). During gatherings, many Hispanic adults converse primarily with other adults, and children do not necessarily participate in these interactions. While viewing TV, adults may not comment on what is occurring. Also, parents may not always ask children for their interpretation of events or evaluations of their emotions. For example, when there is a choice of actions to be taken, adults do not necessarily ask children to voice their preferences (Heath, 1986). This practice is often common in mainstream classrooms (Trumbull et al., 2001). Children have responsibilities at home, such as caring for younger siblings while the parent is occupied with another task or is absent, and it may be that the child's ability to negotiate or voice preferences varies from situation to situation, depending on the extent of the child's responsibilities. It is common that a child who is more fluent in English than a parent has to take on greater responsibilities such as translating during transactions with monolingual adults. Interpreting for parents in certain situations, however, may not be appropriate. Health- or education-related situations, for example, are not appropriate because children are not mature enough to understand the content being discussed.

Hispanic children are exposed to a wider vocabulary related to names for different relatives and family relationships. The emphasis on the words for family names reflects the importance given to the family as a unit. In fact, many Hispanic children are raised to give a higher priority to cooperating with family members than to achieving as individuals. In distressful situations, the family remains cohesive. Naturally, the degree of family cooperation varies from situation to situation, but it appears stronger among Hispanic families than among Anglo groups (Guendelman, 1983).

Many Hispanic parents do not ask their children to repeat facts or to foretell what they will do. Thus, it may be uncommon for any adult to ask a child to recount what happened on any occasion during which both of them were present. It would be more natural for the child to do so if she or he were recounting the event to someone else who was not present (Heath, 1986). This is particularly important to understand, because in the U.S., mainstream teachers frequently ask children to verbalize conversations and information that was previously shared by the teacher and children. This strategy, which allows the teacher to check the student's comprehension and assimilation of the material presented in the classroom, may be unfamiliar to Hispanic children. This type of elicitation method is not unusual in several of the current language proficiency tests mentioned in Chapter 2 (i.e., the Language Assessment Scales and the Idea Language Proficiency Test). If a child of Hispanic heritage has difficulty recounting what is known to both interlocutors, it is important to keep in mind that this difficulty could be due to lack of exposure to or experience with the practice, rather than being symptomatic of a language-learning disability. However,

retelling in writing what was taught is not unusual in Hispanic countries. In exams, students may be tested on their retention of what was presented in lectures or taught with written materials. Therefore, the U.S. practice of having a student retell almost verbatim what the teacher or professor has said might be a way of assessing how well the student has assimilated the information, but this assessment may be more relevant if it is done in writing.

In addition to communication that is manifested in words, "nonverbal communication" in the form of gestures and intonation needs to be accounted for. Langdon (1992a) found that nonverbal features of communication patterns among Hispanics fall into two main categories: (1) those relating to the person's identity and relationship to others, and (2) those relating to the meaning of what is being said. Some nonverbal communication features of interpersonal relationships are

1. An appreciation of the uniqueness of an individual that is expressed by referring to the person's *alma* ("soul") or *espítiru* ("spirit"). A mainstream Anglo or more acculturated Hispanic might feel that this characterization is too sentimental.

2. A respect for individuals because of their advanced age or experience. For example, a mechanic with a great deal of experience may be referred to as "maestro" (master) (Condon, 1986). It is advisable for clinicians to address a parent, adult, or older patient with the formal "Ud" (you) and never with the familiar "tú" form. Addressing a younger child with the "tú" may be appropriate, but there may be variations in the use of "tú" from Hispanic culture to Hispanic culture. In some Hispanic groups, parents refer to their child as

"vos" (a variation of "Ud"), a form that is common in Argentina, for example.

3. The observance of certain conventions for greeting and leavetaking. Handshaking is commonly done upon greeting someone, both among men and women. Occasional hugging and kissing is appropriate when the persons know each other.

4. The observance of certain conventions for conversation. Initiating a conversation with personal questions rather than with business talk is common, because many persons of Hispanic backgrounds may interpret opening a conversation without a personal note as being rude.

5. An awareness of lasting and close relationships. Among Hispanics, family takes precedence over everything else, even over a job, school, or friendships. In the Anglo world, the emphasis is often on remaining loyal to a job, even if is stressful to the family.

6. The use of expressive physical gestures. Hispanic children's use of gestures as they speak may be much greater than that of non-Hispanic children. This use of gestures should not be necessarily be interpreted as a communication disability (Kayser, 1990).

Some nonverbal features of communication relating to the meaning of what is being said include

1. The concept of "mañana" (tomorrow). The word "mañana" does not necessarily mean "tomorrow," but may indicate the future. Anglos are much more time-bound, more driven by schedules and deadlines than Hispanics are (Condon, 1986). Hispanics often comment that it is difficult for them to adjust to the rigidness of schedules in the Anglo world. For many Hispanics,

people and their needs take precedence over precise schedules or appointments (Penfield, 1989). In some Hispanic families, strict adherence to schedules takes second place to socialization with friends and relatives, even when the schedules involve medical treatment. A missed appointment may be due to a lack of transportation or to possible economic repercussions, however. For example, a day or a few hours away from work for a medical or clinical appointment may mean lost wages (Rodríguez, 1983). Also, an appointment may be missed because of failure to understand the urgency of the problem or the need for repeated visits (e.g., for a speech and language or hearing evaluation). Visiting a clinician for therapy that requires regular appointments may be particularly difficult for some parents to understand because progress is often slow and may not be immediately apparent. It is important for the clinician to explain the intervention clearly, and, on a regular basis, to set expectations. Lack of transportation may also be an issue for parents attempting to comply with regular visits.

2. The observance of politeness conventions. Hospitality is wholehearted and terms denoting politeness may be somewhat exaggerated, such as in the phrase "Está Ud en su casa" (the literal translation, "You are in your own home," really means "Please feel as if you were in your own home"). When scolded, children are forbidden to look at adults; also, when talking with adults, they may look away to show their respect. Out of politeness, a patient may not openly disagree with the professional, but may pretend to follow the prescribed recommendations—even when there is no language barrier.

3. The nonliteral interpretation of language. The use of "Sí, como no" ("yes, indeed") does not mean that the person agrees with what is said, but rather is an acknowledgement that the person is attentive and listening.

The nonverbal characteristics mentioned above have also been observed in other CLD populations such as Asian-American populations (Cheng, 1991). Although teachers and SLPs must necessarily have an increased awareness of some nonverbal features that may occur in their communications with Hispanic persons, remaining aware of subgroup and individual differences is essential.

African-American Perspectives

As with any group, being African-American should not be equated with specific characteristics, as each individual is different. In general, a strong sense of family and kinship is also common among this group. In the early days of settlement in America, men and women slaves had to work on the plantation and their children were left to the care and upbringing of older siblings or adults. Leigh and Green (1982) report that despite the separation of families during their transport to the United States in the seventeenth century, the sense of family bonds and community has always remained strong. Even today, where a great number of African-American women are heads of the family, attachment to the community continues to be strong. Approximately 43% of families with children are headed by single African-American women as compared with only 13% of non-Hispanic white populations (McKinnon, 2003).

Willis (2004) recommends that assumptions related to "appearances" should be avoided when interacting with an African-American family. Specifically, do not address an individual by his or her first name unless permission has been given, do not make assumptions about the fact that the head of the family is a female or is unwed, and do not assume that there is dysfunction because the family is poor. Overall, families attempt to make children aware of their heritage and history, and decisions are often made that take into account the benefit for an entire group. Discipline is somewhat stricter among these families as they need to teach their children about self-respect as a way to learn to appreciate the rights of others. The importance of family is emphasized by adults who may "translate" their position in the family by making statements such as "momma's sister is my aunt"—because it helps children appreciate their family circle and where they belong (Willis, 2004, p. 161).

African-Americans may speak one or more dialects of English depending on the region in which they live. Whether or not Ebonics should be taught in the schools has raised a great deal of controversy. The Oakland decision in 1997 to consider Ebonics another language and respect those who speak it has been often misinterpreted. This issue was discussed in Chapter 3. For a review of various aspects of this controversy, the reader is referred to Perry and Delpit (1998). Communication among African-Americans is considered to be passionate and animated. "Conversational style is provocative and challenging, and the intensity is focused on the validity of ideas being discussed" (Kochman, 1981, pp. 30–31). At times, volume and pitch may show greater variation than in the mainstream culture. African-American speakers tend to maintain eye contact more directly when speaking than when listening. The use of more frequent gestures may also be noted. African-Americans touch their children more frequently and for longer periods of time. Just as with many linguistically and culturally different groups, older persons are held in respect. Parents and older persons are generally shown more respect than in the mainstream culture. Somewhat like Hispanic persons, members of African-American groups may not always adhere to strict timelines.

Asian-American and Pacific Islander Perspectives

There is a wide variation in this group because persons of Asian and Pacific backgrounds constitute a large geographic, historical, linguistic, religious, and cultural group (see Chapter 1). For further details, the reader is referred to general resources such as Chan and Lee (2004), Cheng (1991, 1996), and Pang and Cheng (1998). See also specific resources such as the discussion of the Vietnamese in Zhou and Bankston (1998), and the discussion of the Koreans in Yum (1987) and Wang (1983).

The family is an important institution for this group. Respect for the past, elders, and ancestors are key to most members. Even though respect is shown to all members of a given family, the older son may be more valued than daughters. Each family member is addressed in a manner that reflects the person's role. Paternal grandparents receive the highest level of authority and respect followed by the father, mother, oldest son, middle daughter, and youngest son (Chan & Lee, 2004). The woman is traditionally considered to be in charge of the house, and that includes the raising and education of the children. Relationships between parent and child often may supersede each spouse's ties. Infants receive a great deal of attention and children often share their parents' rooms and beds during preschool and even during early school age, a practice that is emerging even among mainstream Euro-Americans today.

The young child is typically not put under any pressure or forced to keep rigid schedules, but early toilet training is not uncommon.

More discipline is imposed as the child grows up. Just as in other cultures such as the Hispanic culture, it is common for older siblings to care for younger ones. As they grow older, children are guided to behave and complete responsibilities. If children misbehave, parents may react by teasing or using verbal reprimands. It is the mother who plays the role of the primary disciplinarian. Verbal praise is uncommon and speaking favorably of the child in public is viewed as being very inappropriate.

Understanding both verbal and nonverbal communication styles is important. For example, some persons from Asian backgrounds do not openly disagree or agree with what is being said. Referring to Vietnamese immigrants, Chu (1990) comments: "In America, you value freedom of speech; in Vietnam, we value freedom of silence" (p. 2). Often, silence may be a sign of interest and respect. Facing a speaker may signify to persons of Asian backgrounds some hostility or impoliteness, and in order to convey the opposite, eye contact is often avoided. Gestures that are commonly accepted in one culture may be viewed by another culture in a diametrically opposite fashion. For example, the American gesture of waving "good-bye" to a child may signify "come here" (Chan & Lee, 2004). Also, when persons use the crossing of the index and middle fingers to signify "good luck" or the "OK" sign, it may be interpreted as an obscene gesture. Many persons of Asian backgrounds may smile, but this facial expression has a different meaning than the one commonly interpreted by the mainstream Euro-American culture. Smiling may denote embarrassment, or a reaction to a compliment, or acceptance of a proposal. Persons from Asian backgrounds may

PERSONAL STORIES

A Personal Reflection

Verbal praise and speaking favorably of a child in public is not typical of Asian cultures. But this childrearing style is not necessarily exclusive to such cultures. Moreover, it may be a characteristic of families who believe children should have a strict upbringing, or may be a product of the mentality of older generations. My parents, who were of Eastern European descent, rarely praised my brother's or my accomplishments to other people. Only when they moved to United States and had lived here for 10 years, did they begin to praise our accomplishments to friends and acquaintances. Therefore, the influences of a new culture can also influence a family's childrearing style.

maintain a greater distance when interacting with each other, but shaking hands is common among members of the same sex.

Native American Perspectives

As with any group, families from Native American (including Alaskan Native) backgrounds may be representative of either the more traditional or more "acculturated" subgroup. Additionally, there may be differences across various Native American groups. The reader is referred to Chapter 1 where assimilation and acculturation issues were discussed in greater detail. The Native American family includes family members as well as "fictive-kin" that may include nonfamily members. Childrearing responsibilities may also rest on grandparents, other family members, and elders in the community. Their inclusion in discussing a student or client's communication disability is important for ensuring a more successful outcome. Some persons in this group may display what appears to be a "lack of affect" or "passive attitude" with regard to problems or illness. Struggles and difficulties are often viewed as

part of life and such a perspective may explain this seemingly "indifferent attitude" (Joe & Malach, 2004).

From an early age, Native American children are taught to be self-reliant. Miller (1979) documented that Native American children were able to dress themselves much earlier than white or African-American children (age 2.8 as compared with 3.7 and 4.0, respectively), and also they were able to complete chores earlier (age 5.4 as compared with 6.1 and 6.3, respectively). Socioeconomic factors may force some members of the family to leave their families behind to start a new life in another city (Joe & Malach, 2004). Children learn from their parents and families by observation and not necessarily through verbal mediation. Avoiding eye contact and not asking direct questions shows respect, which is something that professionals need to consider during their interactions with this group.

Table 4-1 presents a summary of the main characteristics discussed in this chapter regarding childrearing and family interactions in Anglo-American, Native American, Hispanic, African-American, and Asian-American groups.

TABLE 4-1   Childrearing and Family Interactions across Various CLD Groups

Anglo-American	Hispanic	African-American	Asian-American	Native American
Family is defined in a narrow way. Emphasis on individualism.	Nuclear and extended family is very important.	Nuclear and extended family is important.	Each member has specific role. Family is very important.	Family includes larger number of members. There is a broader family nucleus.
Elders do not share home.	Elders are cared for and respected.	Elders are respected.	Elders are respected.	Elders are more respected.
Child's self-help is fostered. Parents follow child's lead.	May be more relaxed about child development.	Strict with childrearing.	Child-parent bonding is important; this directs child.	Children are self-reliant.
Timelines are used.	Time is not always essential.	Time is not as essential.	Time is relatively important.	Time is settled.
Emphasis on competition.	Emphasis on group effort.	More emphasis on the given situation.	Depends on the situation. Collectivistic.	Not as competitive.
Emphasis on directness.	Not as direct. Saving face is important.	More emphasis on collaboration.	More indirect. Emphasis on nonverbal communication.	Not as direct. Saving face is important.

FAMILIES' AND CHILDREN'S EXPERIENCES IN ATTAINING LITERACY AND ACCESSING FORMAL EDUCATION AND VARIOUS HEALTH CARE AND COMMUNITY AGENCIES

Recent immigrant children, adolescents, and adults come from a variety of socioeconomic groups; they have varying levels of formal education and, therefore, have varying experiences with educational institutions, agencies, and medical establishments. Understanding their backgrounds, knowledge, and experiences is very important for ensuring that the process of assessing and planning intervention for their educational and medical needs is successful. Chapter 3 provided some examples of the educational strategies used in some countries within the Hispanic world, in Vietnam, and in China and Taiwan. However, it is very difficult to capture all variables only by reviewing some of the literature provided. Therefore, an interview with the family, student, or adult client is important. Figure 3-5 provided some guidelines for gathering such information. The attainment of literacy varies widely from country to country. Some facts about world literacy are presented in Figure 4-2.

The data shown in Figure 4-2 indicate that there is a very low literacy rate in developing countries especially. The concept of "literacy" can have various definitions. In the early 1990s when I conducted a survey with the National Office of Literacy, the person in charge informed me that "being literate" may mean that individuals could complete a form with data on personal information, or that they could respond in writing about their country's culture and history (National Office of Literacy, personal communication, April 1990). Furthermore, as shown in Figure 4-2, it is

- One billion people, or 26% of the world's population, are nonliterate adults (UNESCO, 1998).
- Women make up two-thirds of all nonliterates.
- Ninety-eight percent of all nonliterates live in developing countries.
- In the least developed countries, the overall illiteracy rate is 49%.
- Fifty-two percent of all nonliterates live in India and China.
- Africa as a continent has a literacy rate of less than 60%.
- In sub-Saharan Africa since 1980, primary school enrollment has declined, going from 58% to 50%.
- In all developing countries, the percentage of children aged 6–11 not attending school is 15%. In the least developed countries, it is 45% (UNESCO, 1998).

The number of people speaking lesser-known languages is 1.25 billion, or 20% of the world's population.

- The average adult literacy rate among that population is an estimated 31%.
- The average adult literacy rate in their mother tongue among speakers of lesser-known languages is an estimated 12%.
- In twenty-six countries, more than 90% of the total national population speaks lesser-known languages. The average literacy rate in these countries is 63%.
- In twenty-one countries, less than 1% of the total national population speaks lesser-known languages. The average literacy rate in these countries is 93%.
- Of the world's nonliterate population, an estimated 476 million people are speakers of lesser-known languages. In other words, approximately 50% of all nonliterates are minority language speakers.

There is a correlation between income and illiteracy.

- Per capita income in countries with a literacy rate of less than 55% averages about $600.
- Per capita income in countries with a literacy rate between 55% and 84% is $2,400.
- Per capita income in countries with a literacy rate between 85% and 95% is $3,700.
- Per capita income in countries with a literacy rate above 96% is $12,600.

FIGURE 4-2 *Facts about Literacy in the World.* (Adapted from *International Literacy Day, September 7, 2001, Washington, D.C.* [n.d.]. Retrieved October, 12, 2005, from http://www.sil.org/literacy/LitFacts.htm.)

evident that there is a high correlation between literacy rates and income. In addition to having this information, it is important for an SLP to consider whether a given country provides its citizens free vs. paid access to education. For example, in certain countries primary schools may be compulsory, but secondary education may be optional and only available with paid tuition.

The facts listed in Figure 4-2 indicate that 26% or one-quarter of the world's population is illiterate, two-thirds of those who are illiterate are women, and 98% of those who are illiterate live in developing countries. India, China, and Africa have the lowest literacy rates of all. Twenty percent of the population speaks lesser-known languages, and several of those languages do not have scripts. More detailed definitions about literacy and its oral and written connections will be provided in Chapter 6.

Anglo-European Perspectives

Access to education is of extreme importance in the United States. Public education is free to any child and is compulsory until age 16. The majority of students attend public schools, but there are a number of secular and religious schools available as well. Even though local governments have jurisdiction over schools they have to adhere to federal guidelines as well as to regulations such as those in No Child Left Behind (NCLB, 2002). Parent participation is highly encouraged and is part of the "culture." For students placed in special education, the role of the parent is essential, beginning with their participation in the Individual Family Service Plan (IFSP), and, during school years, in the Individual Educational Plan (IEP). Parent involvement may include volunteering in the classroom or in school activities as well as participating in associations where school administration and staff discuss various aspect of the school management.

Understanding teachers' expectations and classroom rules is key to successful teaching and learning. Some students who were raised using different behavioral criteria may have greater difficulty adjusting to the American norms. Even students raised in the mainstream need to adjust to the school culture. Each teacher and classroom has its "own climate." Some classroom behaviors may be more general than others. A list of school expectations and typical classroom routines is reported in Figure 4-3.

Reviewing school expectations and classroom rules is a helpful strategy for all students regardless of their linguistic and cultural backgrounds. To ensure that all students understand these guidelines, teachers should periodically review expectations and rules. Many students who were raised in other countries and attended schools in other locations may be accustomed to the different rules and expectations that occur at all educational levels—from primary to college and graduate levels.

Box 4-1 describes how, as a graduate student, I interpreted some of those rules and routines.

The previous comments were centered on educational issues. However, children and adults with various communication disorders often need to interact with both education and

Preschool
- Show-and-tell
- Clean-up
- Story time

Elementary Grades
- Reading group
- Workbooks
- Working on cooperative activities
- At first learning to read, later, by Grade 4, reading to learn

Middle and Upper Grades
- Recount past events and experiences in a predictably logical order
- Make oral presentations
- Learn to look for and compile information using specific instructions
- Know how to obtain information
- Sustain and maintain social interactions in a group
- Adjust to different styles of being tested
- Provide opinions on a given issue or subject
- Comprehend and take notes during lectures
- Adapt to various teaching styles and expectations in upper grades
- Produce more written work at higher grades
- Organize work and become more independent learners

In All Grades
- Listen attentively
- Play "the school game" by knowing the rules
- Follow teachers' oral and written directions

Some Typical Classroom Routines
- When the teacher wants us to be quiet, he/she...
- When I want to ask the teacher something, I...
- If I know the answer to a question, I...
- If I don't know the answer to a question, I...
- If I need help, I...
- I talk quietly when...
- When the teacher talks, I...
- When I finish my work I...

FIGURE 4-3 *Some Typical School Expectations in the Mainstream Culture.* (Adapted from Morine-Dershimer, 1985.)

BOX 4-1

A Graduate Student's Experience with Educational Expectations

Even though I had been an excellent student in undergraduate school in Mexico, I failed to perform as expected in graduate school in the United States. Different standards and expectations did not permit me to succeed. I was used to exams where students were asked to "repeat" what had been said in class (this style of education was practiced even in college). The scene was quite different when I took exams during graduate school in the U. S. Exams assessed the student's ability to "apply" what had been discussed in class and in the assigned readings. Had I been given a hint that this was the performance expected of me, I would have performed with greater success. The lesson I learned was that, in order to prepare them for the best way to demonstrate their true knowledge, students need clearer guidelines for how to meet a school's expectations.

medical professionals. Currently, there are many American-born individuals who do not have medical insurance coverage and, in case of medical need, they must know how to access information to receive the appropriate services. The latest statistics indicate that 15.7% of people in the U.S. are without any medical coverage. That proportion is higher for African-Americans (19.1%) than it is for Hispanics (32.7%) and Native Americans (29%) (U.S. Census Bureau, 2005).

Being a native speaker of English does not always facilitate or guarantee access to medical agencies, as variations in coverage may exist from region to region. However, overall, understanding medical agencies' billing systems and procedures with regard to what may or may not be covered by medical insurance continues to be a challenge as charges are often not very clearly delineated. It is not unheard of that a couple might have family coverage, yet still consume a great deal of time in accounting for what is or is not covered by insurance. Therefore, seeking the appropriate medical assistance is only one of the barriers to solving health-related issues. The other is obtaining the "know-how" to ensure that payments are adequately accounted for by the insurance. The negotiation between indi-

viduals and agencies is complex even when persons speak the same language, and is many times more complex for those individuals who are not familiar with the system and the language.

Hispanic Perspectives

Members of the Hispanic culture have varying attitudes toward education and schooling that depend on social class (Ogbu, 1987). Middle-class immigrants adapt more easily to new institutions and to the operation of schools. But, as Trueba (1989) points out, the constant flow of immigrants may obscure the true extent to which Hispanic parents accept and support their children's formal education. Some families are eager to learn English and maintain Spanish. Others continue to speak Spanish, but are unsure of the value of learning English. Still others may be opposed to bilingual programs because learning "more English" will enhance their children's adaptation to the new culture and society.

Hispanic parents encourage their children to learn, but they do not always know which competencies to emphasize. Those who have failed in school may promote more the values of family tradition and culture. In their research, Maestas and Erickson (1989) found that parents helped their children with schoolwork if they were given specific instructions to follow, and they made their children feel responsible for their own learning. In addition to supporting their children's learning, Hispanic parents wish their children to be polite (Rodríguez & Olswang, 2003). "Educación," which is translated literally as "education," is interpreted not only as formal education but as adequate behavior and moral standing (Goldenberg & Gallimore, 1995; Trumbull et al., 2001; Zúñiga, 1988).

Hispanic parents respect teachers highly. Often they feel that "teachers know best" and educational decisions are the school's job (Gallegos & Gallegos, 1988). Many Hispanic parents' preoccupations at parent-teacher meetings are more about behavior than about their children's performance, at least initially. Recent immigrants tend to believe that schooling will provide better opportunities for the next generation, and they encourage their children to learn English so that they will better settle in the new country (Romo, 1984; Suárez-Orozco, 1987). Many Hispanic parents feel strongly that their role is more in the realm of moral and social development and would not necessarily welcome suggestions concerning those areas from school-based personnel (Trumbull et al., 2001). In working with students with special educational needs, parents often do not understand the process and don't feel capable of supporting their children's progress. Parents from other minority and even mainstream groups may share these feelings. However, Brisk (2005) suggests that: "High and reasonable expectations for academic achievement, support for native language development as well as English, and assistance in cultural adjustment so that students do not reject either culture should be included among the goals on which schools and families need to share and collaborate" (p. 93).

Although Mexican-born individuals have fewer years of schooling than do those born in the United States, even second-generation Mexicans may have a negative view of school. Hispanics of Mexican descent have the lowest proportion of high school degrees than do other Hispanic groups (50.2%), Cubans (74%), or Puerto Ricans (66.8%) (U.S. Census Bureau, 2003). Therefore, among Mexicans, few might remember successful public school experiences. Despite this fact, they desire a good education—even a college education— for their children. Research by Suárez-Orozco and Suárez-Orozco (1996), and Goldenberg, Gallimore, Resse, and Garnier (2001) has shown that, because of second-generation Mexican families' own negative experiences with school, they may demonstrate diminished educational aspirations for their children. Therefore, parents' expectations may be raised if, in addition to parents, educators also attempt to foster students' academic performance. Creating parent-mentor programs and workshops has proved to be very successful in enhancing CLD parent participation in school-related matters (Trumbull et. al., 2001).

Until 30 years ago, there was an inequality between women and men's educational attainment in most cultural groups—with the greatest differences being noted for Hispanic and African-American groups. Even though such inequality still exists, the differences in attaining literacy is comparable across genders in most of the Hispanic world, with some exceptions such as Bolivia and El Salvador. However, educators need to always understand the family's point of view. An experience with a Hispanic family, for example, helped me understand the reason for a female student's lack of motivation to learn (see Box 4-2).

> **BOX 4-2**
>
> ### An Attempt to Connect Formal Education with Family Values
>
> A second-grade Hispanic girl, the oldest of four children (the rest were all boys), was not achieving in school. Extensive testing indicated that she had no learning disabilities. When she applied herself, she was able to perform quite well. At home, this girl was a great helper, and her mother trusted her with many household responsibilities. The girl's parents encouraged her to do well in school because they, themselves, did not have very much formal schooling. The child appeared to strongly identify with her mother; she wanted to be like her and showed no motivation to apply herself at school. To motivate her, the school staff assigned her to a Spanish-speaking aide whom she liked; this adult served as a model for her by also working in cooperation with her family. Follow-up indicated that the student eventually began liking school and did well academically.

A review of the literature on Hispanic parents' participation in their children's schoolwork found that mothers were more involved than fathers (Delgado-Gaitán, 1992; Diaz, 2000; Goldenberg & Gallimore, 1995). Personal contact is one of the most effective ways to communicate with Hispanic parents and also other CLD populations. Sending notes and asking parents to fill out forms is not as effective. Trumbull et al. (2001) illustrate this point: "Some parents or guardians don't like filling out forms that ask for a huge amount of personal information because they question whether confidentiality can be assured or they don't know the answers to certain questions. As a result, children may go without services to which they are entitled, such as free lunch, and school officials may draw unwarranted conclusions about parents' degree of concern for their children's welfare" (p. 37).

Like any other immigrants, Hispanics settle in a community where they have some social networks, friends, relatives, or both who can serve as "brokers" in finding resources. And, when a member of that newly arrived immigrant has a disability, the network can offer some support and guidance. During my career as an SLP, I have worked with numerous families who have often made the comment that they moved to the United States because "in their home country there were no resources for the child" with a given disability. However, these families are also troubled by their legal status, which also complicates their situation. They may be hesitant to provide information that may reveal their migratory status. Professionals working with these families need to be familiar with undocumented persons' access to eligibility for specific programs. Collaborating with rehabilitation counselors, lawyers, and social workers is necessary.

African-American Perspectives

Support for education is strong among many families even though it may not be as apparent due to the frequent substandard schooling that African-American children receive. Formal education is considered as a path to a better life. However, Willis (2004) reports that 53% of African-Americans live in inner cities where there may be higher crime rates and unemployment, and inadequate housing, resources, and school standards. Some families feel resentful and may distrust available resources because those resources have not met their needs. Drug trafficking is one the primary causes of homicide among young African-Americans aged 15–34 (85%) as compared with the overall population (13%). African-Americans are twice as likely to be in prison than Hispanics (16.6% vs. 7.7%) and six times more likely than the mainstream.

A recent report by Frankenberg, Lee, and Orfield (2003) indicates that the South and West have more schools that are interracial (where approximately 50% of the student body is nonwhite) than does the rest of the country. The researchers found that schools in general are becoming increasingly segregated. In addition, they noted that only one-sixth of African-American students are educated in the South and West, and only one-fourth receive appropriate education in the Midwest and the Northeast. The largest urban schools in the nation tend to be essentially multiracial and have limited white-student enrollment. Segregation is also noted in suburban districts, except for the Southern states. The researchers found that during the 1990s, African-American students' attendance at majority white schools decreased by 13 points—to a level lower than in 1968. For more details, the reader is referred to McKinnon (2003).

Access to health care facilities is comparable to the mainstream where it is necessary to negotiate the intricacies of Medicare and other benefit and insurance groups. However, for the poor, accessing a clinic or a hospital is more difficult. Many delay seeking medical care until an illness occurs; then families go directly to the emergency room instead of accessing a network of physicians. This situation is also common among other poor mainstream uninsured and CLD populations. Additional difficulties include lack of health education. For example, medications may not

be taken when needed, and patients may overmedicate or discontinue treatment prematurely. In some instances, health care programs for African-American persons may be more successful if sponsored by a church group (Bonder et al., 2001).

Asian-American and Pacific Islander Perspectives

Education is highly valued among most Asian groups and the teacher is viewed in high regard. Differences in parents' attitudes towards education and teachers vary depending on the group's acculturation, their socioeconomic status, their formal education and, last but not least, individual differences. "Traditional families" and recent immigrants tell their children to listen to their teachers. In many of their countries of origin, students are reminded to be quiet, to stand and bow when the teacher enters the classroom, and to not look the teacher directly in the eye as a sign of respect. Learning takes place in a more passive mode, as children are not encouraged to ask questions—and, when teachers formulate questions, the questions are taken from classroom lectures and from textbooks. Students are expected to take notes and memorize them. This is very different from the average mainstream class where discussions and collaborative work is emphasized (Cheng, 1991). Just as with the Hispanic cultures, coming to school for a conference may signify that the child is misbehaving, something the family may be ashamed of and is not ready to face. Understanding these aspects is important for interpreting children's behavior and their parents' reactions when they are asked to join a school conference.

Nevertheless, parents also feel responsible for guiding their children toward school achievement. Children demonstrate responsibility by trying their best in school. Performing well ensures greater opportunities for success in education and occupation, and brings higher social status to the family as well as economic benefits (Chan & Lee, 2004). Although there may be variations across the great diversity of Asian cultures, schooling and respect for teachers is very important. Relationships between teaching and learning in Asian-Pacific populations (as well as some educational implications) are reported in Table 4-2.

Teachers are expected to lecture and direct the students. The teacher is the one who knows best; he or she is the authority and it is considered disrespectful to engage in discussions or debates with the teacher. If teachers do not assign homework, it may signify to parents that they are not doing a "good job." Students do not volunteer questions or comments unless encouraged to do so. It would mean they are "showing off." Even when a student does not understand a lesson they may not ask teachers for help. Students may read to acquire facts without using the acquired knowledge to make inferences, or synthesize or apply the information. Just as in the Hispanic culture, parents believe they do not know as much as teachers. Students work cooperatively and help each other in class and they may not understand the concept of cheating because they want to help their peers.

Parents do not see the value of joining the Parent-Teacher Association (commonly known as the PTA) or any educational group. Teachers working with Asian-American and Pacific Islander students should be aware of all of the facts just presented when determining whether a student may or may not have a learning difficulty. For example, if a student does not volunteer it does not mean that he or she does not have the answer to the question. The student may not ask questions because he or she believes the teacher should not be questioned. What may appear to be cheating may just be the cooperation of peers to obtain answers.

Native American Perspectives

Children of Native American and Alaskan Native backgrounds may find adjustment to a typical "American" classroom difficult. Students attending typical classrooms experience similar challenges to the ones experienced by students who were sent to boarding schools in the past. One of the main difficulties is students' adjustment to the competitiveness very apparent in most mainstream classrooms. The following is recounted by one teacher who taught in a remote village in Alaska: "In Yup'ik culture the 'group' is important. There is little, if any, competition in the Yup'ik culture. When the Western school system entered the picture, the unity of the group slowly shattered. Children were sent hundreds—often thousands—of miles away to be schooled in boarding schools where they were forced to abandon their own language for the foreign English with its accompanying foreign ways. They learned the Western value of competition. They learned to be individuals competing against each other instead of a group working as a unit. There were seldom, if any, times when they were allowed to help each other; this would have been construed as 'cheating'" (V. Dull, in Nelson-Barber & Dull, 1998, p. 95).

Although there are variations from tribe to tribe, teachers should tolerate more silence or no interaction from students. As previously discussed, nonverbal communication such as eye contact may be interpreted differently by both mainstream and Native cultures. The child or person might not look directly at the speaker or listener, but this does not signify lack of respect. In certain Native American

TABLE 4-2 Teaching and Learning in Asian-Pacific Populations (and Educational Implications)

General Asian/Pacific-American Values Concerning Education

Asian/Pacific-American Themes	*Educational Implications*
Schooling is a formal process.	Teachers are to be respected and not to be treated casually. Teachers are to be treated formally.
Teachers are to be respected and obeyed.	Students may not ask or answer questions out of respect for teachers. Students may believe in rules like "Speak only when spoken to." Students may appear to be passive to teachers.
Teachers are important authorities.	Students may not question the authority or knowledge of teachers because that would be disrespectful even if the student believes the teacher has given incorrect information.
Humility and modesty are important values.	Students may be reluctant to volunteer in class and may not offer new ideas to a class discussion in fear of looking like they are "showing off."
Cooperation is an important virtue. Harmony is valued.	Students may help each other on their homework. In addition, students may feel it is important to help each other with classwork and may not understand the concept of cheating. Students may also encourage each other by providing answers.
Schooling is a serious process.	Students are expected to be on task and work hard at their desk. They may not believe it is acceptable to let students walk around the room.
Teachers have "knowledge" and should impart it to students.	Teachers may be expected to lecture much of the time. Students may not have skills to engage in inquiry, discussion, or Socratic methods because the teacher is expected to explain to students what to do. Students may not engage in discussions with teachers because that would be disrespectful.
Parents trust teachers.	Parents may not be active in PTA or other educational groups. Parents may believe they do not know as much as teachers. If students are successful, then parents may not understand the importance of PTA and parent-teacher conferences.
Parents believe in developing technical skills in students.	Teachers may believe in developing a well-rounded person. However, parents and students may see the importance of cognitive development in fields like math, science, and English. Parents may believe other subjects like physical education, auto mechanics, and chorus should be included only if there is time. In addition, parents may not understand the emphasis teachers place on self-esteem, creativity, and independence.
Students should be obedient.	Students may be on task and exhibit behaviors of high-achieving students. Though they may not understand the lesson, they will not ask teachers for help.
Reading for information is important for providing facts and lessons.	Students may read for facts, but may not have the initial skills to infer, synthesize, and apply information.
Teachers are expected to give students homework.	If teachers do not give students work to be done at home, teachers are not doing "good" job.

Source: "Educating the Whole Child," by V. O. Pang, 1998. In V. O. Pang and L. Cheng (Eds.), *Struggling to Be Heard: The Unmet Needs of Asian Pacific-American Children* (pp. 292–293). Albany, NY: State University of New York Press. Reprinted with permission.

cultures, specific knowledge might be the prerogative of certain persons in the community. For example, Trumbull et al. (2001) report that certain knowledge may be acquired or passed on by the eldest son of a spiritual leader. A review of various effective teaching strategies and research carried out with various Native tribes can be found in Tharp and Yamauchi (1994). In their review, the authors discuss the use of Instructional Conversations (IC) (Goldenberg, 1993) that emphasize more interaction between teacher and student, and student and student—and that prescribe more small discussions on a given topic. The authors propose that the classroom in which the IC is most likely to occur would be one where the ratio of students to teachers is small. The teacher might float among individual and small group activity settings or might be stationary but approachable. The teacher would offer responsive instructional conversation as needed, while allowing students opportunities to initiate and terminate those conversations. It would appear that a more interactionist approach to teaching may facilitate learning, and that this is an approach that might be helpful in any classroom.

HOW STUDENTS/CLIENTS AND THEIR FAMILIES UNDERSTAND AND REACT TO VARIOUS EDUCATIONAL AND MEDICAL DISABILITIES

Accepting a given disability may be difficult for any family, but particularly more difficult for immigrants. Some examples of general and special education programs available in a few other countries outside the United States were described in Chapter 3. As noted, services in special education are scarce in those countries (China, Taiwan, Vietnam, Mexico, Cuba, and even Puerto Rico).

The United States is the leading nation in the world in recognizing various language and learning disabilities of children of younger ages, and in researching various intervention approaches which are generally limited in other parts of the world. Therefore, some CLD families may not be acquainted with resources that can be used to identify and remedy some of the disabilities that often surface when children attend school—difficulty with reading and academic performance, for example. Ultimately, however, a family's reaction to a handicapping condition affecting a child or an adult is a personal matter. Some parents find it easier to understand that their child has a "handicap" if it is more "visible"— such as with blindness, deafness, cleft palate, or cerebral palsy. It is more difficult for a family to accept that their child might have a learning difficulty—because with such disabilities, there is no "apparent physical problem," and the child may be performing as expected in the home environment. Families also have varying attitudes toward caring for an adult who is suffering from an acquired disability, and they have varying opinions about the issues of death and dying. For example, some families want to care for the adult in the home while others accept the option of using long-term health care facilities. Professionals working with students/clients who have congenital or acquired disabilities need to reflect on their own attitudes about various disabilities and to also understand the families' and clients' points of view. In several cultures, a congenital handicap may be interpreted as being caused by an external, nonmedical factor (Cheng, 1991; Meyerson, 1983, 1990; Weddington, 1990). A speech disorder such as stuttering has an effect on the emotional well-being of most individuals. Different groups have differing views toward this disorder; therefore, it is important to "be prepared to open a dialogue with clients and families to ascertain their beliefs and feelings about stuttering" (Ratner, 2004, p. 294).

Even though the United States is one of the leaders of Western medicine, certain groups may distrust the system. For example, the Hmong have been shown to be suspicious of authority. The story of Lia and her unsuccessful treatment of seizures is well known to the Hmong community. In her case, medications did not remedy her problem. Furthermore, her family was unable to understand what was said to them. Her story is described in detail in Fadiman's book, *The Spirit Catches You and You Fall Down* (1997). In addition to suspicion, other barriers to successful treatment are the role and sex of the provider. For example, discomfort may occur when a male physician examines a female or vice versa, or when bodily symptoms and functions must be shared with persons who are essentially strangers even though they may be nurses or physicians.

Treatment of the seriously ill or dying patient has to be carried out with the collaboration of the health professionals involved—and, when appropriate—with the collaboration of the family and the patient. More often than not, care providers will attempt to save a seriously ill or dying patient using drastic measures unless they are otherwise advised. Very often, patients will have written their wishes on how to proceed in case of impending death. For example, to respect the wishes of a seriously ill 85-year-old woman, no drastic measures may be taken to prolong her life. Instead, the services of a hospice might be adopted. Thus, it is important to take the patients' and their families' wishes into consideration. In some CLD populations, the participation of the extended family is important, as well as the presence of a priest or minister who can administer last rites. Flexibility on the part of health professionals and an understanding of the patient's unique needs are therefore necessary.

Anglo-European Perspectives

Anglo-Europeans support an accurate and realistic understanding of health difficulties and believe for the most part that illnesses usually have a cause. No one cause, however, can explain a given handicap or illness. Several external factors, such as disease or the environment—or simply random factors—could explain a given problem. For the most part, "Western medicine, as practiced in the United States, has traditionally separated disorders of the mind and body and relied on scientific and technical information for diagnosis and treatment" (Hanson, 2004, p. 98). However, in recent years, more groups are considering naturalistic and holistic approaches. In keeping with the mainstream culture, the patient is encouraged to learn as much as possible about his or her illness. Treatment is usually dispensed, and the patient is held responsible for attending to some of the treatment, for example, changing dressings independently, or injecting insulin. This is not the case in other cultures where the patient's family plays a more active role (Luckmann, 2000). Although there is great variation among Euro-Americans in how they express pain, most members of this group will seek assistance when they feel ill.

Patient satisfaction with the treatment may depend on a particular setting. For example, the treatment received in a small community hospital may be different than that of a large research hospital. With the ever-increasing diverse background of patients and health care providers, any encounter between patient and service provider could be difficult, especially when the patient requires residence in a long-term facility. "Caregivers and residents become a close community/family with extended relationships, which may be enjoyable or difficult and may continue day after day. In addition, the personal cultures of the caregivers may radically conflict with those of the residents" (Luckmann, 2000, p. 81).

Hispanic Perspectives

Having worked extensively with this population, I have found that parents tend to "accept" their child's "visible" disability more readily than they would a "hidden" disability, such as a language-learning disability or mild general retardation. Some parents interpret these disabilities as being caused by external factors. For example, Meyerson (1983, 1990) reported that several Chicano mothers attributed their children's cleft palate to an eclipse during pregnancy, whereas other mothers attributed the problem to a "susto,"—a "frightful experience" during pregnancy. Most frequently, mothers use terms such as "mal puesto" [witchcraft] or "mal ojo" [evil eye], or name some wrongdoing during their pregnancy—when they try to account for the reasons for their children's disabilities. Among Cubans, a child's physical and mental problems are often attributed to "empacho" [indigestion], "desmayo" or "desvanecimiento" [a fainting spell], "decaimiento" [lack of energy], or "barrenillo" [obsessive thinking] that occurred during pregnancy (Queralt, 1984).

Belief in folk medicine as part of the medical treatment process is common among some less acculturated Hispanics. In describing the healing process, Hispanics often refer to "curanderos" [healers] and "espiritistas" [spiritualists]. Negroni-Rodríguez and Morales (2001) describe how some persons in Puerto Rico believe that everyone has spirits who can protect them, and the "espiritistas" communicate with those spirits. Healers use a combination of intense concern, rituals, herbs and herbal teas, oil massage, amulets, and prayers. Some Hispanic families seek medical care from physicians for physical problems and psychological support from healers. A family's attitude toward disability tends to depend on the family's socioeconomic status. The higher a family's status, the more it tends to cope with their child's mental retardation by "hiding her or him from society" (Smith-DeMateo, 1987). Moreover, many families from rural areas are likely to accept the fact of the disability as an "act of God." Specific Hispanic groups respond to pain differently. Gordon (1997) reports that some Mexican-Americans do not display their physical pain as much as Puerto Ricans do, for example.

Children who are slower in developing or have a "more visible" handicap are often referred to by their families as "enfermito" [sick one]. When their children are identified as having language-learning disabilities, some families may equate this problem with cognitive impairments. It takes time for parents and families to understand the difference between the two terms. Research on the manner in which stuttering has been viewed by the Hispanic culture has yielded some conflicting results (Tellis, 2002). For example, Madding (1995) indicated that Hispanic parents attributed "stuttering" to "the evil eye," whereas other reported that several Hispanic families believed that stuttering could be stopped by having recourse to a "curandero," other researchers, however, disagree. Tellis and Blood (2000) interviewed Hispanic students who did not believe in the powers of a "curandero" for treating stuttering. It is very

---

BOX 4-3

A Mexican-American Man's Reaction to Treatment

At age 68, a second-generation Mexican-American who had gone to school all his life in the United States and was equally fluent in both Spanish and English sustained a dense right cerebral hemispheric stroke with accompanying left hemiparesis and left visual field difficulties. On numerous occasions, he asked about the cause of his stroke and received a detailed explanation with a scientific basis. Four months after his stroke, he inquired whether the clinician thought a folk healer in Mexico could help ameliorate his left hemiparesis. It became clear that all along the patient had wanted approval that would justify his belief in an alternative method for dealing with illness. (Contributed by Gustavo Arámbula, M.A., bilingual speech and language pathologist.)

---

likely that the students who were voicing this opinion came from a more formally educated background as compared with those interviewed by Madding (1995).

Because of a strong sense of family, many more Hispanic relatives visit a sick family member as compared with the European-American family. Also, sick elderly persons tend to be treated at home rather than in long-term facilities. In addition, beliefs and attitudes toward treating illness must be taken into account, as is shown in Box 4-3.

African-American Perspectives

Just as with some other CLD populations, some African-Americans believe that the cause of illness is bad luck or evil spirits, or may be a consequence of disobeying God. Persons with disabilities, even those with mental retardation, are as respected as any other individuals. Willis (2004) reports that for the most part, families will respond positively to interventions once some counseling is offered regarding the possible cause of a given disability, but differences exist from group to group. For example, a first-generation African-American from Senegal or Libya might interpret the cause of a disability

or illness differently depending on his or her own experiences and education. Different health-related vocabulary words may be used and interpreted differently among the various African-American groups. For example, "pain," "anemia," "vomiting," "diarrhea," and "urinate/urine" are interpreted as " miseries," "low blood or tired blood," "throwing up," "running off or grip," and "pass water or peepee" (Cherry & Giger, 1999).

Many middle- and upper-income African-American families use the services of a physician and belong to a health maintenance organization. However, for those who are unemployed or have fewer income resources, access to medical establishment is more problematic. Some may have coverage under Medicare, but it is variable. Because of lack of funds, often families with limited resources wait to seek medical attention until after an illness has occurred. Therefore, preventive medical attention is often not obtained. Many families do not adhere to medical directions and suggestions. Patients either over- or undermedicate themselves with antibiotics.

Willis (2004) advises medical professionals to ensure that families be presented with medical advice that they can easily understand

and follow at home. It is important to ensure that patients understand how to use the medication or equipment provided to them. Follow-up calls are necessary for ensuring that the suggestions of the physician are followed. Willis states, "These suggestions, although made in the context of working with African-Americas of low socioeconomic status, are equally applicable to many families with whom service providers work" (p. 165).

Asian-American and Pacific Islander Perspectives

Many Asian-Americans and Pacific Islanders attribute a child's disability to the mother's lack of an adequate diet, or to events occurring during her pregnancy. Chan and Lee (2004) cite the case of a woman with a Chinese-Vietnamese ethnic background who attributed her daughter's congenital anomalies (fused fingers and a split thumb) to the fact that she had worked as a seamstress during her pregnancy. Another woman from Hong Kong attributed her child's cleft lip and palate to the fact that she had seen horror movies and watched evil gods during the first months of her pregnancy. And another mother—of Korean descent—felt she had caused her son's autism because she had cried profusely at a funeral when she was pregnant, and had also suffered from mood swings during that time. As mentioned for other groups, Asian-American and Pacific Islander populations may believe that disabilities are consequences for misbehavior such as drinking or gambling.

Regarding the understanding of the disability of mental retardation, this condition may have different names among the various Asian-American and Pacific Islander groups. In some cases it may be equated with learning disabilities, while in others it may be equated with emotional disturbance or behavioral problems. Watanabe (1998) reports that when she asked

special educators in China about their treatment programs for learning disabilities and behavioral disorders, they indicated that there were no such programs. Instead, they reported that they had programs for the sensory impaired and the severely cognitively impaired, and for students who were orthopedically handicapped. When Watanabe spoke with educators from other Asian countries such as Japan and Korea, their answers were the same. The author suggests that professionals working with families of Asian-American and Pacific Islander cultures be aware of the families' beliefs and knowledge about various types of disabilities and the disabilities' impact on learning. It is important to build trust with these families so that they may collaborate with special education personnel with greater ease.

The SLP will find that, as with any parent, some parents in this group are reluctant to admit that their child has a problem for fear of feeling that they have not fulfilled their role properly. Working on this issue will be important when planning an intervention program for these children and their families.

Native American Perspectives

Many Native Americans and Alaskan Natives believe that disease is caused by supernatural powers; therefore, seeking the assistance from a healer in addition to using Western remedies is common. However, each tribe, or individual members of a given tribe, may react differently to a given educational or medical disability.

Before a more formal medical and/or educationally based treatment is started, the family may want to engage in a more traditional ceremony. A healer may be consulted prior to any intervention.

Medical care is offered as part of the federal Indian Health Service (IHS). Insurance coverage may also include Medicare, Medicaid, and coverage from private insurance companies. Resources are also available in cities with larger numbers of Native Americans, but Joe and Malach (2004) report that chronic disease such as diabetes and hearing disease are on the rise. For the Native American group a higher incidence of fetal alcohol syndrome and cleft lip/palate is reported (see Table 1-6, p. 17). There are an increasing number of programs established today to treat substance abuse and prevention.

SUMMARY

SLPs who are an integral part of the assessment and intervention team for CLD populations must continually evaluate their own background experiences and that of their students/clients. The knowledge-based information SLPs should have "at their fingertips" includes childrearing practices, communication patterns occurring within families, and an understanding of the student/client's (and their families') previous experiences with formal education and literacy. In addition, knowing about student/clients' previous contact with various institutions such as schools, health care providers, and various other agencies assists in planning a better course for intervention.

The following are three important suggestions for helping SLPs to succeed in providing appropriate services to CLD populations:

1. Learn as much as possible about a given cultural group, but avoid generalizations. However, SLPs should keep in mind that it is impossible to know everything about a given culture. Hanson (2004) comments, "Service providers are cautioned against using this information to overgeneralize or characterize all members of a cultural group as the same. Instead, they are advised to use this knowledge to form a basis for

respectful interaction" (p. 5). Remembering that there are "subgroups" and exceptions within any group is very helpful. Those differences also exist within the culture of the service providers themselves. Members within a group differ because of a number of variables such as experiences, access to education, and attitudes toward gender, age, and various personality types. "A person is not a collection of cultural 'facts,' but rather a bundle of cultural influences and other factors that impact perceptions and sentiments as well as behaviors" (Bonder et al., 2001, p. 8).

2. When relating to CLD students/clients and their families, evaluating their situation and taking "their" perspective should be attempted as much as possible. For example, suggestions to parents on how to assist their children with developing specific language skills and activities should be realistic, feasible, and take into account the parents' resources and time. Evaluating the course of any intervention is important for determining its effectiveness in serving clients. Bonder et al. (2001) describe how a psychologist had to change the focus of her sessions in working with a primarily African-American group who resided in an urban setting and who had been diagnosed with schizophrenia. The initial focus had been on learning new skills that would enable them to become integrated into the community. But the focus of the sessions had to change after the psychologist realized that the group often changed the topic of the session to a discussion of their own experiences in viewing certain TV shows and soap operas. The sessions had to take on a more social tone before the psychologist

could develop plans for discussing the job opportunities and skills that had been the original reason behind the sessions. By adopting this temporary focus of the group, the psychologist was able to make the patients comfortable, and as a result, many of the patients were able to transition into the community much faster.

3. Observing the clients' behaviors and methods of communication should be conducted in as many contexts as possible. When unsure about the meaning of certain behaviors or responses from clients, SLPs should consult with a trusted colleague who has a similar background as the clients. Working with a well-trained language interpreter/

translator (I/T) is also paramount. In the role of a participant-observer, the SLP's perspective is important for understanding clients from various cultural backgrounds. Being involved in such observations promotes ethnographic research that is defined as "educational research based on anthropological constructs that include methods such as field work, interviews, and participant observations" (Nieto, 2004, p. 149). As Nieto mentions, engaging in this type of research enhances better understanding of the best practices for instructing second-language learners.

OUR CLIENTS

Eric, Ana, Jack, Grace, and Leonardo

To remind the reader about each one of these cases, a synopsis of each case is presented. (For more detail about each client's background, please refer to previous chapters.) At the end of each synopsis is a list of conclusions that might be drawn from both the information presented in this book about each client and the concepts reviewed in this chapter.

Eric

Eric is a 4-year-old preschool child born in the United States. His parents are first-generation immigrants from Vietnam. Both Vietnamese and English are spoken in the home. His parents speak Vietnamese to him, whereas his two older siblings communicate in English with him. His parents are concerned because Eric's language skills in both languages are limited as compared with his siblings and other children who are growing up in similar bilingual backgrounds. Eric has been a healthy child. Eric's teacher has reported that he prefers playing by himself. His concentration is limited unless he watches cartoons or videos.

Points to consider:

- The fact that Eric's parents immigrated to the United States when they were teenagers—and that his father has completed two years of college in the United States—indicates that the family (perhaps the father more than the mother) should be knowledgeable about major community resources such as schools and health care agencies. However, they may not be aware that children who have some language difficulties can be assessed through their school district (even though they have two older children).

- We do not know the level of acculturation and assimilation of the family, but we should be careful in misinterpreting nonverbal communication. For example, a smile may not indicate that the parents agree with what is said. Also, silence may need to be interpreted with care, as well.

- Because Eric is the youngest child, it may not be uncommon for him to be "taken care of" by his older siblings; not enough, therefore, may be asked of him.

Ana

Ana is a 9-year-old enrolled in fourth grade who emigrated from Mexico at the age of 5 and who is having difficulty reading in English. She is the oldest of three children. She was raised by her maternal grandparents beginning at the age of 6 months; after five years she was reunited with her parents.

Ana attended kindergarten in Arizona but moved in the middle of that year when her parents found better jobs in California. Ana has learned English quite well but she is behind in reading. All of her schooling has been in English. She speaks Spanish to her parents and to some relatives who live nearby, but she talks to her siblings in both English and Spanish. Her parents insist that only Spanish should be spoken at home.

Points to consider:

- The SLP should interview Ana's parents in order to ask them for their perspective of the problem. Their level of formal education should be determined, and the SLP should inquire about whether anyone in the family has had difficulty learning to read.

- What materials are read in the home? How does Ana participate in reading or being read to? Does the family have an opportunity to visit the library?

- Do the parents feel that Ana has made progress in the last year?

Jack

Jack is a 14-year-old of African-American descent who is has difficulty with subjects such as social studies, English, and writing. Mrs. G., Jack's paternal grandmother, adopted him when he was 2 years old because his single mother could not raise him. Prior to entering School District A (summer 2002), Jack attended a private school for two years. Even though both Mrs. G. and Jack have a Southern accent and speak AAVE, his use of a different syntax and vocabulary do not seem to interfere with his academic learning.

Jack had to remain in the ICU for about seven days after birth due to respiratory distress. His developmental milestones occurred within a normal timeframe except for his speech, which was delayed: Jack did not put words together until he was about 3 years old. His latest vision and hearing screenings were unremarkable (fall 2002). Mrs. G. reports that Jack is on daily medication for anger, anxiety, and agitation. He is receiving counseling to address his emotional issues.

A previous school assessment report written by an SLP and the psychologist indicated some learning difficulties, but their severity did not warrant intervention from special education. Because the results of this assessment were not satisfactory to Mrs. G., she sought an outside assessment by a neuropsychologist. Results indicated that Jack has difficulty with working memory and sequencing skills. Mrs. G. states that Jack has difficulty synthesizing oral and written information. Writing is difficult for him: Jack does not respect rules of grammar and punctuation.

Points to consider:

- Mrs. G., Jack's grandmother, is very well aware of the system. She has the advantage of having the education (she is a nurse) and the "know-how" to reach for the appropriate resources. There is no question that she

(Continues)

(*Continued*)

knows how to seek medical and educational assistance. Jack is being treated for anxiety and she has pursued an evaluation of his learning difficulties. Now she is asking the school district to address his learning needs.

- The school district has not addressed Jack's learning needs because they were not as apparent during his first evaluation by the school. However, Mrs. G. has contacted the school and is asking for a reevaluation.

Grace

Grace is a 60-year-old Mandarin-speaking former businesswoman who sustained a stroke in the right hemisphere of her brain while visiting the United States on a business trip.

Grace was a successful businesswoman prior to her accident. She speaks Mandarin, Cantonese, English, and French. She completed her business degree in China, but spent five years in the United States when she was first developing her business. The languages she speaks most frequently are Mandarin and English. She speaks Cantonese with her relatives. Prior to her stroke she could converse on several topics in all the languages she knew. However, she felt most at ease reading and writing in Chinese and English. She was very proficient in reading and writing English but her strongest area was business English.

Points to consider:

- Because Grace is well educated and she has lived in the United States for five years, she is most likely familiar with the various health care establishments. However, this is not certain because we do not know exactly how long ago this was.

- Grace may not be able to advocate for herself because her speech and mobility skills are limited at this time. She will need a friend or relative to assist in mediating her medical transactions.

Leonardo

Leonardo is a 45-year-old fieldworker from Guatemala who suffered a traumatic brain injury following a dispute with a neighbor. Leonardo is an illegal immigrant who has been traveling back and forth between the U.S. and Guatemala for more than 20 years. He works as a crop picker in several states including Washington, Ohio, Michigan, California, and Oregon. He completed seven grades in Guatemala but was able to get his GED while in the U.S. after attending night classes.

He is able to communicate in English, but even after his years spent in the U.S., he is still much more fluent in Spanish than in English. Prior to his accident, he could read newspapers in both English and Spanish but concentrated primarily on sports and local news. At this time, he can walk but he cannot process what is said to him in either Spanish or English. He is disoriented, he cannot keep track of time, and he forgets daily routines. After spending two weeks in a rehabilitation center he was dismissed and is currently living with some friends.

Points to consider:

- Even though Leonardo has been in the United States for 20 years and he has a command of the English language, we are not sure how much experience he has had with the medical establishment. If his health has been good, he has not had to visit doctors. It is uncertain that he has any coverage other than Medicaid. This is something that needs to be determined.

- Leonardo will need the assistance of a friend to help him navigate through the medical establishment, since he is significantly impaired at this time. Hopefully, it will be someone who has some knowledge of the medical services available and who speaks English fluently. Otherwise, he will have to rely on social workers to guide him and to ensure that he has appropriate language interpreting services. His illegal status should not be a deterrent for receiving appropriate medical services.

Further Readings

Bonder, B., Martin, L., & Miracle, A. (2001). *Culture in clinical care*. Thorofare, NJ: Slack Incorporated.

Lynch, E., & Hanson, M. (Eds.). (2004). *Developing cross-cultural competence: A guide for working with children and their families* (3rd ed.). Baltimore: Brookes.

Pang, O. P., & Cheng, L. R. (Eds.). (1998). *Struggling to be heard: The unmet needs of Asian/Pacific-American children*. Albany, NY: State University of New York Press.

CHAPTER 5

ASSESSMENT PROCEDURES FOR CLD CHILDREN: INFANCY THROUGH ADOLESCENCE

"The assessment process of a culturally and linguistically diverse (CLD) individual (child or adult) requires a multifaceted approach because tests are only a fragment of the whole story" (Author).

CHAPTER OUTLINE

INTRODUCTION

The speech-language pathologist (SLP) assesses the language competence of a main-streamed student by gathering information from various sources (i.e., parents, teachers, family, or other professionals who know or have worked with the student/client) to determine whether a speech-language problem is present. In addition, the SLP's formal and informal interactions with the student assist in making a diagnosis. For older students, language difficulties may be the primary reason for their failure in acquiring reading fluency and reading comprehension skills. Depending on the nature of the concern, consultation with teachers and parents offers the school staff specific strategies they can follow prior to recommending a more complete evaluation. For example, prior to deciding to conduct a more thorough assessment, additional practice may be recommended for a kindergarten student who has not acquired phoneme-grapheme correspondence at the same pace as his or her peers. A third-grader who has difficulty comprehending classroom instructions may be assisted if the SLP can focus the child's attention more regularly and can warn him or her about the number of instructions that will be given. Or, instructions may also be written on the board using key words and some visual aids.

New guidelines of the Individuals with Disabilities Education Act (IDEA) drafted in 2004 indicate that students needing specialized educational services may not be necessarily identified following the "traditional discrepancy vs. performance model." Instead, educational needs of the students should be met through careful planning on the part of all school personnel that includes the teacher, a special educator, and other ancillary staff (which also should include the SLP). The key concept to remember is "Responsiveness to Intervention" (RtI). The focus should be on specialized teaching strategies that could be implemented to enhance the learning of the student. Therefore, a process of collaboration with teachers, special educators, and other school personnel who are qualified to meet the educational needs of all students who are at risk must be undertaken prior to initiating a more formal speech and language assessment. If the student does not improve following the suggested recommendations, the SLP must assess the nature and severity of the problem by using any number of available standardized tests, which often include specific measures of language form, content, and use. The assessment may also include the elicitation and analysis of an oral language sample as well as a written language sample. If the student is eligible for speech-language services, the SLP uses the assessment results and observations to write specific speech-language goals designed to meet the student's communication needs. When working with adults, the goals may be more functional and work oriented.

Circumstances that determine the need for an assessment of younger populations (children and adolescents), as opposed to older populations (adults and seniors), are very different. In the case of a student attending a school program, there is time to decide whether or not to conduct the assessment. This is not always the case for the adult client, who may have sustained a traumatic *injury or stroke, or be afflicted with a sudden neurological disorder. More time and planning may be needed for other communication disorders such as various dementias. Therefore, the assessment processes for the student client and the older client are described in separate chapters. Specific assessment and intervention procedures for adult CLD clients are discussed in Chapter 8.*

This chapter will focus on the pre-assessment and assessment processes. Evaluating assessments and determining the diagnoses of communication disorders in children and adolescents will be discussed in Chapter 6.

Assessment Processes for CLD Students

In a school setting, it is often the SLP who is consulted to determine whether a student should be assessed. My research (1989) found that the reasons given for referring Hispanic bilingual students generally had to do with concerns about the students' language delay in English, Spanish, or both languages—a delay that was accompanied by slow academic progress (Langdon, 1989). Because there is a strong relationship between oral and written language (this will be discussed in Chapter 6), it is important to evaluate both the student's oral and written language skills.

The assessment process consists of several phases. The first two phases include an evaluation of areas related to the student's health history and motor and speech-language development, as well as an evaluation of the student's previous schooling. The first two phases also include a review of accommodations that have been made for the student, which are referred to in this chapter as pre-assessment considerations. The term "accommodations" refers to the teacher and school personnel's efforts toward enhancing the student's learning success. Examples of accommodations include giving the student more time to complete an assignment or an

examination, reducing the amount of required homework, teaching the student specific strategies for more effective recall, and offering individual tutoring. Once the information is obtained in the initial assessment phases, a decision needs to be made about whether a more comprehensive assessment (that includes specific tests) is necessary. Assessment is defined as the process of collecting data about an individual over time—whereas testing, which is a part of assessment, is one piece of the total amount of data that is obtained in order to evaluate the individual and determine a diagnosis.

Testing is assessing an individual's performance on a particular task in one particular situation. The complete assessment process is illustrated with the flower depicted in Figure 5-1. Each petal represents one piece of the assessment (data). In order to complete the flower, each piece of the data on the petals needs to be obtained. Testing is only one of the petals. It is important to "complete" the flower, but testing constitutes only part of it. The stem of the flower can be considered as the evaluation portion of the process and the pistil the final diagnosis. Each leaf represent a piece of the assessment process that includes observations, developmental history, observations, comments from parents and teachers, and student response to accommodations.

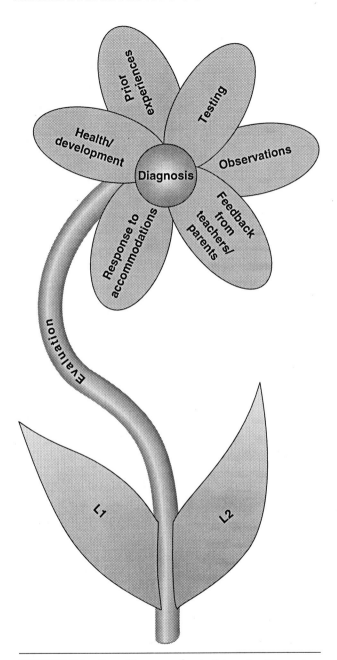

FIGURE 5-1 *Steps Necessary for Arriving at a Diagnosis.*

Pre-assessment Considerations

Prior to conducting a full assessment of a CLD student, the SLP should investigate certain topics that have been discussed in previous chapters, such as (1) the length of the student's residence in the U.S., and (2) the type of educational programs in which the student has previously been enrolled. If the student has resided in the U.S. for less than a year, he or she may simply need some additional time in which to acquire English. The student's school attendance should also be verified. Frequent absences not only disrupt the educational process, but also decrease the CLD student's opportunities for exposure to English. If, however, a student who has resided in the U.S. for less than a year is having difficulties in his or her native language, a referral for a complete assessment may be warranted. Documentation of the types of programs that a student has attended is important for determining whether the student has received optimal second-language instruction that uses the techniques that were described in Chapter 3. For example, questions such as the following should be explored: (1) Has the student been exposed to sufficient comprehensible input during instruction? (2) Has the student had enough interactions with native speakers of English? and (3) Has the program been consistent? Verifying the student's progress over time should be documented as well. Reviewing the student's cumulative records and conversing with parents and previous teachers will assist in gathering more accurate information.

In determining the need for a more in-depth speech-language assessment, the SLP should ascertain whether the student has had previous experience with certain school-related activities as well as with the process of being tested. For example, it is helpful to check whether the student has been exposed to literacy activities at home; whether the family has had opportunities to visit the library and knows how to use its resources; and whether the student has used the Internet as an additional resource for completing homework a given research project (this last question is applicable to older students).

Other areas to check include whether the student has been exposed to the types of assessments that are utilized to evaluate the student's mastery of curriculum content. In certain countries students are tested on what the teacher has said in class; therefore, all information is memorized. Tests consist of essays instead of multiple-choice questions. This is prevalent in European countries as well as in other countries (such as Mexico and Vietnam) that have been influenced by European educational systems.

To determine if a speech-language problem exists, comparing the student with siblings and peers is very helpful. Naturally, each individual is different, but if one child in a family has difficulties and the other does not, this may signal a problem. Students should not be referred for special education because of dialectal differences, however. For example, the use of African-American Vernacular English (AAVE) is not a disorder and only AAVE-speaking students who clearly have an articulation/language difficulty should be referred for an assessment. The reader is referred to Goldstein (2000), who compiled data on phonological, morphosyntactic, and syntactic characteristics of children from various American dialectal as well as other language backgrounds. Goldstein made use of various sources such as Anderson and Battle (1993), Bailey and Thomas (1998), Hyter (1996), Pollock et al. (1998), Seymour and Seymour (1981), and Washington (1996).

A health and developmental history helps determine if the student has a health-related history such as hearing loss or delayed language development in the primary language, or had a difficult birth history. These factors will influence the rate of language development, which has an influence on second-language acquisition. All of the information discussed in this section can be gathered by reviewing the student's cumulative records and by consulting with the student's teachers and family. Obtaining answers to a teacher's questionnaire is also helpful. Questionnaires for parents and teachers (Figure 5-2 and Figure 5-3) provide the perspectives of persons who interact with the student on a daily basis.

The parent questionnaire (Figure 5-2) is divided into four sections which include: (A) Social and Family History; (B) Parent/Family Observations About the Student; (C) School History; and (D) Health and Developmental Information. Figure 5-3 includes information to be filled out by the teacher(s) for two languages (if the student is enrolled in a bilingual program).

The parent questionnaire (Figure 5-2) can be completed at the time of the initial School Assessment Team (SAT) meeting or can be collected during a face-to-face interaction or on the telephone. If the SLP does not speak the language of the student, an interpreter/translator (I/T) can be trained to carry out this task. Depending on the answers provided, the assessment team may decide that further assessment is not indicated at that time. For example, if the child has attended school for only a short time, a full assessment may be postponed—provided that the student's performance at home is comparable to that of siblings or peers.

Some questions require particular tact. Obtaining information on the student's length of stay in the United States is important, for example, but the SLP must realize that some parents may come to the United States without their children so that they can initially establish themselves; they therefore leave the children behind in the care of grandparents or other relatives. The child emigrates later and may consequently experience some difficulty in adjusting to the new family life. Finding out as much as possible about the prior schooling of such children is helpful. If a parent hesitates to give an answer concerning the family's length of stay in the United States, the SLP can reformulate the question by saying, "Have you been in this country for more than two years, and has your child lived with you all this time?" Similarly, to avoid embarrassing a parent who may have had a very limited formal education, the interviewer may ask about the parents' education by saying, "How many years of schooling did you have an opportunity to complete in your country?"

Deciding Whether a More Comprehensive Assessment Is Necessary

If the parents report that the student has had a delay in language development in L1, it is recommended that the SLP conduct a more comprehensive assessment. If the parents report no delays, it is recommended that the SLP verify previous educational experiences and previous teachers' comments. If learning problems are reported, it is recommended that the SLP observe the student in the classroom and provide accommodations to meet the student's needs as best as possible. If the case concerns a preschool child it is important to observe the child in his or her home setting. Reviewing the child's health and developmental history is also important. These observations allow the SLP to compare specific behaviors of the student with the behavior of peers—as well as to verify reports from parents, teachers, or other professionals who know the student. It is also helpful to observe the student's interactions with other adults and peers—in different situations and settings (e.g., classroom, playground, lunch room)—and to document changes over time. Checking progress within a period of four to six weeks is recommended.

Name of Student:_____

Birthdate:_____ Age:_____ Place of birth:_____

Grade:_____ School:_____ Teacher:_____

Name of interpreter:_____ Language:_____

Date:_____

A. SOCIAL AND FAMILY HISTORY:

A.1. How long on the U.S. mainland? Father:_____   Mother:_____ Student:_____

A.2. How many persons living in the household?_____

Name	Age	Relationship

	1	2

A.3. Language(s) spoken to student by (1)   Father:_____

Language(s) spoken to student to (2)   Mother:_____

Siblings:_____

Other relatives:_____

A.4. Father's occupation:_____ Education:_____

Mother's occupation:_____ Education:_____

Parents' proficiency in English: Mother:_____   Father:_____

A.5. Has any family member had any language and/or learning difficulty?   Y   N

Please explain:_____

A.6. Trips to country of origin (indicate length of stay, where applicable):

_____

B. PARENT/FAMILY OBSERVATIONS ABOUT THE STUDENT:

B.1.	Does your child have problems following directions?	Y	N
B.2.	Does your child have problems understanding what you say?	Y	N
B.3.	Do you have problems understanding your child?	Y	N
B.4.	Does your child relate ideas in sequence?	Y	N
B.5.	Does your child express events that will be happening?	Y	N
B.6.	Does your child express events that might happen (predict)?	Y	N
B.7.	Is your child told stories?	Y	N
B.8.	Do you comment about what you read or tell your child?	Y	N
B.9.	Do you and your family read? Please specify what:_____	Y	N
B.10.	Please specify your child's interests:_____		
B.11.	Does your child have behavior problems?	Y	N
B.12.	Does your child have difficulty making friends?	Y	N
B.13.	Does your child have difficulty learning new concepts?	Y	N

(Continues)

(Continued)

C. SCHOOL HISTORY:

C.1. Was your child in school in your home country?   Y   N

  Please explain:_____

C.2. Any problems observed?   Y   N

  Please explain:_____

C.3. Grade attained:_____

C.4. Has your child attended preschool in the U.S. or your home country?   Y   N

  Please explain:_____

C.5. Have there been any school attendance problems?   Y   N

C.6. Have you had to move frequently?   Y   N

  Please explain:_____

D. HEALTH AND DEVELOPMENTAL INFORMATION:

D.1. Problems with vision?   Y   N

D.2. Problems with hearing?   Y   N

D.3. Problems with allergies?   Y   N

D.4. Any significant illnesses?   Y   N

D.5. Any hospitalizations?   Y   N

D.6. Medications in the past or present?   Y   N

D.7. Any difficulty learning to walk?   Y   N

D.8. Any problem learning to talk?   Y   N

D.9. Any problems while mother was pregnant or at time of delivery?   Y   N

D.10. Indicate location of delivery: home, hospital, clinic. (Circle one.) Birth weight: _____

Please explain if answer is *yes* for any of the above questions:_____

_____

_____

Please describe one of your child's typical days (e.g., what he or she does, what he or she plays with).

_____

_____

_____

_____

_____

ADDITIONAL COMMENTS:_____

_____

_____

_____

FIGURE 5-2 *Parent Interview Questionnaire.* (Adapted from Langdon and Cheng, 1992)

Please check all the areas that apply to the student to whom you are referring. Indicate the language(s) with which you notice a difficulty. Thank you.

(Student's L1) (English)

1. Frequently chooses to play alone _____ _____
2. Is usually quiet _____ _____
3. Chooses to sit in areas outside the mainstream of activity (i.e., in the back of the room) _____ _____
4. Frequently fails to follow directions, needs repetition _____ _____
5. Listens, but does not seem to comprehend _____ _____
6. Appears to hear some things, but not others _____ _____
7. Has trouble retaining information _____ _____
8. Frequently misunderstands words _____ _____
9. Gets nervous when asked to respond orally _____ _____
10. Avoids speaking during "sharing" time _____ _____
11. Rarely volunteers to answer questions in class _____ _____
12. Prefers to speak to friends in _____ _____ _____
13. Rarely asks for clarifications _____ _____
14. Frequently speaks in words or short phrases _____ _____
15. Speaks in incomplete sentences _____ _____
16. Gives inappropriate responses _____ _____
17. Uses inappropriate vocabulary to express ideas _____ _____
18. Has difficulty recalling words (hesitates, pauses) _____ _____
19. Is unable to tell a story in sequence _____ _____
20. Draws attention to self by speech _____ _____
21. Speaks in a way that is unclear and difficult to understand _____ _____
22. Omits or substitutes sounds in words _____ _____
23. Speaks in extremely loud or soft voice _____ _____
24. Stutters or stammers frequently _____ _____
25. Has a "raspy" or "hoarse" voice _____ _____

FIGURE 5-3 *Teacher Questionnaire.* (Adapted from Langdon and Cheng, 1992.)

If no previous educational problems have been identified, document the student's progress carefully over a designated time. If progress is not noted despite documented accommodations, a more in-depth assessment is recommended. A flow chart of the process of deciding whether to conduct a more comprehensive assessment is represented in Figure 5-4.

If progress is limited, further assessments are warranted. In this case, the SLP must identify the nature and severity of the problem, the most affected language dimensions (e.g., form, content, or use), and the relationships between the communication problem and other areas (e.g., reading and writing) in the school-age child.

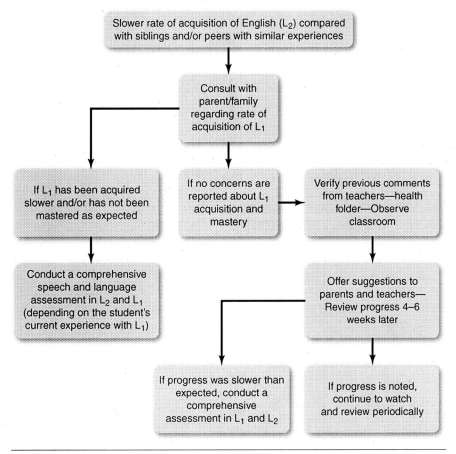

FIGURE 5-4 *Deciding Whether to Conduct A Comprehensive Assessment.*

CONDUCTING A MORE COMPREHENSIVE ASSESSMENT

Once the team has decided that a more in-depth speech and language assessment needs to be conducted, the SLP is faced with several dilemmas. These include the following: (1) Should the assessment be conducted in one or two languages? (2) How should the testing be conducted? (3) If the SLP does not share the same language as the student and the assessment needs to include the student's proficiency in L1, what are the best strategies for

collaborating with an I/T? (4) Since there are very few tests that are available in other languages than Spanish, how should the SLP cope with the dilemma of selecting appropriate tests? and (5) What strategies should be used for obtaining language samples that portray the students' communicative skills in both the primary and second language?

Should the Student Be Assessed in One or Both Languages?

It is not uncommon to base a decision about which language to assess on the results of proficiency tests. A common practice is deciding to assess the student in the dominant language. However, as discussed in Chapter 2, the term "dominance" is misleading. A student may be dominant in a given language but not proficient in any of the languages that he or she speaks. Therefore, assessing a student's language proficiency in only one language provides an incomplete profile of the student's communicative competence. A CLD student should be tested in two languages if one of the following three situations is true:

- The student responds in the native language most of the time when spoken to by the family and/or caregivers.

- The SLP's informal communication with adults and observations of peer interactions indicates that the student can understand the home language, but the student's appropriate responses alternate between the home language and English.

- The student is enrolled in a bilingual program or was enrolled in a bilingual program for at least three years. (Keep in mind, however, that the effect of language loss needs to be considered when interpreting the effectiveness of the bilingual programs.)

Testing communication competence in both languages enables the SLP to determine whether the student's skills in one or the other language are superior for certain language uses. Taking dialectal differences into account is very important as well. Neglecting one language, even the one in which the student has weaker skills, would provide an inaccurate appraisal of the student's general language competence. Testing the student in only one of the languages should especially be avoided whenever such testing appears to be a frustrating experience for the student—for

example, if the student shows signs that the items are too difficult and he or she cannot find words to express his or her thoughts in the language of interaction. All testing attempts should be properly documented, however. Assessing a bilingual student will take much longer than assessing a monolingual child. From my 1989 survey of 13 bilingual SLPs, I discovered that it took the SLPs an average of 5.75 hours to complete an assessment of a bilingual child that included analysis of the referral information, contact with the student, analysis of the data, the writing of the report, and participation in the Individual Educational Planning (IEP) meeting. By contrast, it took only an average of 3.5 hours to complete an assessment of an Anglo student.

Alternating from one language to the other may be appropriate when the student's language skills in both languages are very weak (Chamberlain & Medeiros-Landurand, 1991), but testing one language at a time is likely to produce a clearer picture of the student's language performance in each. Research is limited on which language to test first when conducting a bilingual assessment, however. Experience suggests that it is best to begin the testing with the language that is most familiar to the student. Determining this familiarity should be based on (1) a review of the student's cumulative records, (2) results of preliminary proficiency tests, and (3) reports from teachers, parents, and caregivers. Although it is important to acknowledge every response of the student, even if it is not in the language being tested, the student should be encouraged to respond as much as possible in the language being tested. In some situations, it is a good idea to conduct the assessment in one language and, if some items were missed, reassess those items in the other language after the student has completed a segment of the test. For example, on one occasion a kindergarten child from a Spanish-speaking background responded with greater success when she was asked to identify and name colors in English. She was also able to count from 1 to 20 with greater fluency in English than Spanish because those concepts had been explicitly taught in English.

There is little research-based information on how much time should elapse between testing in one language and testing in the other. Testing the student on different days may be a better procedure, however. If students are assessed on the same day, there may be carryover from one language to the other. For example, Pollack (1980) found that young bilingual children performed better than expected in English because they had been tested in Spanish earlier that same day.

How Should the Assessment Be Conducted?

Because testing and assessment of educational achievement is more frequently practiced in countries in the Western Hemisphere than in other countries, some immigrant children may lack experience in being tested. Yet, as the American Educational Research Association (1985) noted, "For a nonnative English speaker, and for a speaker of some dialects of English, every test given in English becomes, in part, a language or a literacy test." In addition, the success of testing may depend partly on the interaction between the clinician and the student. Data on communication between SLPs of varying ethnicity and CLD students are still scant, but Kayser (1989) found indications that Hispanic and Anglo SLPs may use slightly different strategies. For example, in a sample in which all subjects had normal language development, she found that Hispanic SLPs, as compared with Anglo SLPs, were more accurate in their assessment of the

students' skills. Only 10% of the Hispanic SLPs indicated that the children had a language problem—as compared with 60% of the Anglo SLPs. When administering tests, the Hispanic SLPs made sure they repeated some of the directions because they felt the children needed extra support. Both groups of SLPs used expressions of encouragement; however, Anglo SLPs used comments to tease, whereas the Hispanic SLPs used comments to console.

If the SLP is proficient in the student's language, he or she can assess the student in each one of the languages. Collaboration with an I/T is necessary when the SLP is not proficient in the student's language or does not know the student's language. Highlights of the collaboration process are discussed in the following sections. For more details, the reader is referred to Langdon and Cheng (2002), and to a video illustrating this process (Langdon, 2003).

Collaborating with Interpreters and Translators

Even though collaborating with an I/T was advocated by the American Speech-Language-Hearing Association (ASHA) more than 20 years ago (ASHA, 1985), there is still a limited amount of literature that documents the preferred strategies for training and working effectively with I/Ts in the speech- and language-pathology field. Some researchers who have examined this subject include Hwa-Froelich and Westby (2003a, 2003b), Langdon (2002), and Manuel-Dupont and Yoakum (1997). Langdon and Cheng (2002) provide the SLP and the I/T some guidelines for preferred collaboration strategies that have been used in working with the deaf and in the interpreting process during international conferences. These strategies have also been used in the medical and legal fields

(Carr, Roberts, Dufour, & Steyn, 1997; Gile, 1995; Roy, 2000).

The collaboration procedures outlined in the next section can also be applied to nonschool settings, such as when I/Ts collaborate with SLPs in clinics, rehabilitation centers, hospitals, and nursing homes. Additional information will be provided in Chapter 8, which discusses the assessment process for older CLD populations.

Specific Procedures

Collaborating with an I/T requires additional preparation time and training on the part of both the SLP and the I/T. Therefore, it is essential to ask a bilingual individual to serve as the I/T well in advance. The SLP should meet with the I/T prior to a parent conference or prior to the testing/assessment of the student in order to plan the content and format of the interaction. This first phase is referred to as the *briefing*.

The SLP should be present during the testing (i.e., during the administration of standardized tests or adapted test items, or during the elicitation of a language sample) in order to observe the behaviors of the student and the reactions of the I/T. Also, some factors— such as whether to accept or not accept a student's particular answer as correct when it will affect the outcome of a particular test, or when to switch tasks because of a problem with the student's attention—may need further clarification even after a briefing has taken place. If possible, it is wise to have one or more conference sessions (that include all three participants) before the testing date so that the student can become accustomed to having both the clinician and the I/T in the same room. Such a session is particularly helpful if the student is shy, but it may be impractical because of time constraints. This phase of the

assessment process (conference and testing sessions in which the SLP, I/T, and student are all present) is referred to as the *interaction segment*. After the testing/assessment or conference session, the SLP and the I/T should discuss what occurred. This third and last phase of the process is referred to as *debriefing*. After the debriefing, both the SLP and I/T should continue to have an ongoing dialogue about how best to facilitate future contact with students whose language proficiency may have to be assessed and how best to communicate with the students' families.

In summary, the process of collaborating with an I/T should consist of three parts: briefing (B), interaction (I), and debriefing (D). Langdon and Cheng (2002) refer to this sequence as the BID process.

An interpreted or translated/adapted test should not be scored unless it has been normed on the given population and the manual indicates that trained assessors can administer it. Rather, the SLP should make notations about how and when the student was able to provide accurate responses and about when the student had difficulties. Thus far, only limited studies have been conducted to determine the effects of another professional's presence (such as an SLP or psychologist) on students when a test is administered in the student's language by an I/T. Swanson and De Blassie (1979) compared the performance in English of Spanish-dominant bilingual students on the *Wechsler Intelligence Scale for Children-Revised* (WISC-R, 1974) under different conditions, one of which involved collaboration with an I/T. The researchers could not draw firm conclusions because there were no data available on the students' initial language proficiencies. It appeared, however, that the presence of the I/T may have created a "halo" effect, because the scores obtained when the tests were administered through an I/T were higher than those obtained when the tests were administered in Spanish only.

Role of the Interpreter/Translator

It is important that the person who serves as I/T in a speech-language assessment has high oral and written abilities in the languages. Oral proficiency alone is not sufficient. The I/T should also be familiar both with the technical vocabulary used in the field of speech-language pathology and with testing procedures. In addition, both the SLP and I/T should receive training on the best strategies for working together. In no instance should a person with no previous exposure to testing be asked to serve as an I/T. Often, it is erroneously assumed that the need for bilingualism supersedes the need for an understanding of the complexity of testing, particularly in another language. It is therefore preferable to select a person who has training in a field related to speech, language, and hearing (e.g., a teacher, educator, or health professional). The least desirable person is a family member or another student fluent in both languages; such persons have not been specifically trained and, moreover, may inadvertently assist the student with the test.

The interpreting/translating must be as accurate as possible. Since the SLP is not proficient in the language, he or she should discuss, after the assessment, the responses provided by the student. The I/T must remain neutral and cannot become emotionally involved with the case. Interpreting and translating are not easy tasks. Specialized training is necessary before one can become an international conference interpreter for the United Nations, an interpreter for the deaf, or, in some states, a medical and court interpreter. The interpreting/translating process in the educational and clinical fields, such as speech-language pathology or audiology, has

not yet received the recognition that it deserves, however, and is not yet considered a "professional" occupation. With the ever-increasing multicultural and multilingual populations, more trained I/Ts will be needed in these fields.

When Speech and Language Tests Are Available in the Student's Language

This section discusses issues related to the process of oral and written language testing (when tests are available in the student's language).

Oral Language Testing

An assessment typically should include information on language form, content, and use. Traditional speech and language tests in English focus on various dimensions of language form such as phonology, morphology, syntax—and more recently—on phonemic awareness, metalinguistic skills, and pragmatics. Additionally, the ability to follow oral directions and comprehend paragraphs is evaluated in order to assess various levels of language comprehension. Collecting and analyzing language samples from various testing contexts that involve as many different participants as possible assists in gaining information on the student's expressive language skills. For example, the SLP can assess the student's narrative skills by asking the student to tell a story using wordless books, or the SLP can elicit a sample by witnessing the student's conversation with one or several partners, including the parent when relevant. Eliciting naturalistic samples enables the SLP to evaluate the pragmatics of language.

Several tests, such as the *Test of Language Competence* (Wiig & Secord, 1989), the *Test of Problem Solving* TOPS 3 (Bowers, Huising, &

LoGuidice, 2005) and TOPS 2 (Bowers, Huising, & LoGuidice, 2007), and the *Test of Pragmatic Language* (Phelps-Terasaki & Phelps-Gunn, 1992) evaluate the student's ability to verbalize solutions to various situations. The vast number of tests available in English attests to the fact that no one test can capture all the various aspects of language.

Tests in other languages have not kept pace with the explosion of tests currently available in English. Students around the globe who are evaluated in other languages than English are assessed by using locally developed observational ratings and translations of English tests. It is hoped that the SLPs who adapt those tests into their own language do not use the norms provided in the original manuals of the English tests, as they would not be valid for their students.

A number of tests in languages other than English have been developed in the last 30 years, especially tests in Spanish. However, very few have been normed adequately on monolingual or bilingual Spanish-speaking populations. Table 5-1 presents a chronology of tests that have been adapted and/or normed on Spanish and bilingual Spanish-English populations. The *Diagnostic Evaluation of Language Variation-Screening Test* (Seymour, Roeper, De Villiers, & De Villiers, 2003) and the *Diagnostic Evaluation of Language Variation (DELV)-Norm Referenced Test* (Seymour, Roeper, De Villiers, & De Villiers, 2005) are not included in the table but need to be considered. These tests allow for differentiation between typically developing students who speak different dialects of English and students who may have a disorder.

The table lists the tests by name. Specific references for the tests are listed in the References section of this book. The legend indicates whether the test has been normed on Spanish-speaking or bilingual individuals, and

whether it is currently accessible. The legend also notes the particular language area (form, content, use, and dominance) addressed by the test.

As noted from the tests listed in Table 5-1, the majority of tests focus on primarily language form and content. Very few, with the exception of the IPT or the CELF-4 (Spanish version), include a pragmatic assessment component or a scale.

Several tests have been developed in Spain, but the majority are adaptations of the tests in English and include vocabulary that would be more appropriate for the Spanish spoken in Europe. For further information on each one of the assessments listed above, the reader is referred to Langdon and Cheng (2002). The chronology of the development of the tests reflects trends in attitudes toward bilingualism as well as toward language research. For example, the reader will note that many more tests were developed in the 1970s and 1980s and that they had a focus on syntax, grammar, articulation, and vocabulary. Only a few more tests have been updated since then, including new versions of the PLS and the CELF, as well as the ROWPVT and the EOWPVT, and only two have been newly created—the W-ABC and the CPAC-S. There is still a lack of specific tests that focus on the pragmatic skills of bilingual students The high cost of developing tests and the current trend toward English-only instruction in the United States explains why fewer tests are being developed in Spanish.

When using tests that were normed on Spanish-speaking subjects, it is necessary to interpret the results with care and to review the particular population that was utilized in obtaining those norms. For example, the *Pruebas de Expresión Oral y Percepción de la Lengua Española* (PEOPLE) (Mares, 1980) was normed on bilingual Spanish-speaking children in the Los Angeles area.

TABLE 5-1 Chronological Development of Tests in Spanish

NAME OF THE TEST DATE	DATE
Test of Auditory Comprehension (Carrow) (C)	1973#
Screening Test of Spanish Grammar (Toronto) (F)	1973°°
Austin Spanish Articulation Test (Carrow) (F)	1974°°
Dos Amigos Verbal Language Scales (Critchlow) (D)	1974=
James Language Dominance Test (James) (D)	1974°°
Medida Española de Articulación (MEDA) (Mason et al.) (F)	1974°
Bilingual Syntax Measure (BSM-1 & -II) (Burt et al.) (F & D)	1975=
Del Rio Language Screening Test (Toronto et al.) (F & D)	1975°° =
Ber-Sil (Level I & -II) (Receptive Vocabulary) (Beringer) (C)	1975°° ^^
Idea Language Proficiency Test (ITP-I & -II) (Ballard & Tighe) (F, C, U, & D)	1977+++ =
Language Assessment Scales (LAS -I & -II) (De Avila & Duncan) (F, C, U, & D)	1977+++ =
Preschool Language Scale (PLS-4) (Zimmerman et al.) (F, C, U, & D)	1977+++ =
¿Cómo detectar all niño con problemas del habla? (Melgar de González) (F)	1980°
Pruebas Illinois de Habilidades Lingüísticas (ITPA) (Kirk & Van Isser) (F, C)	1980° ^^
Prueba del Lenguaje Oral y Percepción Española (PEOPLE) (Mares) (F, C)	1980° =
Brigance (Brigance) (Bilingüe-Español) (F, C, & U)	1983#
Test de Vocabulario en Imágenes Peabody (TVIP) (Dunn et al.) (C)	1986^^
Assessment of Phonological Processes (APP-S) (Hodson) (F)	1986° +++
Spanish Articulation Measures (SAM) (Mattes) (F)	1987, 1995#
Structured Photographic Expressive Language Test-Spanish (SPELT Level I and Level II) (Werner & Kreshek) (F)	1989#
Clinical Evaluation of Language Fundamentals (CELF-4) (Semel et al.) (F, C, & U)	1995+++
Bilingual Verbal Abilities (BVAT) (Muñoz-Sandoval et. al.) (D)	1998=
Expressive and Receptive One-Word Picture Vocabulary Tests (EOWPVT and ROWPVT) (Brownell) (C)	2001=
Mac Arthur Inventario del Desarrollo de Habilidades Comunicativas (Jackson-Maldonado et al. (C)	2003^^
Contextual Probes of Articulation Competence (Goldstein & Iglesias) (CPAC-S) (F)	2006#
Wiig-Assessment of Basic Concepts (W-ABC) (Wiig & Langdon) (C)	2006=

Legend:
*Difficult to find
** May not be available
+++ Multiple versions
#Not normed /criterion referenced
^^normed on monolingual Spanish-speakers only
= normed on bilingual Spanish-English populations
(F) Form (C) Content (U) Use (D) Dominance

Note: Detailed references for the authors of these tests are available in this book's References section.

The *Test de Vocabulario en Imágenes Peabody* (TVIP) (Dunn, Padilla, Lugo, & Dunn, 1986) was normed on monolingual students outside the United States. The *Clinical Evaluation of Language Fundamentals* (CELF-4) (Semel, Wiig, & Secord, 2005) was normed on bilingual Spanish-speaking students residing in the United States in all regions of the country. Approximately 30% of them lived in homes in which English was spoken 96.8% of the time; other languages spoken were French, Italian, and Portuguese. Even though a test might be normed on subjects with similar characteristics to the student being assessed, the SLP needs to consider not only the test results but also the manner in which the student responded. Analysis of students' responses to the W-ABC (Spanish version) test (Wiig & Langdon, 2006) indicated that the Spanish version was most appropriate when students were exposed at least 30% of the time to Spanish.

Suggestions for the careful use and application of tests is summarized in a paragraph from the CELF-4 Spanish manual and can be applied to any test administration: "It is important to remember that a single test administration does not provide you with sufficient information for diagnosing a language disorder. Evaluating the language skills of a Spanish-speaking student, whether the student is in a bilingual or monolingual environment, is a complex process. For an overall evaluation of the student's language ability, the results of CELF-4 Spanish should be supplemented with a complete family and academic history, parent interview, results of other formal and informal measures, an analysis of a spontaneous language sample, the results of other linguistic and metalinguistic abilities tests, classroom behavioral observations, observations with peers, and an evaluation of pragmatic and interpersonal communication

abilities. If the student is bilingual, the best practice is to evaluate skills in both languages" (Semel et al., 2005, p. 18). In summary, tests are tools that assist us in making evaluations but should not be used to establish diagnoses or program implementation.

The *Diagnostic Evaluation of Language Variation Screening Test* (Seymour, Roeper, J. De Villiers, & P. De Villiers, 2003) and a newer more in-depth norm- referenced test titled *Diagnostic Evaluation of Language Variation* (DELV) (Seymour et. al., 2005) assesses all aspects of language. These tests were created to differentiate language differences from language disorders in children from various regional areas whose speech is different from Mainstream American English (MAE).

Written Language Testing

The number of formal tests designed to assess reading, writing, and academic achievement in other languages than Spanish is still limited. There are several Spanish tests, however, and those that are most commonly used are reported in Table 5-2. A notation identifies whether the tests are administered individually or in groups.

Obtaining a Language Sample

Language sample analysis is an effective tool for assessing a student's language use. It may be a time-consuming process, however, because the sample must be representative of the student's overall communication skills and the scoring may therefore be laborious. More than 20 years ago, Prutting (1983) said, "the language sample is the only procedure which provides an opportunity to assess communication in real live contexts with real live communicative partners who need to communicate. The

TABLE 5-2 Most Commonly Used Reading and Writing Tests in Spanish

Individually Administered Tests	• *Bateria III Woodcock-Muñoz* (2003). Two different batteries (cognitive and achievement) that can be administered in either English or Spanish for ages 2 to 90. Subtests include same areas as the English counterpart, but have been normed on Spanish-speaking and bilingual speakers. The achievement battery includes achievement in several language areas such as receptive vocabulary, verbal analogies, letter-word identification, dictation, understanding directions, story recall and passage comprehension. Math is also included.
	• *Woodcock-Muñoz Language Survey-Revised* (2005). Ages 2 years to adult. The test focuses on language-based areas in each language (Spanish and English), enabling the examiner to determine a language proficiency profile.
	• *Test of Phonological Awareness Ability in Spanish-Speaking Children* (Riccio et al., 2004). The test assesses several phonological skills, such as phonemic awareness, sound manipulation, and rhyming. The test does not include any other phonological skills such as blending or segmentation.
Group-Administered Tests	• *Aprenda 3* (2004). A revised version of previous tests that is based on the Stanford Achievement Test (Tenth Edition). The test includes assessments in reading, mathematics, language, spelling, listening, science, and social science.
	• *Logramos* (2006). The test includes the same measures as the Iowa Test, but is not a translation of this instrument. The test includes areas such as vocabulary, word analysis, reading comprehension, language (identifying specific concepts and detecting correct and incorrect forms), and math (math computation and math problem solving).
	• *Spanish Assessment of Basic Education (2ⁿᵈ Ed.)* (2000). A nationally norm-referenced achievement test in Spanish. The test battery includes tests of Spanish reading, language, and spelling, as well as mathematics.
	• *Reading-Level Indicator & Spanish Companion* (Williams, 2000). This version is a translation of the English test titled the Reading-Level Indicator. When an ELL student from a Spanish-speaking background does not achieve at a desired level, the Spanish version is administered. The test consists of 40 items. The first 20 items assess reading comprehension; the other 20 items are related to vocabulary. The test is designed in a multiple-choice format.

language sample remains a most valued clinical tool" (p. 90). This statement remains valid today; a language sample is very helpful for assessing a student's communication skills—especially when formal tests do not exist or are unavailable, which is the case for many of those ELL students who speak one of 100 different languages within one school district. Patterson and Pearson (2004) recommend that the SLP consider the context and language used by the student. In addition, knowing the student's experiences in each language is important, and taking more than one sample will provide "a more panoramic view of the student's linguistic skills" (Anderson, 2004, p. 205). For example, a child's primary language sample would be collected in Spanish when it primarily relates to the student's experience in the home. English samples would be taken when they relate to a classroom or school context (i.e., a topic that was covered in class or that relates directly to the classroom environment).

The interaction between the SLP and the student must be structured to some extent in order to obtain the desired information. For example, it is unreasonable to say that a student cannot use a particular verb form if the context of the interaction was not conducive for the elicitation of the form. Likewise, it should not be concluded that a student cannot narrate if there was no opportunity to assess that skill and/or the student has had limited experience with this type of linguistic genre.

The number of utterances necessary for obtaining a representative sample of the individual's language skills remains a source of debate; some SLPs recommend as few as 100 utterances, while others recommend 200 or 300. Given the fact that the numerous responsibilities of SLPs leave these professionals with limited time, the number of utterances may not be as important as the variety of topics and contexts. In the case of a bilingual student, more time will be required because a sample in each language is necessary in most cases.

The topics of conversation or activities (tasks) that are used to elicit the sample must be controlled to allow for comparisons of data across individuals with similar experiential and linguistic backgrounds. To address the issue of what topics and tasks are most likely to elicit a typical language sample, Wren (1985) presented several tasks to three groups of English-speaking children aged 6 to 7 years. Two groups had language difficulties and the third did not. Wren was interested in determining whether one or a combination of tasks would yield the most typical language from the children. Wren elicited the samples by means of free play with puppets, storytelling from pictures, explanation of a game (Candy Land), the use of a View-Master (e.g., asking the student to explain which picture was being referred to), preparation for a birthday party (e.g., using props), and a sentence-building activity to elicit sentences with specific words. The birthday activity elicited the most utterances from all three groups, because the SLP asked the largest number of structured questions during the task to elicit specific syntactical structures. More complex language was obtained from the explanation of the game. During this task the control group used the largest number of embedded sentences (sentences that included a dependent clause). The birthday party, stories from pictures, and the View-Master activity were the most helpful in differentiating the language skills of the different groups. These findings support that a variety of activities should be devised in order to obtain a truly representative language sample.

When following professional recommendations for eliciting the most representative sample possible from preschool and elementary school students, the SLP may

- Use puppets and toys, guiding the conversation to create certain situations.

- Use a toy car, and speculate where it might go. If it has a flat, what would happen?

- Create a scene using the topic of a birthday party.

- Use a dollhouse, and comment about what is happening.

- Use broken toys to enhance a dialogue.

- Ask the child what he or she did that same day or the day before; inquire about the child's family, favorite pastimes, or toys.

- Ask the child if he or she knows a story, or wants to retell something seen on TV. If the child cannot read a story aloud then ask him or her to retell it to another child or a puppet. With upper-elementary-level students, use wordless books.

- Request that the child explain the rules of his or her favorite game (board or sport). If the child cannot, explain a game and ask the child explain it to another child.

- Play barrier games to determine how the child follows and gives directions.

- Ask the child to explain how he or she performs different actions, such as: preparing a sandwich or a snack; wrapping a present; sending a letter; using a telephone or cell phone; or using the computer.

Older students may participate in similar activities, but are also requested to provide definitions of words, solve riddles, and explain absurdities. In addition, the SLP creates situations in which the student must use particular language functions, such as negotiation. Thus, the SLP who needs to obtain a language sample from an older student may

- Ask the student to explain the rules of his or her favorite sport or computer game.

- Request comments about a TV show or a movie that the student has seen.

- Ask for definitions of words for abstract concepts such as temperature, peace, invisible, promise, or inform. More information may also be obtained by administering one of the sections included in the CELF-4 test on assessing word definitions (the subtest is available in both the Spanish and English versions).

- Assess the student's ability to detect verbal absurdities such as those included in the *Detroit Tests of Learning Aptitude* (DTLA-4) (Hammill, 1998) ("At midnight the blind man was watching the birds").

- Ask what the student would do if he or she were invisible, had won the lottery, or had magic powers.

- Determine how the student would persuade his or her parents to let him or her take the family car to a party—or ask how the student would persuade friends to order one particular brand of pizza.

- Inquire about the student's plans upon graduation from high school, or ask what he or she needs to know to be successful in a particular career.

- Analyze the way in which the student retells the content of a story read aloud.

- Request that the student make up a story using a wordless book.

Enabling the Student to Demonstrate His or Her Knowledge

Test results constitute only one avenue for the assessment of a student's language competence. As mentioned earlier, tests need to be supplemented with feedback from persons such as teachers and parents who interact with the student on a daily basis. Also, observation of the student in the classroom and playground provide additional information on various aspects of language, such as the processing and comprehension of more academically oriented language, as well as social communication skills.

Dynamic assessment techniques allow the SLP to obtain a clearer picture of the student's language competence. This follows Vygotsky's (1962) concept of evaluating the student's language competence by comparing the student's present and potential language attainment, which he refers to as the "zone of proximal development," or ZPD. To obtain such information while administering test items, the SLP can first administer the items according to the guidelines of the test manuals. After completing the test administration, the SLP may readminister items on which the student responded incorrectly by using one or several of the following strategies, depending on the type of task: (1) rewording the instructions, (2) offering further explanations of what the student should pay attention to, (3) providing more examples of the same types of items that are being tested, (4) providing more time for the student to respond, and (5) explaining to the student how to maximize recall of certain information presented either orally or in writing. Strategies may also include helping the student employ visualization techniques or find keywords in a text that can aid comprehension. However, when scoring the performance of the student, the SLP should adhere to the guidelines of test administration and interpretation as specified by the various test manuals.

Gutiérrez-Clellen (2004) describes the use of dynamic assessment in evaluating bilingual Spanish-English students' narrative skills and story comprehension. A technique used by Gutiérrez-Clellen, Peña, Conboy, and Pasechnic (1996) consisted of a test-teach-retest approach and two mediation sessions where students were taught how to differentiate relevant from irrelevant information, and how to formulate ideas more clearly. Pre- and posttest gains were obtained in five steps: (1) the students summarized the story facts; (2) the students made inferences about the story; (3) the students organized the information they had obtained and selected the "best" inferences for the story facts; (4) the students evaluated their answers to the questions, and (5) the students restated their answers with an increased accuracy and precision (as a way for the researchers to evaluate the students' performance). This technique enabled the researchers to differentiate those students who were able to benefit from the mediating sessions from those who had more difficulties. The technique has been used with English-speaking children (Gillam, Peña, & Miller, 1999; Miller, Gillam, & Peña, 2001) as a way to assess story productivity, which includes

total number of words, C-units (defined as "communication unit," which consists of an independent clause plus a modifier such as "and," "but," "that," and others), number of clauses per sentence; episodic structures (how many episodes or parts of an episode are included); story components (setting, character information, temporal order, causal relationships); and story ideas and language (complexity of ideas, vocabulary, dialogue, and creativity) (Gutiérrez-Clellen, 2004, p. 252). The student's progress in providing a more cohesive story, and the student's ability to switch between tasks and to transfer various learning strategies from one task to another is measured.

When analyzing the narrative or expository discourse of CLD students, extra caution needs to be taken in differentiating true language impairment from lack of language exposure (Gillam et al., 1999). Gillam et al. indicate that, based on their experience, the utilization of wordless books such as Mayer and Mayer's *One Frog Too Many* (1975) and *Frog, Where Are You?* (1969), are most helpful (1999). The purpose of the mediation sessions is to explicitly teach the child about episodic structure and the importance of adding on characteristics of the various characters in the story. The next level is to make the student aware of the need to be more explicit about the various characters and situations in the story. At the end of the session, the student is asked to verbalize what he or she has learned and what strategies he or she will utilize in providing a more cohesive narrative in the future.

After having conducted two mediation sessions, Gillam et al. (1999) explored five basic questions (p. 40):

1. Was the child able to form a more complete and/or more coherent story with examiner support?

2. How hard did the examiner have to work in order for the child to make positive changes?

3. Did the child pay attention to and include more elements of the story when the examiner used interactive teaching?

4. Once examiner support was withdrawn (as was done with the second story) was the child able to transfer newly learned strategies?

5. Was learning quick and efficient or was it slow and labored?

Those students who respond rapidly to the mediated learning seem to have fewer problems than those who showed few/limited changes following a similar process.

To assess ability to use expository discourse, Gillam et al. suggest using even-numbered items from the *Elementary Test of Problem Solving* (Zachman et al., 1992). Table 5-3 provides the format suggested by the authors.

The student's responses are analyzed using an adequacy scale that includes categories ranging from detailed to no responses, descriptions of grammatical complexity, number of clauses, type of complex sentences, and grammatical acceptability.

Complex sentences are those that include one main clause in addition to one or more coordinated or subordinated clauses. As a result of mediation, progress in using more complex sentences and semantic complexity is desired. Items of the SLP's own choosing or from the *Elementary Tasks for Problem Solving Kit* (Zachman et al., 1990) can be used during the mediation sessions. The student's progress is measured by administering the even-numbered items on the *Test of Problem Solving* (Zachman et al., 1992). Pre- and posttest changes are recorded and notations are made about how

much effort was put forth by the SLP in attaining the gains made by the student. These gains are quantified using the *Modifiability Scale* devised by Gutiérrez-Clellen and Quinn (1993). The scale measures the examiner's effort and the child's responsiveness and includes four categories: Extreme (3), High-Moderate (2), Moderate (1), and Slight (0). In addition, the ability to transfer the skills is rated on a 3-part scale: Low (0), Medium (1), and High (2).

Dynamic information that assesses the student's ability to respond to some accommodations can also be obtained through informal assessment during the testing session. As an example, a story might be read to the student at the beginning of the session and the student may be asked to retell the story following the reading. After providing extra assistance to ensure that the student understood the sequence of story, he or she is asked to retell the story at the end of the session. This provides informal, but helpful, information on how well and fast the student can acquire and process new information.

The student's interactions with different persons and in a variety of settings can be observed with the assistance of different staff members who interface with the student, as well as with the assistance of the family and parents. In analyzing the student's responses, the SLP makes notations about those modifications that were helpful in improving performance. In addition, the SLP can make the following observations:

- Could the student perform better when input was shorter and the sentences were less complex?

- Could the student retain information as stated, but if so, did he or she have difficulty with inferences and hypotheses?

TABLE 5-3 Expository Discourse Assessment Procedure

Procedures	Analysis of Responses
Administer pretest: *Test of Problem Solving* (Zachman et al., 1992) (even-numbered items)	Adequacy Scale—
	Detailed—exceeds expectations
	Complete—meets expectations
	Incomplete—partially complete
	Ambiguous—unclear or imprecise answers
	Incorrect—the answer is wrong
	No response—the child makes no attempt to respond
	Grammatical Complexity—
	Number of clauses
	Type of complex sentences
	Grammatical acceptability
Select 1–2 examples for mediation from the cards in the *Elementary Tasks for Problem-Solving Kit* (Zachman et al., 1990) or make your own tasks	Determine how to mediate for story structure using
	Intentionality—What will be taught?
	Meaning—Why is this structure important?
	Planning—How will child approach the task?
	Transfer—What is this related to? How can the child remember?
Retest with the odd-numbered items from the *Test of Problem Solving* (Zachman et al., 1992)	
Summarize	Child learning during MLE
	Pre-post changes
Implications for intervention	What helped the child learn?
	How can this support be integrated within classroom contexts?
	How can support be targeted during intervention?

Source: From "Dynamic Assessment of Narrative and Expository Discourse," by R. B. Gillam, E. Peña, and L. Miller, 1999, *Topics in Language Disorders*, *20*(1), p. 45. Copyright R. B. Gillam, E. Peña, and L. Miller 1999. Reprinted with permission.

Were the responses/comments made during testing and language sampling pragmatically appropriate?

- Was the student easily distracted by noise? Was attention better on a one-on-one basis than in a group or classroom situation?

- How did the observations made during the one-on-one interaction with the SLP compare with those made by other staff members and the family?

- Was there a difference in any of these areas across languages?

By focusing on the student's ability to comprehend and process oral language in the various contexts, and by using the different mediating strategies, the SLP can describe more accurately the response mode and behavior of the student. Also, because the assessment is a compilation of test results, observations, and other measures, the SLP is able to identify what the student can or cannot do, and to report conditions that promote better responses. Before the date of the Individual Educational Planning (IEP) meeting, the SLP may also want to include the student in a small group that matches the student's needs and observe his or her progress over time. This method is very relevant given the fact that the current interpretation of IDEA 2004 is to determine whether or not "the student responds to scientific, research-based intervention as part of the regular special-education evaluation procedures" [Sec.614b].

When There Are No Tests Available in the Student's Language

In the vast majority of cases there are no normed tests available in languages other than English and Spanish, and the few that are available in other languages are mostly translations/adaptations of English tests. Given that it is important to determine the linguistic proficiency level of a student in his or her primary language, the most practical approach is to implement the strategy described in this section. In any case, collaboration with a well-trained interpreter/translator (I/T) is crucial. Langdon and Cheng (2002) provide two options:

First, during the initial session, assess the student with a set of English tests. Request the assistance of an I/T during a second session; readminister the items missed in the student's language and prepare a careful translation of those items. Ensuring that the level of the translated item corresponds to the same level of difficulty in the student's primary language is important, and level of difficulty is often connected to how familiar the word is. For example, "compel" translates into Polish uses the word "zmuszac," which is more commonly used and heard in Polish than "compel" is in English. Two words can be used as translations of "gigantic" in Polish: either "gigantyzny," or "kolosalny." When a test has been adapted to another language, norms should never be used, even though the majority of the test might have been administered in English. A qualitative description would, however, be appropriate. For example, indicate that the student could answer 25% more items correctly when the item was adapted to the student's language, or that there was no difference in the student's responses whether the item was administered in English or in the student's primary language.

Second, the assessment can be supplemented with informal measures such as asking the student to follow oral directions or to engage in a conversation with the I/T. However, prior to the interaction, planning the topics of conversation or methods for eliciting the language sample should take place. If the student has attended formal education in the language assessed, he or she can be asked to read a passage from a reader or book at the student's level, and follow this with carefully designed comprehension questions. The student can also be asked to retell the content of what he or she read. A writing sample can also be obtained. When tests are not available in the student's language, the SLP will need to rely on the

I/T's knowledge of the language. The analysis of the language sample should enable the SLP to make judgments about the student's proficiency in various aspects of language including form, content, and use.

SUGGESTED PROTOCOLS FOR TEST ADMINISTRATION AT VARIOUS AGE LEVELS

Questions and dilemmas often arise regarding the best protocol to use in assessing CLD students of various ages. In the following section, protocols are suggested. Naturally, variations will need to occur depending on the child's age, experiences, and cognitive development. Table 5-4 includes a list of formal and informal assessment tools that can be used.

For example, for a very young child assessment should occur in a familiar environment, such as the child's home, whenever possible.

REPORTING TEST RESULTS AND ASSESSMENT FINDINGS

The administration of "standardized" measures alone does not provide an adequate basis for concluding that a mainstream student—much less a student with a different linguistic and cultural background—has a language-learning disability. Test results alone should not be the sole driving force for determining any student's eligibility for special education services—even though (because of the mandates of the 2001 No Child Left Behind legislation) "testing" is currently one of the sole measures used for

TABLE 5-4 Suggested Assessment Tools for CLD Students of Various Ages

AGE LEVEL	ASSESSMENT TOOLS In all cases obtain a development and health history.
Infant (0–3 years)	• Spanish translation of Rossetti Infant-Toddler Development Inventory • Mac Arthur Inventory of Communication Skills (Spanish) • Play-based assessment • Observation of parent/caregiver interactions When assessing in other languages, obtain an inventory of the child's receptive vocabulary and expressive language—including consonant and vowel inventories. In all cases, be sensitive to individual styles of parent-child interactions as well as expectations.
Preschool (3–5 years)	• PLS-4 (Spanish version) • Bilingual Spanish-English versions of ROWPVT and EOWPVT • W-ABC (Spanish) • Play-based assessment • Language samples that assess form, content, and use of language (Refer to previous section for ideas on strategies for obtaining a representative sample.) • Observations of the student with peers and significant others. For other languages, observe child interacting with peers and adults. Language samples should be obtained in as many contexts as possible.

TABLE 5-4 (*continues*)

AGE LEVEL	ASSESSMENT TOOLS In all cases obtain a development and health history.
Elementary (6–11 years)	• PLS-4 (Spanish version because norms are available for ages up to 6–11) • Bilingual Spanish-English versions of ROWPVT and EOWPVT • PEOPLE and/or CELF-4 Spanish • For 5- to 7-year old children, use the W-ABC (Spanish version to assess knowledge of basic concepts.) • Observation of student in various contexts • Language samples • Selected subtests of Brigance (Spanish version) • Rapid automatic naming and phonological awareness tasks listed in CELF-4—including sequences (numbers, letters, days of the week, months of the year) • To assess pragmatic skills and social interactions, use the pragmatic protocol included in the CELF-4, and make observations while obtaining and analyzing the language sample, (Refer to Table 5-3) • Written language tests (select among those listed in Table 5-2) • Use of wordless books • Use pragmatic protocol from CELF-4 For other languages, adapt tasks that assess oral directions, word associations and sentence memory, adapt familiar sequences: days of the week, sequences of numbers, the alphabet, and rapid automatic naming. Language samples should be obtained in various contexts.
Secondary (12–17 years)	• CELF-4 Spanish • Observation of student in various contexts • Language samples • Selected subtests of Brigance (Spanish version) • Rapid automatic naming and phonological awareness tasks listed in CELF-4, including sequences (numbers, letters, days of the week, months of the year) • To assess pragmatic skills and social interactions, use a protocol such as the one included in the CELF-4, and make observations while obtaining and analyzing the language samples • Written language tests (select among those listed in Table 5-2) For other languages, adapt tasks that assess oral directions, word, associations, and sentence memory. Adapt familiar sequences: days of the week, sequences of numbers, alphabet, and rapid automatic naming. Language samples should be obtained in various contexts. Use wordless books and obtain discourse related to expository texts.

evaluating student performance (NCLB, 2002). Therefore, test results need to be adequately interpreted to outline relevant dispositions regarding not only eligibility for services, but also paths for intervention. The results need to be interpreted in light of the student's experiences; observations of the student in various contexts; analysis of the language sample(s); and input from the parents, teachers, and persons who know the student best. Furthermore, because of the SLP's expertise in language, SLPs should assist the school team in interpreting the assessment as it relates to development of academic learning. For example, if a student has difficulty processing auditory information, it may impact his or her ability to understand what he or she reads. Furthermore, this deficit will have an effect on his or her writing skills as well as social interactions. If a student has word-finding difficulties, it will affect the student's ability to present orally in class and the student will need some accommodations such as knowing how to write notes that assist in ensuring the flow of a presentation.

Classifying all the data that is obtained as auditory input (i.e., oral language comprehension/processing) and verbal output (i.e., language expression)—although an artificial method of classifying the communicative process—facilitates the reporting of observations and the identification of strengths and weaknesses. Thus, norms can be reported as part of the findings, but with cautionary notations that indicate how the student's background and language experience differ from the normed population for any given test. As an example, if a student obtained a low score on the *Preschool Language Scale* (PLS-4) in Spanish, it could be that he or she may not have had experience in demonstrating knowledge of colors, because those concepts were taught in English. Also, the student may not have had experience in describing objects or events in Spanish, but can perform this activity in English. Thus, prior experience with and exposure to specific tasks needs to be evaluated, and this can be accomplished by interviewing parents and teachers.

A description of the student's mode of response to the interaction, answers to individual test items, and responses to modified administration and/or mediated sessions assists in providing a more accurate portrait of the student's strengths and challenges with regard to speech, language, and communication. Table 5-5 lists some tasks and tests that encompass the various areas in the area of listening and oral language comprehension/processing that should be addressed in a report.

Listening and Oral Language Comprehension/Processing

It is important to evaluate the way in which the student processes oral language in order to identify specific situations in which the student can perform as expected and those in which the student has difficulties. Specific tests that focus on different aspects of language comprehension in Spanish, and suggestions for alternative tasks to use when no tests in a given language are available, are listed in Table 5-5.

The tasks will need to be prepared ahead of time with the assistance of a well-trained I/T. To ensure that the items are correctly adapted to other languages than Spanish, a back-translation into English is necessary. I realize that these recommendations require a great deal of time on the part of the SLP and the I/T and that they cannot be carried out for urgent cases. However, if it is possible, preplanning on the part of the SLP and of others in the same district is invaluable when assessing students who speak other languages.

Verbal Output (Oral Language Expression)

Analysis of language samples, assessment of vocabulary and concepts, and assessment of articulation skills are discussed in this section.

TABLE 5-5   Tests and Subtests that Assess Various Areas of Listening and Oral Language Comprehension/Processing*

AREA	NAME OF TEST/SUBTEST
Ability to follow oral directions	• Subtests of the Brigance Diagnostic Assessment of Basic Skills (Spanish Version)
	• Conceptos y Siguiendo Direcciones (CELF-4) (Spanish)
	Other languages: Adapt oral directions that include two, three, and four steps in the student's language.
Receptive vocabulary	• Test de Vocabulario en Imágenes Peabody: Adaptación Hispanoamericana (TVIP)
	• Receptive One-Word Vocabulary Tests (Bilingual Editions) (ROWPVT)
	• Receptive subtest of the W-ABC (Spanish)
	Other languages: Vocabulary and comprehension of concepts can be evaluated by analyzing the language sample.
Oral text comprehension	• Story Comprensión (PEOPLE)
	• Entendiendo Párrafos (CELF-4) (Spanish)
	Other languages: Select a book in the student's language, read a passage, and request that the student respond to factual as well as hypothetical questions.
Sentence repetition/memory	• Sentence Memory (PEOPLE).
	• Recordando Oraciones (CELF-4) (Spanish)
	Other languages: Devise sentences that are increasingly longer and more complex.

*The tests in this table are available in Spanish. The table also offers suggestions for assessment in other languages.

Analysis of Language Samples

Documenting the mediated sessions that were suggested earlier in this chapter (Gillam et al., 1999; Gutiérrez-Clellen, 2004; Gutiérrez-Clellen & Quinn 1993) are helpful for differentiating students with and without language disorders. However, extra caution must be taken when considering the student's experiences and type as well as amount of exposure to English. The advantage of these techniques is that they document progress over time. However, there may be students who have not attained sufficient proficiency in English to benefit from mediated sessions, and it is necessary to analyze these students' language skills in their current, more dominant languages. Therefore, obtaining a language sample in both English and the student's first language and comparing them allows the SLP to determine if a problem exists in only English (because of limited exposure to English), or if the problem also exists in the primary language. However, experiences and cultural differences need to be considered. For example, the child may not be used to conversing with adults other than relatives and friends of the family—or the child may have been raised to listen rather than respond when an adult is speaking (as may occur in the families of some children of Asian backgrounds). Therefore, input from the I/T—as well as from parents or adults who know the child well—is invaluable for assessing whether or not there is a problem.

The following describe the various skills that are at the core of all obtained language samples:

- Mechanics of language interaction (discourse): initiating conversations, topic maintenance (e.g., responding to questions by keeping the topic going, following a sequence of ideas, adding information [elaboration], asking for clarification, taking the listener's point of view)

- Using language for a variety of purposes: gathering information, explaining, retelling/recounting, informing, and understanding abstractions (e.g., thinking beyond current visible referents, integrating old and new experiences)

- Form and content: using syntax and grammar correctly, using a variety of sentence types of varying degrees of complexity, using vocabulary correctly, having adequate articulation skills to convey intended meaning to any listener

- Individual communication style: expressing ideas in an appropriate manner (time delay between comment/question posed by the interlocutor), pausing, hesitating (beginning to say a word but only uttering the initial sound or syllables), repeating words/phrases, and using circumlocutions

Comments on student performance should include a notation about the rapport between the SLP and the student, as well as a notation about any peer relationship observed during the collection of the language samples. A list of contexts (and associated languages) in which the samples were obtained increases the information available on the topics that were covered.

Assessment of Vocabulary and Concepts

Frequently, the breadth of knowledge of students experiencing language and learning difficulties is limited. This is often reflected in the student's overall comprehension as well as in the student's comprehension of vocabulary and concepts such as "what constitutes a category?" (e.g., food, animals, professions, quantity, or emotions). Although bilingual individuals may have a reduced vocabulary in each of one of the languages that they speak, language-disordered and learning-disabled students have a significantly lower-than-expected vocabulary as measured by various test instruments and observations.

A few formal instruments are available for measuring the vocabulary of primarily Spanish-speaking students. Two different tests that use pictures can be used to measure the expressive vocabulary of bilingual Spanish/English-speaking students:

1. The bilingual version of the *Expressive One-Word Picture Vocabulary Test* (EOWPVT) (Brownell, 2001a). (The student can respond in either Spanish or English. Norms are based on the combining of responses provided in either language.)

2. The CELF-4 Spanish (*Vocabulario Expresivo*) (Semel et al., 2005). (For evaluating younger children's understanding of basic concepts, it is helpful to use the W-ABC Spanish [Wiig & Langdon, 2006].)

Other ways of measuring vocabulary include asking the student to provide definitions (*Definiciones de Palabras and Clases de Palabras* subtests of CELF-4 Spanish) (Semel et al., 2005), or associate words that go together, such as the auditory association task in the PEOPLE (Mares, 1980).

Analyzing the language sample will provide an additional perspective on the student's vocabulary use. For example, it is helpful to analyze the pattern of responses and determine whether the student has a repertoire of concrete words, but lacks knowledge of more abstract words. When analyzing the type of vocabulary used by the student, the context of conversation or interaction needs to be considered. The student may have a larger vocabulary in his or her native language for relating events that happened in the home or outside of school—as compared with the vocabulary he or she uses for explaining a topic that might have been learned in school. For example, the student might know "horno" (oven) or "abanico" (fan) in Spanish, but be unfamiliar with those words in English. Therefore, it is recommended that the SLP describe and compare the type of vocabulary used by the student in each context across languages.

Phonological Assessment

There are many more tests available in English for assessing articulation and phonological skills in children than any other language. The number of such tests in other languages than English is much more limited, including those that assess dialectal differences in English. Articulation tests developed in Spanish in the 1970s and 1980s include the *Austin Articulation Test* (Carrow, 1974), the *Medida de ArticulaciónEspañola* (MEDA) (Mason, Smith, & Hinshaw, 1976), and the *Melgar Articulation Test* (Melgar De González, 1980). Only three tests have been developed in the last 25 years and include the *Hodson Assessment of Phonological Processes*, which is currently being revised (Hodson, 1986), the *Spanish Articulation Measures* (SAM) (Mattes, 1995), and very recently, the *Contextual Probes of Articulation Competence* (CPAC-S) (Goldstein & Iglesias, 2006), which has been helpful in defining phonological patterns in Spanish-speaking children.

In the first three tests developed in the 1970s (that are mentioned above), consonants and vowels are assessed by means of single words in which sounds occur in different positions. In all instances, the target sound is tested in a single word, and there are no opportunities to consider the sound in other words or in connected speech. For example, The *Medida de Articulación Española* uses the word "árbol" (tree) to assess the final /l/ in a word, whereas the *Melgar* test uses the picture of "pastel" (cake). The SLP notes whether the student articulates the sound correctly.

There are problems with traditional tests. First, the student may not be familiar with the word tested or may not recognize the picture. For example, the word "árbol" may be familiar to the student who speaks a Mexican dialect, but not to the Mexican-American child who may call the word "palo," instead. These same children may use "quequi" (Americanized word for cake) rather than "pastel." Thus, the SLP has to resort to asking the student to imitate the word and may obtain limited data on the student's production of this /l/ sound in the final position. Second, the student may not pronounce the sound correctly because of the phonological configuration of the word. For example, a student may omit the final /l/ sound because of difficulty in pronouncing the /l/ in "árbol," but not in "sol" (sun).

In their tests, Hodson (1986), Mattes (1995), and Goldstein and Iglesias (2006) focused on phonological processes or error patterns rather than on single errors in phoneme production. In Hodson's test, for example, the final /l/ is assessed with the words "árbol" and "azul" (blue). In Mattes' test, the assessment is made using the words "mal" (bad) and others such as "caracol" (snail), "sol" (sun), and "árbol." The student is given more opportunities to produce the phoneme. The Hodson test lists 10 principal processes—such as consonantal omissions, syllable reduction, stridency, glide, and labial, velar, and nasal deficiencies. Mattes' test only comprises seven basic processes, such as initial consonant deletion and final consonant deletion, but also lists eleven additional possible processes. The Hodson test permits only consideration of single words; the Mattes test permits the evaluation of phoneme production in connected speech as well. The CPAC-S includes words that have been used previously to assess the phonological skills of various populations including typical monolingual Spanish-speaking children, monolingual Spanish-speaking children with phonological problems, and typical bilingual Spanish-English speaking children. The examiner can analyze the student's production of words and classify their articulation in any of 17 different patterns. For example, cluster reduction, liquid simplification, and stopping. Analyzing the student's Spanish dialect is strongly recommended in order to avoid making incorrect assumptions about his or her articulation.

In an earlier work published by Goldstein (2004b), the researcher recommends collecting (separately for each language) information on the student's sound production, syllable types used, and number of syllables per word. In order to make a determination about whether the student's development is proceeding adequately, norms for each language, as well as patterns that emerge as a consequence of exposure to two given languages, must be considered. These data are readily available for language combinations such as Spanish-English and various dialects of English, though the data is limited for other languages.

Specifically, Spanish and English share 15 phonemes. Spanish has five consonants that do not exist in English whereas English includes nine consonants that do not exist in Spanish. In assessing bilingual normally developing children with phonological disorders, Goldstein (2004b) described various studies which concluded that both groups demonstrated greater accuracy of production for those phonemes that were shared than for those that were unshared. Research on normally developing and phonologically disordered African-American students came to similar conclusions (Stockman, 1996). The influence of dialect needs to be factored into the assessment in order to avoid a misdiagnosis. For example, typical features of Spanish spoken in the Caribbean are the deletion of some syllable segments (such as pronouncing "dos" as "do" or omitting the nasal /n/ of a preceding vowel (pronouncing "jamo" instead of "jamón").

Fluency Disorders

In a recent review of fluency disorders in bilingual Spanish-speaking individuals, Ratner (2004) suggests using measures such as the *Stuttering Severity Instrument-3* (SSI) (Riley, 1994). Ratner bases her recommendation on the fact that "there are indeed no cross-cultural or cross-linguistic differences between speech and nonspeech behavioral characteristics of stuttering" (Ratner, 2004, p. 300). The author advocates that the SLP consider the attitude of the speaker toward his or her own speech. A checklist for evaluating fluency-related problems in Spanish is available in a questionnaire included in Puyuelo, Rondal, and Wiig (2000, p. 80–83). The checklist covers areas such as the history of the individual's speech difficulties, the student/client interview, and dysfluency measures obtained by analyzing language samples and observing secondary symptoms such as head and facial tensions, body posture, breathing, phonation, articulation, and prosody.

Assessing Specific Processes

Although several of the items just mentioned do provide some information on the student's cognitive and memory skills, the administration of specific items provides further information on these aspects of the student's performance that have ramifications for his or her classroom accommodation needs (Semel et al., 2005). The following are some of the criterion-referenced tasks that provide further information about such areas: (1) phonemic awareness tasks that are particularly helpful to administer to those students who have reading, decoding, and spelling difficulties; (2) word association tasks that ask the student to come up with words that belong to a certain category (such tasks provide information on the student's attention, memory, and retrieval deficits); (3) Rapid Automatic Naming tasks, or (RAN), that provide information on the student's ability to name random sequences of figures and colors (such tasks provide information on the student's speed and organization of thought; Wolf, Bowers, and Biddle (2000) have demonstrated that individuals with dyslexia have difficulty performing this type of task); and (4) working memory subtests that measure the student's ability to repeat random digit sequences of increasing length, both backward and forward.

The Spanish version of the CELF-4 provides tasks that measure each of these skills. Although phonemic awareness is not related to reading skills in languages that are not alphabetical (refer to Chapter 7), administration of the word association, Rapid Automatic Naming, and digit-span tasks (repeating numbers forward and backward) may provide the examiner with valuable information on the student's ability to perform on these tasks. Having such

information also enables the examiner to make comparisons to the student's performance in English. However, caution needs to be exercised when interpreting the results. It could be that the student does not perform as well in the native language due to language loss and not necessarily due to a language-based disability. The RAN task yields best results for children who are at least 5 years of age. Studies have indicated that the RAN is sensitive in identifying "naming speed" deficits and possible dyslexia in subjects who spoke several languages (Wiig, Langdon, & Flores, 2001; Wiig, Zureich, & Chan, 2000).

SUMMARY

In this chapter we reviewed some general guidelines for assessing CLD students whose native language might not be English or who might speak a different dialect of English or a different dialect of their own language. Topics covered included discussions of whether the assessment should be conducted in one or two languages, strategies for how to conduct testing, and how best to collaborate with an interpreter/translator if the SLP does not speak the student's language. The chapter included a review of available oral and written tests in primarily Spanish; provided suggestions for how to obtain and analyze a language sample; and suggested some ideas for how to handle cases where there are no tests available in the student's primary language. Included in the chapter were recommendations on using dynamic assessment procedures that encourage the student to demonstrate his or her knowledge. The testing process was also discussed, and specific age-appropriate tests were recommended. The final section of the chapter discussed the process of reporting tests results and observations.

OUR CLIENTS

Eric, Ana, Jack, Grace, and Leonardo

Because we are discussing assessment issues pertaining to preschool and school-age children, we will turn our attention to Eric, Ana, and Jack. We will revisit our two older clients Grace and Leonardo in Chapter 8.

At the end of each client synopsis is a list of conclusions that might be drawn from both the information presented in this book about each client and the concepts discussed in this chapter.

Eric

Eric is a 4-year-old preschool child born in the United States. His parents are first-generation immigrants from Vietnam. Both Vietnamese and English are spoken in the home. His parents speak Vietnamese to him, whereas his two older siblings communicate in English with him. His parents are concerned because Eric's language skills in both languages are limited as compared with his siblings and other children who are growing up in similar bilingual backgrounds. Eric has been a healthy child. Eric's teacher has reported that he prefers playing by himself. His concentration is limited unless he watches cartoons or videos.

The following points and suggestions are based on the information presented in Chapter 5:

- Because both his parents and teachers are concerned, it is a good idea to conduct a more formal assessment at this time. Since Eric understands and communicates in English and Vietnamese, the assessment should be conducted in both languages.

  Materials and contexts for English can include tests such as the PLS-4 (English version), a language sample using a storybook, and play with puppets and toys (while the SLP guides the conversation to include certain contexts).

  As suggested in this chapter, some ways to elicit a language sample might include (1) using a toy car, and speculating where it might go (then vary the situation: if it has a flat, what would happen?); (2) creating a scene with a birthday party; (3) asking Eric what he did that same day or the day before; and (4) inquiring about the Eric's family, favorite pastimes, or toys.

  Transcribe the language sample and analyze it by documenting pragmatics, syntax/grammar, use of vocabulary/concepts, and phonology. For more detailed information on comprehension and use of certain concepts, use the W-ABC (English) and use Vietnamese for those concepts that were missed.

- Obtain a baseline of expressive vocabulary using the EOWPVT.

- Following the assessment in English, collaborate with a well-trained interpreter and translator and request that those items that were missed on the PLS-4 in English be readministered in Vietnamese. Subsequently, obtain and analyze a language sample using the contexts just mentioned. Complete an assessment procedure in Vietnamese that is parallel to the one performed in English by analyzing the language sample and readministering the EOWPVT. Ensure that the interpreter stay to assist in transcribing and analyzing the Vietnamese language sample.

Ana

Ana is a nine-year-old enrolled in fourth grade who emigrated from Mexico at the age of 5 and who is having difficulty reading in English. She is the oldest of three children. She was raised by her maternal grandparents beginning at the age of 6 months; after five years she was reunited with her parents.

Ana attended kindergarten in Arizona but moved in the middle of that year when her parents found better jobs in California. Ana has learned English quite well but she is behind in reading. All of her schooling has been in English. She speaks Spanish to her parents and some relatives who live nearby, but she talks to her siblings in both English and Spanish.

The following points and suggestions are based on the information presented in Chapter 5:

- There may be several reasons why Ana is not reading well. She may have difficulty with grapheme-phoneme correspondence only and/or reading comprehension difficulties. Assessing her oral language skills both languages will yield important information.

- If the SLP is bilingual in Spanish, the clinician can conduct this assessment alone. It is best to select tasks that can be duplicated in the two languages. Each language should preferably be assessed on different days. Suggested assessments for Ana's age include (1) using core tasks from the CELF-4 (English and Spanish versions); including the RAN and word associations that assess automaticity; (2) administering phonological awareness tasks that assess Ana's skills in that area (this should be done for English only, since she has had only English reading instruction for the past four years); and (3) administering other tasks that could include the bilingual version of the EOWPVT or a language sample elicited from the materials and contexts mentioned previously. To obtain the language sample, the SLP could do the following:

  - Request Ana's comments about a TV show or a movie she has seen.

  - Ask for definitions of words for abstract concepts such as temperature, peace, invisible, promise, or inform. The SLP could obtain more information by analyzing the definition section included in the CELF-4 (both Spanish and English versions).

  - Tape and analyze Ana's narration (in both English and Spanish) of a wordless book.

Jack

Jack is a 14-year-old of African-American descent who is has difficulty with subjects such as social studies, English, and writing. Mrs. G., Jack's paternal grandmother, adopted him when he was 2 years old as his single mother could not raise him. Prior to entering School District A (summer 2002), Jack attended a private school for two years. Even though both Mrs. G. and Jack have a Southern accent and speak AAVE, his use of a different syntax and vocabulary do not seem to interfere with his academic learning.

Jack had to remain in the ICU for about seven days after birth due to respiratory distress. His developmental milestones occurred within a normal timeframe except for his speech, which was delayed: Jack did not put words together until he was about 3 years old. The latest vision and hearing screenings were unremarkable (fall 2002). Mrs. G. reported that Jack is on daily medication for anger, anxiety, and agitation. He is receiving counseling to address his emotional issues.

A previous school assessment report written by an SLP and the psychologist indicated some learning difficulties, but their severity did not warrant intervention from special education. Because the results of this assessment were not satisfactory to Mrs. G., she sought an outside assessment by a neuropsychologist. Results indicated that Jack has difficulty with working memory and sequencing skills. Mrs. G. states that Jack has difficulty synthesizing oral and written information. Writing is difficult for him: Jack does not respect rules of grammar and punctuation.

The following points and suggestions are based on the information presented in Chapter 5:

- It is important to make an assessment that evaluates Jack's oral language skills. His ability to comprehend and process language in various contexts—as well as his to ability to express ideas—should be documented. Toward this end, the following tasks are suggested:

  - The *Peabody Picture Vocabulary Test* (PPVT-III-B).

  - *Clinical Evaluation of Language Fundamentals* (CELF-4, English). Specific subtests should be used, including (1) Recalling Sentences, (2) Sentence Formulation, (3) Word Definitions, (4) Understanding Spoken Paragraphs, (5) Rapid Automatic Naming (RAN), and (6) Word Associations. Because Jack does use standard English when communicating with teachers, there is no need to administer the *Diagnostic Evaluation of Language Variation* (DELV) in this case.

(Continues)

(Continued)

- Other informal tasks that should be administered are part of the CELF-4 and include the following: (1) having Jack recite the days of the week and months, (2) having Jack read a paragraph out loud and answer questions about the content, and (3) having Jack complete tasks that require use of phonological skills (identifying the initial and final sounds of certain words, providing words that rhyme, and segmenting words into syllables). Finally eliciting a language sample from Jack during spontaneous conversation and by using a wordless book such as Mayer's *One Frog Too Many* is recommended as a way for the SLP to assess grammar, syntax and use of language.

Further Readings

Goldstein, B. (2004a). *Bilingual language disorders in Spanish-English speakers.* Baltimore: Brookes.

Roseberry-McKibbin, C. (2002). *Multilingual students with special language needs: Practical strategies for assessment and intervention.* Oceanside, CA: Academic Communication Associates.

Trumbull, E., & Farr, G. (2005). *Language and learning: What teachers need to know.* Norwood, MA: Christopher Gordon.

C H A P T E R 6

ARRIVING AT A FINAL DIAGNOSIS FOR LANGUAGE PROBLEMS IN CLD POPULATIONS: INFANCY THROUGH ADOLESCENCE

"From 1950 to 1980 there were dozens of labels, theories, and training approaches taken up and then discarded on the path to realizing that the majority of learning disabilities are language-based, and that difficulty in using oral and written language remains the single most significant deterrent to educational growth" (Stark & Wallach, 1980, p. 6).

CHAPTER OUTLINE

INTRODUCTION

*T*he quotation above was written 25 years ago but the information still holds true today (Wallach, 2005). It serves as a reminder that there is a strong connection between oral and written language. Many speech and language pathologists (SLPs) have been aware that a large proportion of early oral language development difficulties eventually translate into learning, academic, and social challenges during the school years (Bashir, Kuban, Kleinman, & Scavuzzo, 1984; Bashir & Scavuzzo, 1992). Self-esteem and social relationships are also affected, although the impact varies on a case-by-case basis depending on individual differences and the influence of the family and the environment.

Johnson and Myklebust (1967) were among the pioneers in the field of language-learning disabilities who indicated that phonemic awareness plays an important role in the reading process. Over the last two to three decades, the relationship between oral and written language has been further clarified. For a recent review linking the various issues surrounding connections between oralcy and literacy, the reader is directed to Butler, Nelson, Wallach, Fujiki, and Brinton (2005). Because speech and language development is a natural process, and because recent research indicates that many language and academic challenges are due to early problems with oral language, it is important to identify and work with children who have speech and language difficulties as early as possible. Early intervention that focuses on bridging the gap between oral and written modalities assists students and facilitates their journey through the academic world.

It is challenging to understand these connections with regard to monolingual students. Traditionally, SLPs saw young children with speech and language disorders during the elementary school years, but many of those children also experienced later academic difficulties (reading decoding and often comprehension as well). During the 1980s and 1990s the connections between oral and written language were further defined (Wallach & Butler, 1984, 1994). More recently, numerous research findings have demonstrated the importance of language-based skills in the success of reading; this is summarized by G. Reid Lyon (1998), head of the Child Development and Behavior Branch of the National Institute of Human Development (NICHD). Lyon indicates that approximately 5% of children learn the process of reading effortlessly, whereas 20% to 30% need formal instruction to become readers. For the remaining 60%, the process will be more of a challenge—about 20% to 30% of these children will have serious difficulties in this area.

Children with reading challenges have traditionally been seen by learning-disabilities and reading specialists, with the speech and language pathologist (SLP) peripherally involved in the assessment and intervention process. Because of the close connection between reading and language, it is time for SLPs to take a more proactive role in collaborating in the process. A team approach is warranted—one where the teacher, reading specialist, learning-disabilities specialist, and SLP each has a defined role. Justice and Kaderavek (2004) suggest these service options for

SLPs working with preschoolers and kindergarten-age students who are at risk: (1) indirect services where the SLP offers consultation and collaboration with classroom teachers, and (2) direct service instruction where the SLP works with both large and small groups on areas such as phonological awareness, print concepts, alphabet knowledge, and literate language.

For older students, the charge of the SLP remains to work on the oral aspects of language, including instructing students in phonemic awareness, and building strategies to improve memory for the processing of oral language. The classroom teacher's main charge is to provide instruction in academic areas that include reading and writing. Both professionals share the task of exposing the students to various domains of literate language such as abstract and figurative content, formal oral contexts, and academic as well as metalinguistic aspects (Ukrainetz & Fresquez, 2003). Assessing and planning programs for students who come from culturally and linguistically diverse (CLD) populations is exponentially challenging. This is because research on the connections between oral and written language that occur within and across various languages is still limited.

CONNECTIONS BETWEEN ORAL AND WRITTEN LANGUAGE

Understanding, speaking, reading, and writing are reciprocal skills. Lack of adequate comprehension of oral or signed language will affect speaking and language expression. It will also affect reading comprehension and written language performance. The guidelines of No Child Left Behind (NCLB) require the attainment of various reading and writing standards for various grades. Each state publishes specific guidelines for each grade in each of these four areas: listening, speaking, reading, and writing. Table 6-1 includes samples of standards for kindergarten, third grade, sixth grade, and ninth and tenth grades that are taken from the California standards in the areas of listening, speaking, reading, and writing. Since each state has its own standards for each grade and for each academic area, it would be difficult to give examples for every state; the California standards are therefore used in Table 6-1 as a

representative example. Under IDEA 2004, all students need to be prepared to take state assessments that determine proficiency in academic areas (Mandlawitz, 2006).

The listing of standards for the various grade levels outlines a progression of demands on students to increase their ability to read and understand more abstract, complex, and diverse material. For example, in third grade, students need to generate and respond to essential questions, make predictions, and compare information from several sources. By ninth grade, students need to integrate what they have read and understood about the organizational patterns, arguments, and positions included in the text. The above requirements, which are expressed using terms such as "generate," "respond," "predict," "compare," and "contrast"—are based in language and critical thinking. Thus, to achieve in academic subjects the student needs to have a strong language base.

At the same time, requirements for successful writing skills become increasingly demanding. Students in kindergarten are required to write a

TABLE 6-1 A Sample of California Standards for Listening, Speaking, Reading, and Writing for Selected Grades

GRADE	LISTENING	SPEAKING	READING	WRITING
K	Understand and follow one- and two-step oral directions.	Share information and ideas, speaking audibly in complete, coherent sentences.	Students know about letters, words, and sounds. They apply this knowledge to read simple sentences. Students identify the basic facts and ideas in what they have read, heard, or viewed. They use comprehension strategies (e.g., generating and responding to questions, comparing new information to what is already known).	Students write words and brief sentences that are legible.
3rd	Students listen critically and respond appropriately to oral communication.	By using proper phrasing, pitch, and modulation, students speak in a manner that guides the listener to understand important ideas. Students deliver brief recitations and oral presentations about familiar experiences or interests that are organized around a coherent thesis statement.	Students understand the basic features of reading. They select letter patterns and know how to translate them into spoken language by using phonics, syllabication, and word parts. They apply this knowledge to achieve fluent oral and silent reading. Students read and understand grade-level-appropriate material. They draw upon a variety of comprehension strategies as needed (e.g., generating and responding to essential questions, making predictions, comparing information from various sources). The selections in *Recommended Literature: Kindergarten through Grade 12* illustrates the quality and complexity of the materials to be read by the students. In addition to their regular school reading, by Grade 4, students read one-half million words annually, including a good representation of grade-level appropriate narrative and expository text (e.g., classic and contemporary literature, magazines, newspapers, online information). In Grade 3, students make substantial progress toward this goal.	Students write clear and coherent sentences and paragraphs that develop a central idea. Their writing shows that they consider the audience and purpose. Students progress through the stages of the writing process (e.g., prewriting, drafting, revising, editing successive versions). Students write compositions that describe and explain familiar objects, events, and experiences. Student writing demonstrates a command of standard American English and drafting, research, and organizational strategies.

	Oral Communication	Reading	Writing
6th	Students evaluate the content of oral communication. Students deliver focused, coherent presentations that convey ideas clearly and relate to the background and interests of the audience. Students deliver well-organized formal presentations employing traditional rhetorical strategies (e.g., narration, exposition, persuasion, description).	Students use their knowledge of word origins and word relationships, as well as historical and literary context clues, to determine the meaning of specialized vocabulary and to understand the precise meaning of grade-level appropriate words. Students read and understand grade-level appropriate material. They describe and connect the essential ideas, arguments, and perspectives of the text by using their knowledge of text structure, organization, and purpose. Students read and respond to historically or culturally significant works of literature that reflect and enhance their understanding of history and social science. They clarify the ideas and connect them to other literary works.	Students write clear, coherent, and focused essays. The writing exhibits students' awareness of the audience and purpose. Essays contain formal introductions, supporting evidence, and conclusions. Students progress through the stages of the writing process as needed. Students write narrative, expository, persuasive, and descriptive texts of at least 500 to 700 words in each genre. Student writing demonstrates a command of standard American English and drafting, research, and organizational strategies.
9th–10th	Students formulate adroit judgments about oral communication. They deliver focused and coherent presentations of their own that convey clear and distinct perspectives and solid reasoning. They use gestures, tone, and vocabulary tailored to the audience and purpose. Students deliver polished formal and extemporaneous presentations that combine the traditional rhetorical strategies of narration, exposition, persuasion, and description.	Students apply their knowledge of word origins to determine the meaning of new words encountered in reading materials and use those words accurately. Students read and understand grade-level-appropriate material. They analyze the organizational patterns, arguments, and positions advanced. Students read and respond to historically or culturally significant works of literature that reflect and enhance their understanding of history, and social science. The student is required to be able to make appropriate analysis of the text in order to analyze interactions between main and subordinate characters in a literary text, trace an author's development of time and sequence (including the use of complex literary devices such as, foreshadowing and flashbacks), and analyze the way in which a work of literature is related to the themes and issues of its historical period (historical approach).	Students write coherent and focused essays that convey a well-defined perspective and tightly reasoned argument. The writing demonstrates students' awareness of the audience and purpose. Students progress through the stages of the writing process as needed. Students combine the rhetorical strategies of narration, exposition, persuasion, and description to produce texts of at least 1,500 words each. They write biographical narrative or short stories, responses to literature, and persuasive compositions. They produce legible work that shows accurate spelling and correct use of the conventions of punctuation and capitalization. The writings reflect appropriate requirements, including title page; correct presentation, pagination, spacing, and margins; and integration of source and support material (e.g., in-text citations, use of direct quotations, and paraphrasing) with appropriate documentation (e.g., references).

Source: Adapted from the California State Department of Education, 2007.

few sentences, whereas third-grade students are asked to write a sample that has a certain organization and purpose, and that takes the audience into consideration. The various stages of revising written material are also integrated in the process. By ninth grade, students need to produce papers that integrate information from various sources and that are organized in various formats, such as narrative and expository text formats. It is important to be able to witness a student's progression through the process of reading and writing in order to define more precisely those areas where a student might have difficulty. Understanding a student's progress allows the professional to (ideally) intervene before it is too late. Demands on language expression are greater as students advance in grade. As an example, by ninth grade, students need to make oral presentations that are formal and that follow certain formats.

Kindergarten through third grade is when students gain reading fluency and comprehension. Beginning in fourth grade and thereafter, students increasingly depend on written language in order to acquire and demonstrate knowledge in various subjects such as social studies, mathematics, and science.

Successful Reading Processes

"Reading is a highly complex capability that depends upon the mastery and coordination of many component skills. By adulthood, most of us read so quickly and effortlessly that introspection is a poor guide to what is going on as we do so" (Snow, Scarborough, & Burns, 1999, p. 50). Two areas are at the core of the reading process: decoding and language comprehension. The process is represented in Table 6-2.

Decoding is achieved through successful knowledge of the alphabet and sound/letter (symbol) correspondence (Snow, Burns & Griffin, 1998). In languages that are not alphabetic, the reader needs to memorize thousands of logographs such as those used in Chinese and in Japanese. Making connections between the written and spoken word does not imply ability to comprehend what is read. In some languages, connections between the sound of letters and their written forms have a relatively direct relationship. For example, in Spanish, there is a direct relationship between the sounds of letters and their written representation. When there is very close relationship between sound and letter, the language is considered to be "transparent." For example, Spanish and German are considered to be transparent languages, whereas English and French are less transparent. Thus, "comida" is spelled as pronounced, although the word may have a different meaning depending on the context. It may signify "meal" or "eaten" (i.e., for something eaten that is of the feminine gender such as "naranja" [orange], but not of the masculine gender such as "carne" [meat]). In English, by contrast, a word that sounds like "bord" may be spelled as "board" or "bored"—and the spelling changes depending on the context. Therefore, sound/letter correspondence does not enable the reader to make a reference to meaning unless the context is known. Although contextual cues are necessary in both situations, meaning in English is dictated by both spelling and context. There are examples in English where spelling does not change and the meaning is conveyed by the context—as for "glasses," "mean," or "change."

Depending on the complexity of the language, the successful reader needs to learn specific rules for when sound-letter association is not immediately predictable. For example, in English the /f/ sound can be transcribed as /f/, /ph/, or /gh/. Similar rules exist in French where many vowels and diphthongs can contribute to changing the meaning of a word. For example, a word sounding like "mer" can be spelled in three different ways: "mer" (sea), "mère" (mother), "maire" (mayor). Intonation may also influence the meaning of what is

TABLE 6-2 Components of Successful Reading

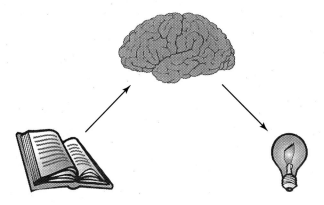

DECODING	COMPREHENSION
• Knowledge of the alphabet/sound-symbol relationship (or the knowledge of different logographs).	• World knowledge assists in this process.
• Phonemic awareness.	• Metacognitive skills are important (e.g., monitoring meaning and connecting it to what has already been said in the text).
• Awareness of the linguistic unit for a given language.	• Student understands the structure of a given text (narrative vs. expository).
• Attention and memory necessary.	• Attention and memory necessary.

conveyed in certain languages. In Vietnamese, for example, the word "ma" may have different meanings depending on the intonation of the word. It may mean "ghost," "cheek," "but," "horse," or "young rice plant." Diacritic signs enable differentiation between all the various meanings.

Although phonemic awareness has been recognized as the focal point in reading for several decades, it is only in the last 10 years or so that more systematic research has concentrated on the significance of phonemic awareness and its impact on the reading process. Texts and single journal articles such as those written by Butler and Silliman (2003), Catts and Kamhi (2005), Lyon (1998), Scarborough (1998), and Snow, Scarborough and Burns

(1999) discuss this topic in great detail. Phonemic awareness is defined as the ability to recognize and manipulate the phonemes within a word. Phonemic awareness is one of the metalinguistic skills needed for decoding words successfully. It is not a natural skill and is usually acquired through instruction. Other metalinguistic skills, such as phonological awareness, involve the "manipulation" of sounds and syllables to ensure successful decoding. These skills include blending (being able to put sounds and syllables together) and segmenting (the opposite of blending, more prevalent in the writing process). The order of difficulty for performing these metalinguistic skills in English is listed in Figure 6-1. This order is similar in Spanish

1. Rhyming—"Do 'bike' and 'like' match?"
2. Phoneme Matching—"Do 'bike' and 'book' begin with the same sound? Do 'dog' and 'pig' end with the same sound?"
3. Phoneme Isolation—"What is the first sound in 'tape'? What is the last sound in 'time'?"
4. Phoneme Deletion—"What sound would be left if you took the /l/ sound away from 'lake'? What sound would be left if you took the /m/ sound away from 'make'?"
5. Blending Phonemes—"What word would you get if you put the sounds /t/, /ei/, and /k/ together?"
6. Segmenting Syllables—"How many syllables are in the word 'elephant'?"
7. Phoneme Counting—"How many sounds do you hear in the word 'bone'?"

FIGURE 6-1 *Phonological Skills: Order of Difficulty from Least Difficult to Most Difficult.* (Adapted from Trumbull and Farr, 2005.)

(Gorman & Gillam, 2003). Other languages will be reviewed in a different section of the chapter.

Successful reading comprehension is enhanced by world knowledge or information about a particular subject. Having experience with the subject matter also facilitates understanding of what is read. For example, seeing a movie or video based on a novel will facilitate the comprehension of the novel's plot, just as watching an experiment may clarify a scientific concept. Inferences are built upon having knowledge of the world and being able to interpret what is said/signed or read. Linguistic components of this process include phonology, syntax, and pragmatics, and not hearing or producing sounds correctly will interfere with communication. Meaning is conveyed by the system of semantics. At a basic level, morphemes convey meaning—such as /ed/ to distinguish the present from the past in English, or /el/ and /la/ to differentiate genders in Spanish. Meaning is further conveyed by words (vocabulary) as well as by combining words into larger segments, all translated by the syntax of the language. Different conventions are used in oral language than in written language. This is addressed in a different section of the chapter.

To read with comprehension, the successful reader completes a number of metacognitive operations that are summarized by Ehren (2005). First, organizational patterns of the text are recognized, such as an opening paragraph with main ideas and a topic sentence, both of which assist in comprehending the content of the text. Second, features of the text are recognized; these assist in answering questions about the author's purpose, and about connections between major and minor points in the text. Thus, a narrative piece is organized differently than is an expository text. Narratives are written to entertain; they require the reader to understand multiple perspectives and varying points of view. Ideas are connected with conjunctions such as "and," "then," and "so." Expository texts are written to inform, and different genres have varying structures although the focus is on factual information and ideas. "Connecting words" in this genre include "because," "before," "after," "when," "if," "then," and "therefore." For a more extensive discussion and review on differences between narratives and expository texts, the reader is referred to sources such as Graham and Bellert (2004), Catts and Kamhi (2005), and Westby (2004).

All of these strategies are part of the metacognitive processes that include working memory skills. These skills enable the reader to remember and manipulate the information that is read; that is, to recall and retain what is read and simultaneously process and integrate incoming new information. Other strategies used by effective readers are self-questioning techniques. Questions are asked about what the information tells and how the information connects to what the reader already knows. In addition, effective readers make a "mental review" of what they have read while making connections to already known material; effective readers are continually asking themselves if what they are reading "makes sense."

Poor readers have difficulty with decoding and with metalinguistic and metacognitive skills. Westby (2004) reviews three main types of reading difficulties: (1) dyslexia, (2) language-learning disabilities (LLD), and (3) Attention Deficit Hyperactive Disorders (ADHD). Students in the first category (dyslexia) primarily have difficulty with the decoding process. The second group of students includes those who have language-based difficulties such as a lack of phonemic awareness, difficulty understanding the meaning of words, and an inability to perceive structure and cohesion across sentences as well as in the general organization the text. The third category, students classified as having ADHD, may have the same difficulties, but they also have problems in the metacognitive domain. Thus, they have difficulty recalling and connecting what they are reading to what they know or what they have already read.

Ehren (2006) identified 12 cognitive underpinnings that can influence the successful completion of a task requiring application of successful reading strategies. The areas include the following: understanding a given assignment; motivation; attention; memory; understanding background information; perceiving organization, main ideas, and use of context; paraphrasing; being able to analyze a text; monitoring a text; strategic orientation; and world-level processing. A couple of examples for each area are listed in Figure 6-2 (they are not listed in any order).

Several strategies can be helpful for assisting those students who have various reading, decoding, and comprehension difficulties. Students with comprehension difficulties can be exposed to written assignments that mirror the particular text structure of what is being read. Also, reading various types of texts to students while using sets of visual organizers assists students in developing their understanding of the organization of a given text. Students with reading comprehension difficulties need assistance in developing strategies for detecting main ideas and for making predictions based on what is already known in the text.

Chapter 7 discusses other strategies that assist in this process.

---

1. General (understands class assignments and is motivated)
2. Attention (focuses on material or task at hand; persists in devoting cognitive energy to reading tasks)
3. Memory (holds information in working memory to complete a task; stores information in organized schemata)
4. Background information (has personal experience; understands underlying concepts)
5. Organization (connects related ideas; places ideas in the correct hierarchy in relation to each other)
6. Main idea (identifies the distinguishing features of an idea; differentiates big ideas from small ideas)
7. Use of context (recalls relevant topics; notices any helpful visual aids)
8. Paraphrasing (is aware that there is more than one way to express a thought)
9. Text analysis (notes relationships of text components; knows the macrostructures of texts)
10. Monitoring (is aware that comprehension is a goal of reading; knows when a communication breakdown has occurred)
11. Strategies orientation (sees the potential application of information; recognizes similarities of situations and settings)
12. Word-level processing (segments words into morphemes; knows the meanings of prefixes, suffixes, and roots)

FIGURE 6-2 *Cognitive Underpinnings of Reading.* (Adapted from Ehren, 2006.)

Successful Writing Processes

"The written word long outlasts the spoken word, and thus the importance of the quality of one's written language cannot be underestimated throughout the life span" (Larson & McKinley, 2003, p. 99). People are often judged according to the way they write. For students to become better writers, they need to write more—and the best way for them to do so is by completing authentic writing activities. This may be accomplished by having students write for at least 20 minutes every day (ASHA, 2001).

Writing is a complex process that demands a number of skills, such as motivational, cognitive, and memory skills (see Figure 6-3). One of the primary skills required for the writing process is related to the motivational/affective domain. The successful writer must be motivated to write, and should have set goals. For example, I was motivated to write this text because I wanted to share my knowledge about and experience of assessing and working with multilingual and multicultural populations. Keeping a certain readership in mind (i.e., graduate students and practicing clinicians in the field) framed the goal. To achieve writing goals, the writer needs to draw on working memory skills such as phonological and semantic memory. The writer also must draw on long-term memory skills, which include (among others) topic knowledge, linguistic knowledge, and the ability to follow the structure of a particular genre.

A narrative, an expository text, and a poem have very different formats. A narrative should include a setting, an initiating event, a reaction, a goal/plan, attempts at action, a consequence of the action(s) taken, and a resolution. In addition, the readership must be considered. Narratives for young children include more pictures; there are fewer words per page and the vocabulary and syntax are controlled. A

textbook should include a preface and several chapters that include headings, tables, and figures. Textbooks may be written for a specific readership such as students, novice professionals, or experienced professionals.

The cognitive underpinnings mentioned for reading are applicable here. Attention, memory for graphemes, syntax and ideas, organization, and monitoring strategies must be maintained while the outcome is translated onto paper or entered on the computer. The goal of writing the piece should constantly be kept in mind. The planning phase is followed by the generation phase, and completed with the revision/editing phase that may take a great deal of time depending on the scope of the writing project.

Several strategies can be applied in completing this process. To secure that the text is cohesive, the writer can use several planning and monitoring strategies such as those in the SCAN approach. In this approach, the writer is asking himself or herself: (1) Does it make **s**ense? (2) Is it **c**onnected to my central idea? (3) Is **a**ddition of more detail necessary? and (4) Do I **n**otice errors? Other approaches include the POW method (**P**ick my idea, **O**rganize my notes, **W**rite and say more) that is followed by a method using specific mnemonics that vary for particular genres. For example, for a narrative: W-W-W-W What +2 How+2 (Harris, Graham, & Mason, 2003). This is translated into the following process: **W**ho is the main character? **W**hen does the story take place? **W**here does the story take place? **W**hat does the main character do or want to do; **W**hat do other characters do? **W**hat happens then? **W**hat happens with the other characters? **H**ow does the story end? **H**ow does the main character feel? **H**ow do the other characters feel? Several other strategies that instruct students in the writing process can be found in Graham, Harris, and MacArthur (2004), and Westby and Clauser (2005).

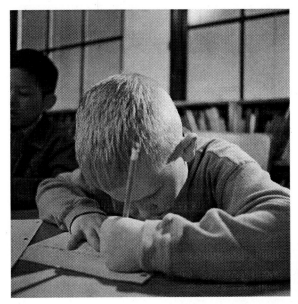

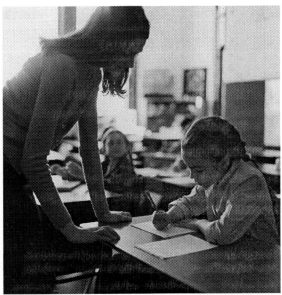

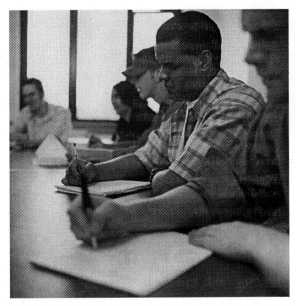

FIGURE 6-3 *Writing Requires Motivational, Cognitive, and Memory Skills.*

Contrasts between Oral and Written Language

Oral and written language depend on the form (phonology) and structure (syntax) of a given language. To have a successful conversation, the listener and the speaker must have the ability to process and comprehend one another. During a conversation, nonverbal communication (eye contact, intonation, proxemics) plays a

TABLE 6-3 Similarities and Differences between Oral and Written Language

SIMILARITIES

ORAL LANGUAGE	WRITTEN LANGUAGE
Both rely on form, content, and use of language. Both modalities require attention and memory. Development depends on opportunities for exposure. Both assist in facilitating communication.	

DIFFERENCES

ORAL LANGUAGE	WRITTEN LANGUAGE
Most of the time it is learned naturally.	Most of the time it needs to be taught.
Special skills are needed to interrupt the process.	Can be interrupted at any time for the most part.
The stream of speech is transient and cannot be captured unless the speaker agrees to repeat.	Print is permanent and cannot usually be referenced to clarification of meaning.
Clarification of a message is possible.	
One is relatively limited in deciding what to listen to.	It is more subject to selection.
Gestures, facial expressions, intonation, and rhythm give richness to oral language.	Gestures, facial expressions, intonation, and rhythm have few representations in print. That is, nonverbal communication needs to be spelled out and translated with punctuation such as exclamation, question, or suspension marks.
Messages are sometimes delivered in incomplete sentences. Some information may be missed due to shared knowledge.	Sentences are required for meaning. Print requires more rigorous word use and word order to deliver a clearer message.
Word order is more predictable and depends on the structure of the language.	Various syntactic structures are possible depending on the particular topic or piece—for example, "quickly he ran to the fence," or "and off the fence they jumped."
Conversations are less organized.	Written language needs to be more organized. The writer needs to alert the reader about the content.
Oral communication involves two or more persons.	Reading is an individual activity for the most part.

Source: Adapted from Purcell-Gates, 1989.

role in interpreting the meaning of what is said. Speakers have an opportunity to ask for clarification. Reading and writing are primarily solitary activities, but can become interactive if there are two people or more reading the same selection, or when more than one reader reacts to a written piece. Listening and speaking to someone is not always a selective activity and needs to be interrupted at a mutually agreeable moment.

Reading and writing are usually performed during the reader's and writer's selected times. The process may be interrupted any time. Similarities and differences between oral and written language are listed in Table 6-3.

The reading and writing process encompasses several common processes. The successful reader or writer must have a conceptual representation of words, phrases, sentences, and paragraphs. These are mentioned in Table 6-3 as depending on form, content, and use of language. Both processes require various cognitive underpinnings that include, among others, attention and memory. Under the area of memory, the listener, reader, or writer needs to be able to recall meanings of words and sentences. To process information successfully, only relevant information needs to be retained. In order to read with comprehension and write successfully, both readers and writers must keep in mind all along the organization of the text and use self-monitoring strategies to recall and connect information. Background knowledge about a given topic on the part of the reader or writer is helpful. Such knowledge is more important in the writing process than in the reading process. Both activities are generally solitary; although in the case of reading, there may be exceptions.

CROSS-LINGUISTIC PERSPECTIVES

Language transfer across languages was discussed in Chapter 2. However, not all areas that are considered important in the reading/writing process transfer from one language to the other because of the varying structures of different languages. Although phonological awareness appears to be central to several languages, it might not explain all of the possible underlying problems that may cause a reading difficulty in a second language.

For languages such as Spanish and English, which are alphabetical, phonemic awareness plays a role in the reading decoding process. However, phonemic awareness does not necessarily place similar demands on the reader across two languages. Specifically, in Spanish stress is at the syllable level, whereas in English

stress is more at the phonemic level. This explains the reason that English-speaking children perform better at detecting the first phoneme of a word as compared with Spanish-speakers (Jiménez & García, 1995). However, extensive research on the relationships between English and Spanish phonological skills such as rhyming, phoneme matching, sound identification, sound deletion, segmentation, and blending indicates that the skills develop in a parallel fashion in both languages (Gorman & Gillam, 2003). Gottardo (2002) found that phonological processing skills in Spanish were related to English reading acquisition in a sample of 85 children aged 5 years to 9 years. In summary, several studies conclude that the best predictors of success in reading in both English and Spanish are phonological awareness skills, and having these skills in Spanish influences a positive transfer to learning to read in English. These findings have implications for assessment and intervention issues in bilingual Spanish/English-speaking individuals.

Differences in transfer with regard to writing systems vary across languages. Mandarin, Cantonese, and Japanese (Kanji script) use a meaning-based writing system in which the language unit is represented as a morpheme. When languages rely on sound-based writing systems, the units might be syllables, such as in Japanese (Kana) or Tibetan. When languages rely on phonemes, the subcategories might be consonantal or alphabetic as in Arabic and Hebrew, which use consonants only. Greek and Roman alphabets, on the other hand, use both consonants and vowels (Cook & Bassetti, 2005). Information about various scripts is presented in Table 6-4.

Even though two alphabets may be the same, the type of phonological awareness varies from language to language. For example, Italian children outperform English-speaking children

TABLE 6-4   Examples of Various Scripts

Writing System	Language Unit	Script	Orthography (Examples)
Meaning-based	Morpheme	Hanzi	Mandarin and Cantonese
		Kanji	Japanese
Sound-based	Syllables	Kana	Japanese
		Tibetan	Tibetan and Bhutanese
	Phonemes	Arabic	Arabic and Persian
	Consonantal	Hebrew	Hebrew
	Alphabetic	Greek	Greek
		Roman	English and Italian

Source: Adapted from Cook and Bassetti (Eds.), 2005.

in segmentation (Cossu, Shankweiler, Liberman, Katz, & Tola, 1988). The authors found that instruction may play a role in promoting the children's phonemic awareness level. Moreover, those students who were taught through a phonics approach in reading performed higher on phonemic segmentation than children who were taught through a whole-word approach.

Because reading has been studied mostly in English, the term "dyslexia" has been defined in terms of the sound structure of the English language, and has been interpreted as relating primarily to difficulty with phonological awareness tasks and word decoding. However, as indicated by the preceding discussion about the relationship between oral and written language, it is apparent that phonemic awareness is not the central source of reading difficulties in many languages that rely on a linguistic unit and script system that is different from English. Furthermore, the term "dyslexia" refers to various types of disabilities depending on the country and/or language

considered. For example, dyslexia in the United Kingdom refers to individuals who have difficulties with reading and writing. In Russia, different terms are used to denote reading difficulties (dyslexia) and writing difficulties (dysgraphia) (Smythe & Everatt, 2002; Smythe, Everatt, & Salter, 2004). Because the same terms refer to different types of disabilities, these authors propose that the definition of dyslexia be expanded in the following manner: "Dyslexia is a difficulty in the acquisition of literacy skills that may be caused by combination of phonological processing and visual and auditory system deficits. Lexical confusions and speed of processing difficulties may also be present. The manifestation of dyslexia in any individual will depend upon not only individual cognitive differences, but also the language used" (Smythe & Everatt, 2002, p. 73).

Learning another writing system may be more or less difficult for speakers of a given language depending on several parameters:

(1) whether the linguistic unit of a given language is consonantal or phonemic (e.g., learning to read in English for someone who speaks Spanish will be easier than for someone who speaks Farsi because English is an alphabetical language whereas Farsi is a consonantal language); (2) whether the language uses a script that is new to the individual reading it (e.g., both languages may be phonemic but the script may be different; this presents a problem for someone who, for example, reads French and is learning Cyrillic); and (3) the level of transparency (e.g., level of grapheme/phoneme correspondence, as in, for example, Italian and Spanish).

Other differences to consider are the various processes used in recalling the spelling of a word. In English, readers look at a word and try to recall if it "looks" right. When they need to ensure that a given word is spelled correctly, they will write down each letter that corresponds to a given sound. In Italian, Spanish, or German, which are considered transparent languages because each phoneme is generally represented by a given grapheme, this process is not used. In Chinese and Japanese, which use logographs, the writer may use "finger tracing" or drawing to recall the spelling of the character.

Differences in directionality of reading must be considered as well. Several languages are written horizontally, but there are other variations in direction. As examples, for Hebrew and Arabic the direction is left to right. Writing in Chinese is oriented vertically. Cook and Bassetti (2005) report that the directionality of reading and writing in a given language has implications for interpreting sequence. For example, advertisements in English or French, which depict a sequence, go from left to right, whereas the opposite is true for advertisements in Hebrew and Arabic. Children who are asked to place in a sequence cards that depict actions taking place will follow the order used in reading and writing. Arrows that depict "before" and "after" point up and down in Chinese, instead of left and right in English or in another language that reads from left to right.

Several considerations need to be taken into account when students who speak other languages than English experience difficulty learning to read and write. These considerations include primarily the linguistic unit, which can be alphabetic, consonantal, or morphemic; the type of script; and the orthography. Therefore, when assessing bilingual individuals whose languages use different scripts, Everatt, Smythe, Ocampo, and Veii (2002) suggest using the following battery of tasks and skills as assessment tools, because strengths and weaknesses do not manifest themselves in the same way across two different languages: (1) basic skills such as the correct use of the alphabet, numbers, and days of the week sequences; (2) the ability to read words and nonwords; (3) the ability to spell words and nonwords; (4) phonological segmentation and assembly skills; (5) auditory short-term memory and auditory discrimination; (5) visual tasks such as copying, visual recall of shapes, and visual sequential memory; and (6) Rapid Automatic Naming skills (pictures, numbers, and letters). Table 6-5 lists some "dos" and "don'ts" suggested by Geva and Wade-Wooley (2003) for assessing CLD students who might have dyslexia.

Some Cross-Linguistic Contrasts

It is important to consider that bilingual students and adults may not pronounce some English sounds correctly due to variations in the existence of consonants or the positions of those sounds in the respective languages. In assessing the student's or client's phonology,

TABLE 6-5 Dos and Don'ts for Assessing CLD Students for Whom Dyslexia Is Suspected

Dos	Don'ts
• Assess as many areas known to be related to dyslexia as possible.	• Delay assessment until the student has reached an "appropriate" level of oral language proficiency.
• Assess both languages whenever possible.	• Assume that word recognition and word attack skills are unimportant.
• Monitor progress and learning over time.	
• Look beyond language proficiency.	• Assume persistent language and reading difficulties "will catch-up" if ignored.
• Provide direct instruction in reading.	• Seek to establish a discrepancy between ability and performance to justify the label of "reading disability."
• Consider the student's transfer skills from the first language.	• Assume that persistent difficulties merely reflect "negative" transfer from the first language.
	• Use test norms based on the child's first language.

Source: Adapted from Smythe and Everatt, 2002.

the SLP must be aware of similarities and differences in sounds between the two languages. In addition to sound differences, it is important to consider contrasts between the languages with regard to the placement of sounds within words. For example, Spanish has the /st/ cluster (e.g., "estatua")—but not in the initial position as in English (e.g., "statue"). Selected consonant sounds that may cause problems in English for some CLD students are listed in Table 6-6.

The pronunciation of various vowels and diphthongs must also be considered. For example, Spanish has only five vowels and five diphthongs. Chinese has fewer vowels than English and because it is a tonal language like Vietnamese, the meaning is provided by the pronunciation of the tone. Word order also varies from language to language. See Table 2-1 for a list of the scripts of languages most frequently spoken by English Language Learners (ELL) students. The table also shows the word order of those languages.

DEFINING THE LANGUAGE AND SPEECH DISORDERS OF CLD STUDENTS

This section will include definitions for language and speech disorders, beginning with language disorders. A CLD student may have a speech disorder or a language disorder, or both.

Language Disorders

A language disorder may manifest itself at different ages and stages in the course of a child's development. For example, an infant may have difficulty in acquiring an oral system of communication, while an elementary-school-age child may be able to express basic needs, but has problems in narrating a story with a logical sequence due to difficulties in formulating more complex ideas. Typically, this child may also have reading and writing problems. An older student may have learned basic reading skills, but has difficulty with

TABLE 6-6 Selected English Consonants That Are Challenging for Second-Language Learners

Consonant	Spanish	Vietnamese	Hmong	Korean	Chinese	Arabic	Russian
/b/	3	3	1		2		
/ch/		1					
/d/		3			2		3
/g/	3	3	1		2	1	3
/j/	1	1	1				
/k/	2	2					2
/p/	2	2				1	2
/sh/	1	1		1			
/th/		1		1		1	1
/ð/	1	1			1	1	1
/v/	1	3		1	1	1	
/z/	1	1		1	1		
/r/	1			1		1	
/s/				1			

Legend:

(1) Often a problem

(2) May be a problem at the beginning of words

(3) May be a problem at the end of words

Source: Adapted from Echevarria, Vogt, and Short, 2004, and Swan and Smith, 2004.

more complex material. When ideas are more embedded in the text, this student may have difficulty integrating the information so as to make inferences, formulate hypotheses, and make predictions. Also, the student may have weaknesses with regard to comprehending more figurative language, such as metaphors, idioms, and humor. In the younger student, comprehension difficulties may be apparent in the way he or she follows oral and written directions, or appears to integrate the essence of a class discussion.

In some cases, a language disorder is a manifestation of a traceable condition, such as hearing or vision impairments. It could also have a neurological basis, such as cerebral palsy, or it could be the result of autism, a syndrome, or mental retardation. In most cases, however, the source of the problem cannot be easily detected, and the lack of a clearly identifiable cause makes it even more difficult for parents to accept that their child has a problem. The parents—and often teachers as well—of many second-language learners attribute their child's problem to the process of second-language acquisition. In addition, if the student manages to decode words (often without really understanding the text), parents with limited literacy in English or even in their own language find it difficult to understand the reason for the student's lack of success in school. It is a particularly delicate process to approach parents when problems are not identified until the student is in upper elementary grades or higher. The literature on what constitutes a language disorder in monolingual English-speakers is abundant. Some recent sources on this subject include Butler and Silliman (2004), Catts and Kamhi (2004), and Paul (2006).

Research on the language disorders of students of primarily Spanish-speaking backgrounds dates from the 1970s and 1980s, and includes literature by Ambert and Meléndez (1985), Linares-Orama (1977), and Langdon (1977, 1989). The research on the various linguistic aspects of language disorders (with a particular emphasis on bilingual Spanish-English speaking students) is described in greater detail in Goldstein (2004b). One difficulty in summarizing the findings is that those who conducted the existing research focused on the various areas of language (i.e., phonology, grammar and syntax, and discourse) in only one of the languages (typically the first language). However, some major trends in all the current research indicates that students who have a language disorder in one or several discrete areas (phonology, grammar, use of language) in one language may not necessarily have identical difficulties in the other, depending on the structure of the language, the length of exposure to the language, and the student's use of and experiences in the given language. However, the overall conclusions are that the student with a language disorder does not advance in language development in the second language as well as his or her peers who have similar experiences and the same first language—and that there is also a lag in academic performance that is due to reading and writing challenges.

Thus, the language disorder of a CLD student may manifest itself in areas similar to those in which a monolingual English-speaking student's language disorder is manifested—however, specific contexts in which each language is used need to be considered. Thus, the student may perform differently in the second

language than in the first language. As an example, Langdon (1977) found that bilingual, language-disordered students and their normally developing peers made similar errors in English. However, the group that was identified as language disordered made more errors than the other group. Thus, the number of errors rather than the type of errors could differentiate the groups. Paradis (2005) found similar results in a study that evaluated the ability of young children aged 4 to 10 to use different morphological features of English. The children came from various first-language backgrounds. The results indicated that the children made similar errors as those made by native speakers. It was therefore concluded that assessing morphology might not differentiate the two groups effectively and that additional assessment in other language areas in both the second and first language is necessary. For example, in the area of Spanish syntax and grammar, Restrepo and Gutiérrez-Clellen (2004) found that students with language impairments made frequent article omissions and gender agreement substitutions, and Bedore and Leonard (2001) noted that the number of agreement errors were more prevalent in students with language impairments. Some of these observations are similar to those found by Ambert (1986). In my research (Langdon, 1977), I found that the bilingual Spanish-English students who were suspected of having a language disorder made significantly more errors in a task where they were asked to process, retain, and retrieve information in Spanish. Analysis of the narratives of Spanish-speaking children with language impairments further indicates that these students have more difficulty with cohesion, substitution of pronouns for referents, and the ability to retain and express episodic information (Gutiérrez-Clellen, 2004). Therefore, a language disorder needs to be assessed in both languages to gain a more valid picture of the student's competence. Moreover, differences in the language structures of each one of the two languages should be carefully analyzed when conducting the assessment.

Speech Disorders

Two possible disorders that may be diagnosed in CLD students include articulation/phonological disorders and fluency.

In previous sections we reviewed some contrasts between seven of the most frequently spoken languages spoken by CLD populations as they learn English. It is important to note those contrasts and to consider variations in dialects within American English as well as dialects within other languages. As mentioned by Goldstein (2004b), the goal of conducting a phonological assessment is to determine if the phonological system is developing normally in each one of the student's languages. If development in only one language is not on a par with that of other monolingual or bilingual speakers of the same language, the observed differences are not due to a disorder, but rather reflect a difference. It is necessary to take into account both the influences of dialect and the norms that are typical for individuals who speak a given language as they learn a second language. For example, it is not atypical for Spanish speakers or speakers of another language to apply some of the first-language rules when communicating in English. First-language influences can be noted not only for consonants but also for vowels. For example, a Spanish speaker might add a vowel to an /s/ cluster—[sk] as in "eskool"—or omit an /s/ at the end of word because he or she speaks different dialect of Spanish. Not atypical are the Vietnamese and Korean speakers' problems pronouncing /r/, which is not in their

language repertoires. To review the challenges speakers of several languages may encounter, the reader is referred to Swan and Smith (2004).

An understanding of the fluency disorders of bilingual speakers is just emerging. More information is available relating to bilingual Spanish-English speakers than to speakers of other languages. The level of severity of the fluency disorders (stuttering) of bilingual individuals tends to vary a great deal for the two or more languages that the individual may speak. Ratner (2004) indicates that the level of severity may be either similar or different for each language; therefore, she advocates assessing fluency in both languages. Stuttering may also involve different parts of speech or sounds depending on the particular language. Von Borsel, Maes, and Foulon (2001) report that dysfluency tends to be higher in the less-proficient language user. The SLP needs to be cautious about diagnosing a fluency disorder in those students or adults whose difficulty retrieving words that express their thoughts in a particular language may be due to limited proficiency in the language. It is not uncommon for speakers of two or more languages to appear dysfluent when trying to express their thoughts about topics and under conditions that are stressful. In summary, the research on transfer of fluency across languages is inconclusive.

ARRIVING AT A FINAL DIAGNOSIS

In analyzing the results of formal and informal discrete-point tests (oral and written), and in examining language samples in order to arrive at a final diagnosis, the SLP should also consider whether such factors as the student's school attendance, school experience, and type of instruction are affecting the student's language performance. By carefully identifying and exploring the different variables, the SLP can determine if a true problem exists.

An ELL's language disorder may manifest itself in a variety of areas, just as for a monolingual student. With an ELL student, however, certain areas may be affected in one language but not the other, depending on the student's exposure to and use of each language, and depending on the structure of the language. Most likely, however, if an ELL student experiences oral language processing difficulties in the second language at significantly higher levels than other students who have had similar exposure to English, the student might also experience those difficulties in his or her primary/native language. The fact that such a problem might not be evident in the initial stages of the second-language acquisition process is one important reason for assessing a bilingual student in both languages.

When analyzing the language profile of an ELL student who has been assessed in two languages, it is helpful to consider the areas of BICS (Basic Interpersonal Communication Skills) and CALP (Cognitive Academic Language Proficiency). Four different profiles are possible, and within each case, there may be the variations of severity that are shown in Figure 6-4.

1. The student may have adequate basic communication skills in his or her native language, but little abstract-type language skills and weak academic skills in that language. BICS and CALP in English are also very weak. The student needs more time to acquire CALP in L1 if there are bilingual language programs available. Otherwise, the student might be a good candidate for a well-founded program such as the Specially Designed Academic Instruction in English (SDAIE), or a program utilizing strategies outlined in the Sheltered Instruction Observation Protocol program (SIOP) (Echevarría, Vogt, & Short, 2004) discussed in Chapter 3. Any of these programs would assist this student in acquiring further academic skills in English.

2. The CLD student may have weak skills in both BICS and CALP in both languages. In this case, the student may not have had sufficient exposure to explicit teaching in either language, and the profile may reflect a language-learning disability. Knowing about the student's background health and academic experiences will assist in differentiating whether the difference is caused by a lack of adequate language exposure or possibly by a language-learning disability that affects all language areas in both languages.

3. The student has been able to acquire basic communication skills in both languages, but has problems with CALP in both languages. This may occur when a CLD student has been exposed to English, but has not acquired sufficient metalinguistic and metacognitive skills that enhance his or her performance in academically related tasks in either language. Once again, analyzing the student's exposure to adequate teaching strategies and examining his or her progress over time in both oral and written language development will shed light on whether the profile signifies that the student needs more time, or has a language-learning disability.

4. The CLD student may have adequate BICS and CALP skills in the first language, but both BICS and CALP are weak in English. Very likely, the student will

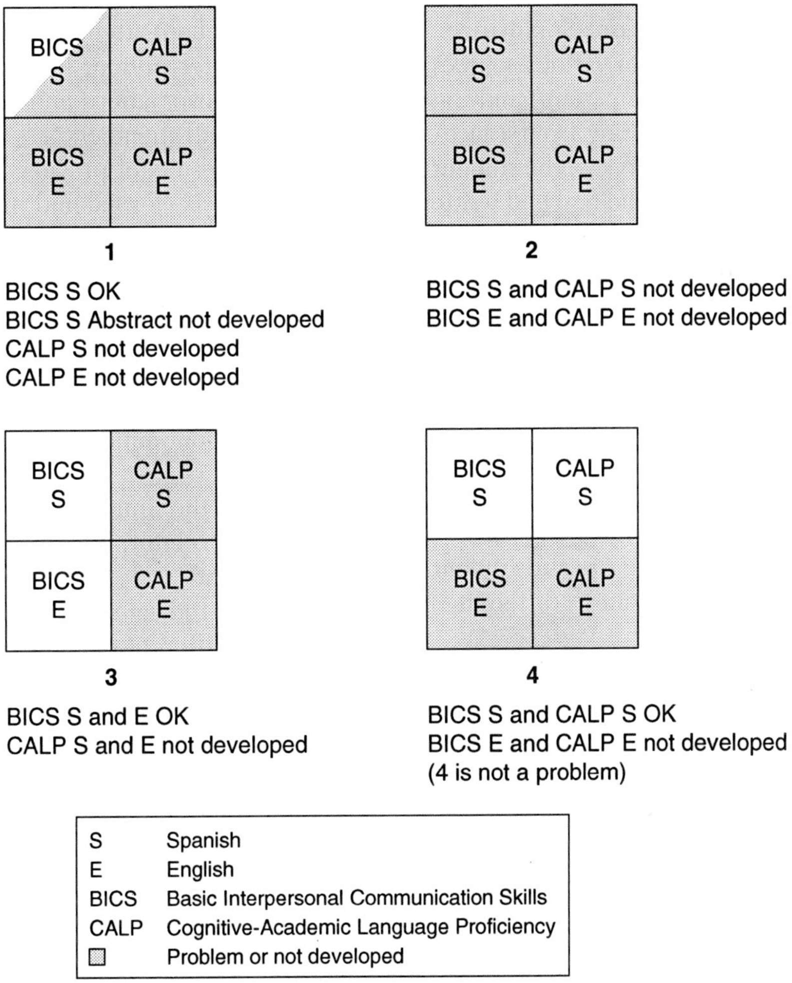

FIGURE 6-4   *Final Diagnosis of a Language Problem.*

benefit from more language exposure and from the explicit teaching of English using strategies such as those mentioned in Chapter 3. Most cases, however, are not as straightforward as this, and do not fit into such neat categories. Nevertheless, the four sets described here and shown in Figure 6-4 are helpful for delineating the language profile of CLD students who may have a language-learning disorder.

WRITING THE FINAL REPORT

Writing the final report on a bilingual student will take almost twice as long as writing one for a monolingual student, because comments need to be made in all the considered areas for each of the two languages. The following is a list of areas that should be considered:

1. **Reason for Referral:** List the reasons that the student was referred for a bilingual assessment.

2. **Background Information:** Summarize relevant information from various sources (i.e., comments from the parent/family, as well as information resulting from a face-to-face or telephone interview, the student's cumulative record, and the oral and written reports of other educational or professional staff). The information should include

   • *Social and family background*

   (a) Place of birth (e.g., home, hospital) and location
   (b) Parents' perception of their child's language performance
   (c) Sibling position and number of persons living with the student
   (d) Languages spoken to the student and by the student to different family members
   (e) Parents' occupation, educational attainment, and proficiency in English
   (f) Information about language development difficulties or learning difficulties of the student and any family member
   (g) Student's experiences at home with literacy—and opportunities for activities outside the home, such as trips to parks, museums, and any outings
   (h) Any trips to the country of origin, including dates and lengths of stay
   (i) Student's school attendance while residing in the country of origin

   • *Health and development background*
   • *School background*

   (a) Programs attended by the student
   (b) Review of accommodation programs that have been meeting the student's communication and academic needs

   (c) School attendance record and any interruptions in education
   (d) Observations and comments from staff members
   (e) Results of previously administered tests (formal and informal)

3. **Testing Procedures and Materials Used:** Indicate if the bilingual assessment was conducted by one SLP, two SLPs, or with the collaboration of an I/T. List the materials used and briefly describe the language/communication areas assessed using particular tests. Make a statement regarding the limitations of the tests and the need to interpret results according to the student's experiences and use of each language. Indicate how testing took place (e.g., on different days or weeks, by testing one language at a time, and/or whether switching between languages was needed to make the item comprehensible). List the results of the tests in your report. As an example, the report profiles of three of our clients (students) will be highlighted at the end of the chapter.

4. **Observations:** Report observations made during the one-on-one interaction with the student, as well as any observations made in the classroom or in other settings such as during recess or lunch.

5. **Verbal Input and Language Comprehension:** Describe how the student processes different types of information (e.g., by following directions, responding to different questions that are based on orally presented material, and imitating sentences). Indicate whether slowing down the pace of item administration, repeating the information, or asking the student to visualize the activity improves the student's performance. Make a notation if

extraneous noise interfered with the student's responses. Integrate the information obtained in the one-on-one interaction with observations made by parents and teachers. Note any differences in the student's proficiency in the two languages.

6. **Verbal Output or Language Expression:** In addition to describing the results of verbal interactions, describe the student's use of vocabulary and concepts, and the student's articulation/phonological skills. Also, report voice quality and fluency, as well as the results of an examination of the student's oral peripheral mechanism (structure and function of the articulators—e.g., tongue and lips—that are necessary for adequate speech production).

7. **Written Language and Related Skills:** Report results of reading fluency and reading comprehension as well as the analysis of a written sample, if appropriate. Reporting observations of the student's performance in math is also helpful for providing a broader perspective of the student's strengths and challenges. For example, the student may have very good calculation skills, but may experience much more difficulty in solving verbal math problems. This information may not be available for the student's first language due to lack of math exposure or experience. However, the classroom teacher(s) can provide information about the student's performance in English in the various academic areas.

8. **Other Tasks:** A separate section may include information on the student's general knowledge as well as more in-depth information on working memory and executive functions. This information can be obtained by using tasks such as those included in the CELF-4 (English and Spanish versions).

9. **Summary and Recommendations:** Write a summary of findings. Indicate the nature of any problem, and describe the rationale for the conclusions. Make suggestions for intervention, and make recommendations for designated programs such as speech and language services and/or resource programs. Base the goals and objectives of these interventions and programs on the school curriculum. Include two or three suggestions for teachers and for parents and families; ensure that the suggestions for parents and families can be easily followed at home. If possible, write those goals and ideas in the report in the parents' language.

Assessing a CLD student is a lengthy process. In reality, the SLP carries out two evaluations for each student. Although supervisors and administrators may question the lengthier process necessary for assessing an ELL student, the average length of an assessment of a bilingual student is indeed almost twice as long as that of a monolingual student (Langdon, 1989).

SUMMARY

In Chapter 6 we addressed the "mechanics" of oral and written language and how it relates to whether a CLD student might have a language disorder. Issues such as when to decide to conduct a formal assessment, decision-making regarding whether the assessment should be conducted in one or two languages, and what materials to use and how to carry out the process were discussed. The purpose of this chapter was to offer the reader a background on important factors that need to be considered when forming a language-disorder diagnosis for students who speak English as their second language.

We reviewed first the processes necessary for successful reading and writing in one language. We also examined the connections between reading and writing—a reminder to all of us that there is a very close connection between oral and written language. Cross-linguistic oral and written characteristics of various languages were reviewed as well. Being aware of these contrasts is important for understanding how various language and learning disabilities may be identified in other languages. We found that not everyone agrees about what constitutes a reading disability, and that this is because of variations in the languages' linguistic units, and in their scripts. To address this problem, it was recommended that language evaluations include a thorough assessment in both languages—one that takes into account the oral and written characteristics of each language (as suggested by the assessment battery proposed by Everatt, Smythe, Ocampo, and Veii, 2002). The chapter emphasized that it is also important to keep in mind that oral and written language strengths and challenges may not be identical across languages because of the different structures of the languages, and because of the student's experience with and exposure to each language. Therefore, other factors such as the student's past health history, language development, experiences, and educational progress—as well as the observations of people who know him or her well—need to be taken into account. Finally, the chapter provided some suggestions on how to form a diagnosis by taking into consideration the development of BICS and CALP, even though not every student might fit one of the four models perfectly.

OUR CLIENTS

Eric, Ana, Jack, Grace, and Leonardo

Now we are ready to write reports on our three youngest clients: Eric, Ana, and Jack. Within the report we will include our rationale for stating that the students have a language-learning disability.

Eric: Bilingual Speech and Language Assessment Report

Reason for Referral:
Eric is a 4-year-old preschool child whose parents speak primarily Vietnamese to him and who is referred because of low expressive skills in both languages.

Background Information:
Eric was born in the United States. His parents emigrated from Vietnam when they were teenagers. He is the youngest of three children; his siblings are 10 and 8 years old. Eric's parents speak English but they still feel more at ease speaking in Vietnamese, and this is the language spoken in the home. Eric's siblings speak English to him and to each other, but they communicate in Vietnamese with their parents and family members with no difficulty. Eric's mother completed high school and works in retail, whereas his father finished two years of college and owns a restaurant.

Eric's speech development proceeded slower than expected as compared with his siblings'. At first, his parents were not alarmed; they felt that because he was spoiled and everyone in the family treated him as the "baby," his speech was understandably slower in developing. However, now that he is in preschool, he clearly appears to be behind other children who are also acquiring English. He prefers to play by himself and he has difficulty concentrating for more than a few minutes at a time unless he watches his favorite cartoons or videos. His health has been good and there are no concerns about his hearing. His parents have mentioned their concerns about Eric's language development to the pediatrician several times, but they were told that often bilingual children are slower to develop language. Because limited progress was noted, they contacted the school district and, with the support of the teacher, requested a formal evaluation.

During an interview with Mrs. HWL, a bilingual speech and language pathologist (but one who does not speak Vietnamese), the parents indicated that the family had spoiled Eric and that part of his delay might be due to his siblings answering for him. They also stated that they felt ashamed that their son was not progressing well and that they blamed themselves for this. When specifically asked about how Eric expresses himself, they stated that Eric speaks in short sentences in Vietnamese and in slightly longer ones in English. However, he is not on a par with other bilingual children in his community.

Eric was present during this interview, which enabled Mrs. HWL to note that he seemed to understand what his parents said to him in Vietnamese, and that he answered them in both English and Vietnamese. Eric was able to play with toys and puzzles very appropriately during a 30-minute period. It was a good idea to meet Eric prior to the assessment to establish easier rapport.

Assessment Process:

The assessment began with a visit to Eric's preschool. Mrs. HWL introduced herself to the class and Eric knew she would be working with him because his parents had told him about it and he had met her previously. Eric did not mind because the classroom has many visitors who work with the children individually.

During her observation, Mrs. HWL noted that Eric followed the class routine well. A schedule on the wall that included the name of the current classroom activity (and that was augmented by visual icons) indicated times for free play, circle time, outdoor recess and snack time, and specific group activities. When the children transitioned from activity to activity, the teacher pointed out their schedule. The teacher used all the best teaching practices: speaking at a slow pace (but not too slow), using visual aids, conducting dialogue with the children, and checking for comprehension during story time by asking a child to point to a picture or to respond to a question. Eric was attentive during small-group activities, but had a difficult time during circle time. He moved in his seat and was easily distracted by the children sitting next to him. When he was asked a question about the book, it had to be repeated because he was not paying attention. During free time, he played by himself and did not seem to seek company from other children. However, he responded to one or two children who came to see what he was playing with.

Materials used for this assessment included a puzzle, a picture book, some cars and a garage, and the PLS-4 in English as well as the EOWPVT. Mrs. HWL felt that a bilingual evaluation was necessary because she had heard Eric use Vietnamese while communicating with his parents during the interview, and also because he seemed to understand what his parents said to him. Mrs. HWL contacted an interpreter she had worked with previously, and requested that she join her in a week to complete the evaluation.

Eric was willing to come with Mrs. HWL into a quiet room next to his classroom. The assessment began by asking Eric to complete a 10-piece puzzle of a car, which he seemed to enjoy. During this activity, Eric was fairly quiet even though he uttered short phrases such as "I like play car" and "My daddy have a car too." However, it was difficult to get him to answer questions about where he might ride with his dad, or about who had brought him to school that day (his father brings him to school).

Eric was asked to complete the PLS-4 in English. After the items were given in English, an interpreter was contacted to assist in administering in Vietnamese the items that Eric did not know in English.

Results:

Eric was attentive during the one-on-one interaction. He responded well to verbal praising and to stickers as rewards.

(Continues)

(Continued)

Results and Discussion:

Observations and performance on the formal tests yielded the following results for English:

- Eric could follow one- and two-step directions.

- He responded to questions like "who," "what," and "where" while looking at a book.

- He had more difficulty responding to the clinician when he was asked a question out of context, such as "Where is your brother?" or "What did you have for breakfast?"

- On the Receptive portion of the PLS-4, he responded correctly to several items: identifying "negative-type statements" (Show me the baby who is not crying); categorizing pictures and objects; identifying quantifiers such as "more" but not "most"; identifying and naming all primary colors; counting to five; and understanding some prepositions. He had difficulty understanding longer sentences like "Show me the white kitten that is sleeping"; understanding inferences; and completing analogies.

- Eric communicated in short sentences such as the one previously described in the play portion of the assessment. Other typical sentences included "I like to eat ice cream," "My dad buy me this one," "Look at the car," "What is that?" and "Where is car?" It was difficult to elicit longer sentences from him. When asked to name pictures (EOWPVT), he could name animals, playground equipment, and some vehicles. He had more difficulty naming examples of categories such as "animals," "fruit," or " drinks."

- No articulation errors were noted in his speech.

After a briefing with the Vietnamese interpreter, a language sample was obtained using both a book for children written in Vietnamese and a toy train. In addition, the test items that Eric did not know in English were readministered in Vietnamese. Patterns similar to those observed in Eric's use of English were noted for Vietnamese. Eric could respond to simple questions but he rarely made reference to the past. The readministration of the items that he had failed in English indicated that he did indeed have similar difficulties in Vietnamese. Eric had difficulty understanding inferences, and when sentences were long he seemed confused and did not know which picture to show. He completed analogies with somewhat greater ease. While responding in Vietnamese, some of his short sentences included English words even though he tried to respond in the language in which the interaction was taking place. Eric could name certain words in Vietnamese but not in English—such as "basket" (cái thúng), "star" (sao), and "grape" (nho)—which is not unusual for a child growing up in a bilingual environment. After a briefing with the interpreter, and after transcribing Eric's sentences, the SLP's overall impression was that Eric's proficiency in English and Vietnamese were comparable. Examples of sentences he used in Vietnamese were "Toy moo-un trung" (I want an egg); "Die zee day" (What is this?); and "Guy ne" (This one). No articulation problems or difficulty with using tones were noted in this context, possibly because Eric's expressive language development is still quite limited.

Summary:

Eric is a 4-year-old child growing up in a Vietnamese-English bilingual environment where Vietnamese is the home language and English is the language of school and community. The concerns of his parents and teachers regarding his language development were justified. A bilingual English-Vietnamese evaluation indicated that Eric was attentive and seemed to try his best on a one-on-one basis. Even though he could respond to some concrete questions and perform several tasks such as categorizing and following some directions, he had difficulty processing longer strings of words in both languages. Difficulty in processing language was reflected in his limited language output. Despite these challenges, Eric communicated in the language in which he was addressed.

It is estimated that Eric's language comprehension is at the 3-year level whereas his expressive language is more like that of a child who is 2 ½ years old.

Eric certainly qualifies for services in speech and language development.

Eric's profile resembles the profile of (2) shown in Figure 6-4.

Ana: Bilingual Speech and Language Assessment Report

Reason for Referral:

Ana is a fourth-grader (aged 9) who was referred for a speech and language assessment because of slow progress in gaining more abstract language in English, and because of reading difficulties in English.

Background Information:

Ana lives with her parents and two younger siblings, aged 5 and 3. The family is originally from Michoacán, a state neighboring Mexico City. She was raised by her maternal grandparents beginning at the age of 6 months; after five years she was reunited with her parents. Ana attended kindergarten in Arizona but moved in the middle of that year when her parents found better jobs in California. She is in the fourth grade in a school where her mother works in the school cafeteria. Ana has learned English quite well but she is behind in reading. All of her schooling has been in English. Ana has always attended the same school. Her teachers voiced no concerns until this year because she was able to complete her work, and because previous teachers attributed some of her difficulties only to her bilingualism.

Ana speaks Spanish to her parents and some relatives who live nearby, but she talks to her siblings in both English and Spanish. Her parents insist that only Spanish should be spoken at home.

Mrs. S., Ana's mother, reported that she, herself, attended only elementary school in Mexico and could not continue her studies because she had to work to help her family. She is taking classes to improve her English and plans to go back to school to eventually receive a high school equivalency diploma. Mr. S. completed high school in Mexico and is attending a community college for training as a mechanic. He is working in an auto shop. Both parents are eager to see their children achieve in school.

Ana's parents read newspapers, magazines, and some books in Spanish. They visit the library every week and encourage their children to take out books in both Spanish and English as well as tapes and movies. The family watches TV together and goes to different places on the weekends—places such as the flea market, amusement parks, and restaurants.

No health or developmental difficulties were reported. Ana's parents indicated that even though they had not seen her for a long time, she had had no ear problems or infections that they were aware of. Since she has lived with them she has had no health issues. The last school vision and hearing screening was unremarkable.

Assessment Process:

Ms. HWL, a bilingual Spanish-English speech-language pathologist, evaluated Ana. In addition to administering tests in Spanish, Mrs. HWL supplemented the school SLP's English evaluation to obtain results in equivalent language areas.

The assessment began in Spanish and ended in English as one language was assessed at a time. However, if Ana responded in the other language, her responses were acknowledged. The following materials were used to assess Ana's speech, language, and communication in Spanish and English:

1. *Bilingual Syntax Measure* (BSM-I)

2. *Bilingual One-Word Receptive Picture Vocabulary Test* (ROWPVT)

3. *Bilingual One-Word Expressive Picture Vocabulary Test* (EOWPVT)

4. *Clinical Evaluation of Language Fundamentals* (CELF-4) (Spanish and English versions) (Selected subtests)

5. A language sample taken during informal conversation. In addition, Ana was asked to make up a story in each language using a wordless book: Mayer's (1975) *One Frog Too Many*

6. *Brigance* (Spanish and English): Reading Decoding and Reading of Paragraphs Subtests

7. Informal writing tasks

(Continues)

(Continued)

Ana was briefly observed in her classroom. The students were asked to answer questions from their social studies book. Ana worked with an assigned peer. The classroom teacher worked with the pair to ensure that they understood the assignment. Ana copied her friend's answers using very neat but labored handwriting.

During the one-on-one interaction, Ana did not have difficulty transitioning from task to task or language to language. Initially, she did not say very much as it took her some time to feel at ease in interacting with the clinician. Overall, she seemed to enjoy the individual attention; this was noted by her smiling. She seemed to try her best and often she asked if she was doing well.

It was easier for Ana when questions were paired with pictures and when she did not have to elaborate on her answers. For example, she formulated responses on the BSM and the Formulated Sentences subtests (CELF-4) fairly quickly. More hesitations and repetitions of words or phrases were noted when she had to narrate the story using the wordless book. These hesitations were more prevalent in English. This is not unusual for a second-language learner. However, persons working with Ana need to continue using visual aids and allow her to take time to respond.

Results and Discussion:

Ana's performance in each language must be interpreted by taking into account the fact that her exposure to each language has been varied and contextually different. Specifically, her formal exposure to English began in kindergarten. She communicates in Spanish with her family and in both languages with peers and siblings. One must also remember that her performance in Spanish may not be as strong in some areas due to language loss. For example, it was difficult to elicit the conditional tense from her in Spanish. This is one of the last grammatical forms that appear in a child's speech and the first one to be lost once the language is not used as often.

Results of the CELF-4 in each language need to be interpreted with care as well. The English version was standardized on monolingual English-speaking students; the Spanish on bilingual Spanish/English-speaking children in the U.S.

Test/Task	Spanish	English
BSM-1	RS: 15/18 Level 5–Proficient	RS: 16/18 Level 5–Proficient
ROWPVT	RS: 63 SS: 73	4th percentile Age: 6–4
EOWPVT	RS: 64 SS: 101	53rd percentile Age: 9–6
CELF-4°		
Recalling Sentences	RS: 62 SS: 9 37th percentile	RS: 42 SS: 6 9th percentile
Paragraph Comprehension	RS: 6 SS: 8 25th percentile	RS: 8 SS: 7 16th percentile
Formulated Sentences	RS: 32 SS: 10 50th percentile	RS: 37 SS: 9 37th percentile
Word Associations	RS: 28 Met criterion.	RS: 24 Did not meet criterion.
Rapid Automatic Naming	Could not be completed because could not recall the names of the figures in either language.	Training did not help her recall the names of the figures. She could perform the color sequences in both languages, but at a lower speed in each language.
Phonological Awareness	RS: 35 Did not meet criteria. Difficulty is indicated for this area.	RS: 50 Did not meet criteria. Difficulty is indicated for this area.
SAMPLE Wordless Book:*One Frog Too Many*	Total: 24 sentences. Nine compound sentences joined with mostly "y," "porque," and "que."	Total: 24 sentences. Eight compound sentences joined with mostly "and," "after," and "because."
Brigance Reading	About primer level—less fluent. Read 7/10 words at primer.	About primer level—more fluent. Read 8/10 words at primer.

Ana maintained the same language of interaction as the clinician and communicated in both languages with almost equal ease. She appeared more confident telling a story (narrative) in English (even though more hesitations and repetitions of words and phrases were noted) than in Spanish. She has definitely reached the Basic Communication Skills level in English (BICS) and is beginning to acquire more of the academic language in English (CALP)—but at a much slower pace than her peers.

Language Comprehension and Processing:
Ana had no difficulty comprehending information presented during a conversation in Spanish or English. However, she had more difficulty remembering information when asked questions in Spanish about orally presented short paragraphs (CELF-4 Paragraph Comprehension subtest). There was less difficulty when the same task was administered in English. Ana missed several vocabulary words on the ROWPVT. She was unfamiliar with words such as "reflection," "eruption," "protection," and "injury" (in both languages). These words are generally learned through academic experience and reading.

Short-term memory/processing difficulties were noted when Ana was asked to repeat sentences of various lengths and complexities in either Spanish or English. She had somewhat less difficulty in Spanish, but her overall performance was weak.

In summary, Ana's comprehension skills in both languages are adequate during conversation. She has more difficulty when she needs to respond to less contextual information or novel information—where she cannot depend on contextual clues.

Language Expression:
At first Ana was somewhat reluctant to converse with the clinician. As she began to feel more comfortable, she was willing to share personal information and continue the clinician's conversation. Comments provided below pertain to both languages.

Pragmatics: Ana was able to maintain the topic of conversation. She was also comfortable initiating and expanding on topics presented during the evaluation. For example, she described (in Spanish) how her family took a trip to the beach in Acapulco. She switched from one language to the other with no hesitation. She could use the two languages for a variety of purposes. She could, for example, denote cause and effect in both Spanish and English: "Ya después el niño estuvo contento porque la rana regresó" (And then the boy was happy because the frog came back) and "The boy was sad because he couldn't find his frog."

Grammar/Syntax: Ana used sentences in each language that varied in length and complexity depending on the context. In Spanish, some typical sentences included: "Y ya después el niño llegó a su casa y se fue subiendo a su cuarto" (And then the boy arrived at his home and he went upstairs to his room), and "El otro con el que se iba a casar lo abandonó porque se iba a morir" (The other one, the one whom she was going to marry, she left him because he was going to die). Ana's grammar and syntax were (not surprisingly) more correct in Spanish. She made some significant errors in English such as using the incorrect form of the past ("they fall down" and "the boy tooked"). These errors are usual for early second-language learners but should not be present in the language of students who have had as much exposure to English as Ana has.

Vocabulary/Content: In Spanish, Ana used words like "abandonó" (abandoned) while describing a fragment of a TV show. She could label items and concepts such as "statue" and "footsteps," and identify the map of the United States. When she did not know the label, she would define the use of the item to some extent. For example, when naming a telescope, she said, "to see things." She was unable to remember the word for "shield" and called it "knight," saying "We have those here in school." In English her vocabulary appeared more restricted and Ana hesitated more while expressing detailed ideas in English. Thus, she repeated words or phrases while searching for terms to express her ideas.

Ana's voice appeared hoarse. She denied having a cold or abusing her voice. The clinician did not have a chance to ask her mother if her voice has the same quality. It is advised that she be checked again. In case of doubt, a referral to an ENT is indicated.

(Continues)

(*Continued*)

Academic Skills:

Ana could not say the alphabet in order in Spanish, but she could in English. She knows most of the days of the week in both languages. She can answer questions about which day was yesterday, tomorrow, before yesterday, and after tomorrow in both languages. She does not know the months of the year. She seemed very confused when asked to detect sounds in various positions of words in either language—except for initial-position sounds. She had difficulty blending and segmenting words. It was very difficult to explain to her the meaning behind the concept of rhyming. The RAN could not be completed because she could not recall all of the shapes in either language despite being trained by the clinician.

Ana is currently reading at about the primer level in both languages. She feels more confident reading in English. When she reads, she can remember the words she has not been able to identify previously. She is also reading with comprehension. She does not guess a word, but tries to decipher it so that it makes sense in relation to the rest of what she reads.

She is also more willing to write and spell words in English than in Spanish. She can write words like "pizza," "book," "brown," " stop," and " baby." She misspelled words like "shoe" (sho) and "grass" (gras).

Summary:

Ana is an almost 10-year-old bilingual Spanish/English-speaking student in the fourth grade who was referred by her teacher because of concerns about her progress with academic subjects (primarily reading). She has received some tutoring but very limited progress has been noted. All of her instruction has been in English.

Ana cooperated and attended well during the one-on-one interaction with this clinician. She appeared to try her best and seemed to enjoy the one-on-one interaction. Results of this assessment indicate that Ana's Basic Interpersonal Communication Skills (BICS) are fairly intact in both languages, but that she has occasional difficulty using grammar in English. However, she has underlying difficulties with working memory and processing that are evident in both languages. These difficulties are more pronounced in English than in Spanish. Ana experiences challenges with recall of auditory information, phonemic awareness, and comprehension of information when she has to rely on auditory processing, which is weak. She performs much better when visual support is provided (Formulating Sentences). Even though she can express herself fairly well, the vocabulary words sampled on a test like the EOWPVT revealed limited vocabulary in both languages. The gap is most likely due to lack of exposure to and experience in the process of reading to learn new material.

Ana was able to talk about different topics and her grammar usage in Spanish was adequate, but errors were noted in English. Her language profile is similar to the one shown in Figure 6-4(3). Her BICS skills are adequate, but not her CALP due to difficulty with processing auditory information and lack of phonological awareness skills. These challenges have impacted her ability to acquire reading fluency skills. Her challenges do not reflect a second-language acquisition problem but signal a language-learning disability which is apparent in Spanish, and more so in English. The prognosis for her progress is good (if she obtains adequate instruction) because she has been able to maintain some of her skills in Spanish, even though she uses the language only at home and only for certain purposes.

Jack: Speech and Language Assessment Report

Reason for Referral:

Jack's grandmother requested a speech and language evaluation. She is particularly concerned about Jack's academic performance. She does not believe he is reading well, and he has difficulty writing essays. Jack attends a seventh-grade public school. Jack was previously assessed by the school assessment team but found to be ineligible to receive services from the special education program.

Background Information:

Jack is a 14-year-old seventh grader of African-American heritage. Mrs. G., Jack's maternal grandmother, adopted him when he was 2 years old, as his single mother could not raise him. Jack was born and raised in Alabama, and he has been living with his grandmother in California for the past four years. Prior to entering School District A (summer, 2002), Jack attended a private school for two years.

Mrs. G. is a nurse in the surgical ward of a hospital. Because she has long hours, neighbors supervise Jack's whereabouts. Even though both Mrs. G. and Jack have a Southern accent and speak AAVE, his use of a different syntax and vocabulary do not seem to interfere with his academic learning.

Jack had to remain in the ICU for about seven days after birth due to respiratory distress. His developmental milestones occurred within a normal timeframe except for his speech, which was delayed. Jack did not put words together until he was about 3 years old. The latest vision and hearing screenings were unremarkable (fall, 2005). Because of her concern, Mrs. G. had Jack privately evaluated by a neuropsychologist. Results of the assessment indicated that Jack has difficulty with working memory and sequencing skills. Mrs. G. states that Jack has difficulty synthesizing oral and written information. Writing is difficult for him: He does not know how to begin an essay, and even though he is beginning to use the computer for editing, he still has difficulty following rules of grammar or punctuation.

Jack likes to play videogames. He plays sports after school. When they have time, Mrs. G. takes him to various ball games. They also enjoy eating out on weekends. Mrs. G. described Jack as a pleasant young man who may not succeed as well he might because learning is difficult for him. She is very concerned about receiving adequate help for her grandchild.

Assessment Process:

Jack was evaluated for almost two hours; the evaluation was interrupted by a short break. The following testing materials/tasks were used to assess Jack's speech, language, and communication skills:

1. *Peabody Picture Vocabulary Test* (PPVT-III-B)

2. *Clinical Evaluation of Language Fundamentals* (CELF-4) (specific subtests)

3. Criterion-referenced tasks from the CELF-4

4. The task of reading a paragraph out loud and answering questions about the content

In addition, a language sample was taken during spontaneous conversation/speech and while Jack narrated a wordless book: Mayer's (1975) *One Frog Too Many*. Jack's narration was transcribed and analyzed.

Observations:

There was no opportunity to observe Jack in any of his classes. However, Mrs. HWL, the SLP, asked each one of his teachers to rate his attention and performance. Most of them indicated that he was attentive and seemed to try his best, but he was getting by with Cs and Ds. During the one-on-one interaction, Jack was cooperative and seemed to try his best. He appeared to enjoy the individual attention and did show interest in the examiner's comments by asking about her work and her fluency in the Spanish language. Jack stated that his favorite subjects were PE and math, and he reported that "nothing" was difficult in school. Currently, Jack is taking math, science, social studies, PE, and language arts. When he graduates, Jack would like to work for the NFL, and if he cannot make the team, he would like to be a policeman. Jack said he likes sports and that he spends a great deal of time talking to friends on the phone.

Jack's attention was good during this one-on-one interaction. His responses to open-ended questions were brief, however, and he responded with limited elaboration. It appeared that the lack of elaboration was not due to an expressive language problem—but rather that it reflected the somewhat contrived situation of having to interact with an adult he did not know well. When he was referring to his friends he used more AAVE but then switched to mainstream English.

(Continues)

(Continued)

Results and Discussion:

Test/Task	Raw Score	Standard Score	Percentile
PPVT-III-B	140	90	25
CELF-4			
Recalling Sentences	74	95	37
Formulating Sentences	42	85	16
Word Definitions	20	95	37
Understanding Spoken Paragraphs	6	80	9
Word Associations	44	Adequate	
Rapid Automatic Naming	Time 105 sec.	Not normal	

Language Comprehension/Processing:
Jack could follow oral directions as long as the information was not too complex, and he carried on a personal conversations with success. He could repeat sentences of various lengths and complexity well within the average range, and he could name months of the year in correct order and answer questions about which one came before or after the other. However, he demonstrated greater challenges when he needed to process orally presented information and respond verbally to what was said (Understanding Spoken Paragraphs). Repetition of the information did not prove to be a helpful strategy for increasing his performance on that subtest. However, visual support such as pictures enhanced his ability to retrieve information. For example, he responded with greater success on the Formulated Sentences portion of the CELF-4 and in composing a narrative using a wordless book.

Jack's challenges were also observed during the psychological examination. Ms. M. (the psychologist) noted that "He scored lowest when answering common-thought questions, suggesting that he has difficulty when information is given orally...."

It will be important to use visual support in order to ensure that Jack follows what is said in class, and to provide greater emphasis on using key words and concepts. Pairing him with a few students during small activities (where he can have time to practice what was lectured in class) would be very helpful for ensuring that he understands the material presented. Thus far, he has been able to perform because, most likely, he has been able to compensate: there are more pictures in his books and he has not been asked to take notes.

Language Expression:
Pragmatics: Jack was pleasant and friendly during the entire time. Although he responded to the examiner's questions and comments, his answers were generally brief. For example, when he was asked to explain why he wanted to be a cop, he said, "there's dangers," but he did not say more. When asked to explain how to play football, he proceeded to talk about how teams get selected to go to the Super Bowl, instead of explaining the game in itself. Mrs. G. has observed similar communication patterns at home. Jack's responses were more elaborate when he was asked to make up a story using pictures, or when he needed to make up specific sentences using pictures (CELF subtest and language sample). His difficulty in retrieving words to express himself was nevertheless evident because his answers were labored. On a few occasions, Jack asked the examiner some questions and showed interest when she told him that she spoke Spanish. He willingly repeated some of the numbers and asked how to use some of the common greetings in that language.

Grammar/Syntax: Jack used sentences that varied in length and complexity depending on the topic. Nevertheless, in his narration using the wordless book, he only used connecting words such as "and," "suddenly," and "so" to link two sentences. Examples include "Suddenly, the frog jumped inside the boat and again he kicked the frog out the boat, and the frog, he could not find the frog." However, he used various verb tenses and connecting words appropriately, as in: "I can't go to baseball unless I finish my homework" and "If only I had come home on time I wouldn't have missed the bus" (Formulated Sentences subtest of the CELF-4). When referring to his conversations with friends, he used sentences such as: "One of my friend, he a bad guy. He done a lot of headaches to him parents, oh boy. They tell him he is grounded and instead, after he finish dinner, and he take him father's car and run away."

In summary, Jack can use various types of sentences and more complex constructions when he has visual support. He experiences more difficulty when he has to explain his thoughts during conversation and when he is attempting to explain something in greater detail.

Vocabulary/Content: Fluency-Voice-Articulation
Jack's knowledge of vocabulary varied. He knew most "concrete" words that he had learned through conversation, or by being exposed to certain curriculum areas. For example, he could identify words like "arctic," "pyramid," "compass," "parallel," and "peninsula," but he had more difficulty with words such as "scholar," "assembling," "composing," or "orating" (PPVT-III). Yet he performed with greater success when he needed to provide a definition of a word after listening to a sentence (for example, for "fable": "My friend said, 'that was an interesting fable'"; for "pedestrian": "The driver asked the class, 'Where did the pedestrian go?'") (Average performance range on Word Definitions of the CELF-4). He knew days of the week and months of the year, but he seemed confused when asked which was the first or last month of the year.

There was no evidence of difficulty with fluency, voice, or articulation.

Other Areas:
A formal reading test was not administered at this time because the Resource Specialist would later administer specific academic tests. A screening indicated that Jack's reading fluency is fairly good, but he has difficulty answering questions about what he has read. He was asked to read the passage out loud. It is possible he could perform with greater ease if the passage were read silently. Mrs. G. reported that Jack does not like to read for pleasure.

Jack's performance on the Rapid Automatic Naming (RAN) was slow as compared with the norm, and he made slightly more errors than would be expected for his age. Slower performance on the RAN signals difficulty with word finding and indicates retrieval deficits, which were noted throughout the interaction. Even though Jack performed in the average range on the academic areas of the *Woodcock Jackson-III* when he was later tested by the Resource Specialist, his performance with regard to curricular materials signals some learning difficulties, which need to be addressed through special intervention.

Summary:
Jack is a 14-year-old young man of African-American heritage who was referred for a speech and language assessment. Jack has had some behavior and academic difficulties. Although he did not qualify for special education services (fall, 2002), Mrs. G., his guardian, is concerned about his academic progress. A private evaluation indicated that Jack has difficulty with auditory processing and working memory.

Jack was pleasant, he tried to do his best, and his attention was good during the one-on-one interaction. Jack performs better when tasks are presented with visual support. He is familiar with concepts that he has been exposed to in class or has experienced, but not with concepts he has read about. It is easier for him to repeat what he hears than it is for him to answer questions that are based on information presented orally.

(Continues)

(Continued)

Jack appears to have difficulty processing information presented orally. When he wants to express more complex ideas there is evidence of word-finding difficulties. His speech is filled with revisions, hesitations, and some word repetitions. He can read fluently, but he does not understand well what he reads. Retelling or repeating the information is not always effective for increasing his comprehension skills.

The challenges noted above are preventing Jack from benefiting from the curriculum. In a lecture he is not able to always understand and assimilate the material—unless accommodations are made such as providing visual support, orally emphasizing key concepts, or providing him the ability to practice in a smaller group where he can read and write about what he is learning. Even though (according to previous testing) there appears to be no significant discrepancy between Jack's current ability and his performance in the classroom, efforts by the team must be made to offer him special assistance, as he will continue to fail without proper intervention. In addition, IDEA 2004 states that students' performance be supplemented with observations from parents and teachers, and that students must demonstrate overall progress in academic subjects. The most appropriate course of action would be to provide Jack the services of a resource specialist, supplemented with the consultation of an SLP.

Jack's difficulty does not stem from a lack of language exposure or experience, nor is it a reflection of the fact that he switches to AAVE. Up until now he has been able to compensate for his learning difficulties. Now that curricular demands are greater and he therefore has to process more complex information, take notes, and write more—he is having more challenges.

FURTHER READINGS

Butler K. G., Nelson, N. W., Wallach, G. P., Fujiki, M., & Brinton, B. (Eds.). (2005). Language disorders and learning disabilities: A look across 25 years. *Topics in Language Disorders, 25*(4).

Cook, V., & Bassetti, B. (2005). *Second-language writing systems*. Clevedon, UK: Multilingual Matters.

Smythe, I., Everatt, J., & Salter, R. (2004). *International book of dyslexia: A cross-language comparison and practice guide*. Hoboken, NJ: John Wiley & Sons.

CHAPTER 7

INTERVENTION ISSUES FOR CLD CHILDREN: INFANCY THROUGH ADOLESCENCE

"For any student, the role of the SLP should be that of a mediator who models strategies to enable the student to become ultimately responsible for his or her own learning. When working with a CLD student, the SLP might need to spend more time and have more patience because of the student's potentially different personal and school/program experiences in English. More intense communication with parents may be necessary as well." (Author)

CHAPTER OUTLINE

INTRODUCTION

In planning an intervention program for a student who has one or more speech-language, communication, or learning disabilities, it is essential to focus on the unique characteristics of the individual. This is even more important in the case of a culturally and linguistically diverse (CLD) student.

A broad range of techniques and strategies are available to enable CLD students with LLD (language-learning disabilities) to become more competent in linguistic and academically related tasks; these techniques and strategies will be reviewed in this chapter. Fifteen years ago I co-edited a book entitled Hispanic Children and Adults with Communication Disorders: Assessment and Intervention (Langdon and Cheng, 1992); what was said in that book is still relevant today: "Data are not yet available that determine conclusively what, when, and how certain strategies work best with CLD students who have language-learning disabilities. However, we have research on the best techniques for assisting students who are learning a second language" (Beaumont, 1992, pp. 357–358). This subject was discussed in detail in Chapter 3. In addition, what Cummins said more than 20 years ago is still applicable today: "Research is unlikely to provide answers to these questions for a considerable period; thus it is crucial for teachers and resource personnel in schools to become their own researchers by systematically observing the effects of assessment and placement decisions on students' development over time—and by sharing these observations with other professionals in order to provide a coherent experiential basis for future decisions. Essentially, this suggestion represents an extension and systematization of longitudinal monitoring techniques" (Cummins, 1984, pp. 268–269). This concern applies to not only CLD students, but also to monolingual LLD students: "Language impairments tend to be chronic and pervasive, yet we rarely get the chance to see how intervention interacts with development over the course of several years. Just as important, we rarely get to see how treatment affects the quality of a child's life as he or she matures" (Fujiki & Brinton, 2005, p. 337).

This chapter will provide suggestions on the implementation of intervention strategies based on as many best practices—or "evidence-based practices," as the term is often used today—as possible. This concept, which originated in the field of medicine, has gained importance in the field of speech-language pathology as well as in other health-related fields (Johnson, 2006). "The term evidence-based practice refers to an approach in which current, high-quality research evidence is integrated with practitioner expertise and client preferences and values into the process of making clinical decisions" (ASHA, 2005c). The committee that wrote this statement mentions several areas that are important for SLPs to consider: the recognition of the needs and values of individuals and their families; the identification of the most informative and cost-effective diagnostic and screening tools; the evaluation of the quality of diagnostic evidence (the committee suggests that SLPs supplement their knowledge and conclusions by consulting sources such as textbooks, journal articles, continuing education offerings, newsletters, and Web-based resources); and the monitoring and incorporation of new, high-quality research findings into the clinical practice. In her tutorial, Johnson (2006) describes specific steps that can be taken to attain some of the goals presented above: (1) posing an answerable question that arises as a result of working with a client; (2) locating diagnostic and other relevant information by accessing several electronic databases; and (3) searching for and examining the results of research studies on the particular topic. Following this search, the clinician needs to judge the quality of the collected information and determine how it applies to the particular client and the context. The process is quite complex and demands the collaboration of researchers and educational professionals. For more details, the reader is referred to Johnson's tutorial (2006), which also gives detailed references.

A large portion of this chapter will be devoted to the description of specific strategies that can be applied to improve the performance in language and academic areas of ELL students with LLD. The topic of intervention in educational and home settings will be covered in the section of the chapter that discusses issues related to language choice.

Speech-language pathologists (SLPs) encounter daily dilemmas regarding the best approaches for counseling parents and families on language choice and on the ways parents can enhance their children's language and communication abilities and academic performance—even when the parents and families do not speak English well. More longitudinal studies are needed to document the best practices for teaching ELL students who have a variety of speech, language, and communication challenges. In the meantime, however, there is enough evidence showing that strategies that have proved to be successful in instructing ELL students without disabilities can be applied to those students who have a language-learning disability. Difficulty in following up the progress of ELL students with LLD is one of the greatest barriers to documenting the effectiveness of strategies. Students, and particularly ELL students, move from school to school and district to district. Practices vary from setting to setting, and the very same strategies that were successful in one classroom are not necessarily used by the next school. More coordination in the implementation of effective strategies within schools, districts, and regions would alleviate this problem.

The general trend is a paradigm shift from reductionistic to constructivistic teaching, and this has resulted in the support of strategies that emphasize the "whole" instead of the "parts"—while focusing on language use rather than form alone. This means finding a balance between working on communication and emphasizing correct use of grammatical or syntactical structures. For example, to enhance correct production of the past tense, the SLP may discuss with the student what he or she did before coming to school, or what the student did the day before, instead of "drilling" the past tense of regular and irregular verbs by using picture cards. In Chapter 3 we discussed several strategies for facilitating the language development of students learning another language. Those same strategies can be implemented with second-language learners who are experiencing difficulty acquiring not only a second language, but also their own language, and quite often, also experiencing academic problems.

STRATEGIES FOR MEETING THE NEEDS OF CLD STUDENTS WITH VARIOUS LANGUAGE-LEARNING DISABILITIES (LLD)

In planning an intervention program for CLD students with LLD, it is essential to focus on the language skills that all students need to succeed in school—and to acknowledge what each learner brings to the learning experience. In addition, the focus should be much more on process rather than on outcomes alone. In the past, there was too much emphasis on methods; there was little emphasis on the process of how students learn and spend time (Whitmire, 2005). Therefore, it is important to design strategies that the student can implement and apply to situations that are relevant to them. In addition, oral and written language intervention should not be conducted separately, and there is a need for language intervention to be functional and contextually based (Fujiki & Brinton, 2005).

A constructivistic approach to learning and teaching (as opposed to a reductionistic approach) encourages emphasis on a whole task rather than on its individual parts. For example, the clinician begins with a whole task (e.g., communication events such as conversing, sharing books, writing letters, negotiating task completions), singles out specific skills (the parts) for development, and then returns the skills to the whole in their modified (e.g., improved or corrected) form. In order to focus on the whole, activities should be situated in a cultural, curriculum-based, and/or communicative context. A constructivistic approach takes into account the students' background knowledge, and the teacher uses inquiry activities and dialogue with students.

The reductionistic approach is unsupported by language acquisition and development research. This approach neglects to take into account the interaction patterns occurring in the child's learning environment. Furthermore, it mirrors the medical model in which one member of a pair intends to "fix" another, a model that often prevents the development of authentic, meaning-centered environments (Herrera & Murray, 2005; Nieto, 2004). The characteristics of the reductionistic approach are contrasted with the holistic/constructivistic approach in Figure 7-1.

As noted in the figure, the more traditional approach focuses on teaching from parts to the whole with an emphasis on learning skills. The approach is more teacher directed, the student is pulled out of the environment, and general strategies focus on right and wrong responses. In contrast, a more constructivistic approach focuses on the whole-part-whole relationship, is interactive in nature, emphasizes collaboration with other professionals, and has goals that relate to functional and divergent responses and that focus on the student's strength. In particular, speech and language goals must be tied to the curriculum because "Performance goals must be the same as the state's definition of adequate yearly progress, including the state's objectives for the progress of children with disabilities, as required under NCLB" (IDEA 2004, Sec 612a, 15).

Effective Strategies

Many of the activities implemented in interactive classrooms for regular education students can be adapted for use with any student, whether monolingual or bilingual. They can also be applied when working with those students with LLD. These activities' adaptability to special education is made possible not necessarily by breaking the tasks down, but by

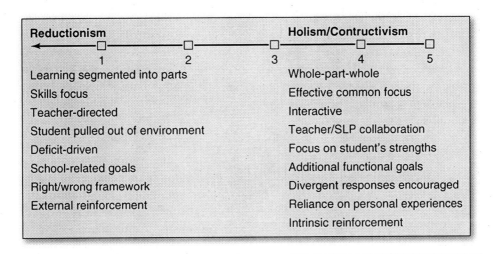

FIGURE 7-1 *Continuum Framework for Activity Design.* (Adapted from Beaumont, 1992.)

providing the instructional support necessary for the students' active involvement. Although the literature has not spelled out the specific outcomes of teaching CLD students with LLD, it is evident that "good teaching" is beneficial to all, including mainstream students. The difference between teaching CLD students with LLD and teaching those without might have to do with how quickly effective teaching strategies are acquired, how effectively those strategies are implemented in appropriate contexts, and how much of the teaching utilizes language repetitions in the classroom.

Crockett (2004) describes five effective principles for promoting positive learning not only for students with language-learning disabilities, but also for higher-achieving students. These principles were originally proposed by Vaughn, Gersten, and Chard (2000):

1. Teachers should identify the elements that need to be learned and demonstrate them with examples.

2. Students need to be taught specific strategies and have multiple opportunities to apply those strategies. Having students participate in small groups where they may interact as tutors on occasions is very beneficial. The small-group interactions enable teachers and students to offer ongoing feedback.

3. Activities presented to students should be meaningful and relevant.

4. Students with reading and writing difficulties benefit from explicit instruction in word decoding and spelling.

5. Regular students do benefit from the effective instruction provided to students with language-learning disabilities. (Crockett, 2004, pp. 464–465)

According to Crockett, Vaughn et al. (2000) pointed out "that none of these instructional principles is revolutionary, and that each holds promise for higher-achieving students. Nonetheless, despite the evidence supporting their effectiveness for a wide range of learners, 'these principles are too rarely implemented in classroom'" (Crockett, 2004, p. 111). These comments serve to remind all involved in education that the evidence for effective teaching does exist, and it is the responsibility of the teaching staff to implement those practices.

Beaumont (1992) described some strategies that can enable a student to travel toward the world of independent learning. These strategies have subsequently been discussed by other researchers (Echevarría, Vogt, & Short, 2004; Farr & Richardson Bruna, 2005; Herrera & Murray, 2005), although they may have been presented in a slightly different form. The strategies are listed below, in no particular order (note that the SLP will need to adjust the activities to the age, abilities, and specific challenges of the student):

- Use authentic, purposeful communication interactions to teach language skills. (If the goal is to increase the ability to sequence, instead of using picture cards to demonstrate the meaning of "first," "second," "third," and "end," involve students in talking about what they did the day or the weekend before. This emphasizes the very same concepts.)

- Plan activities that use whole texts, themes, events, and experiences. (If the goal is to improve the use of regular and irregular verbs in written form, instead of filling in the blank with the appropriate verb form, students can dictate or write a letter to their parents about what they did in class that day.)

- Incorporate students' home/community communication events into activities. (Before discussing a given topic, begin by asking students to share what they already know about the topic.)

- Connect intervention activities to a larger curriculum context. (Put students in small groups and ask them to rehearse their oral presentation of a given topic using flash cards. This prepares them to be able to deliver the same presentation to the entire class. Refer to Table 6-1 for a sample of the curriculum for various grades.)

- During activities, link oral and written language as much as possible. (While discussing a given topic, write down main ideas using a graphic organizer.)

- Create an environment conducive to a wider range of responses. (After reading a short paragraph, ask students to predict what might happen next and write those responses on the board.)

- Integrate form, content, and use in activities within specific categories when possible. (While practicing the pronunciation of a certain sound, write the words that contain the sound on the board, create a short sentence that uses the words, and use the sentence in a hands-on activity. For example, if the sound is the correct pronunciation of /p/, practice words like "pear," "apple," "peach," "plum," "pineapple," "potato," "peas," "grape," etc., and use real fruits and vegetables or plastic replications of those items as props. Then place the items in a basket and have the student practice using the words in a short phrase such as: "I want a....")

- Develop specific strategies the student can apply as often as possible.

  (a) Connect the current task to something the student already knows.

  (b) Direct the student's attention to salient features of the task.

  (c) Use questioning techniques that lead to problem-solving strategies.

  (d) Demonstrate effective *strategies* (as opposed to teaching *skills*, which are not the same thing).

(e) Model mnemonic devices.

(f) Follow the student's cues to know when to intervene and to ultimately transfer the control to the student.

In summary, plan intervention around the goal of effective communication and learning.

The role of the SLP is to be a mediator of the learning process; this role is based on the "intention to transcend the immediate teaching situation" (Wiig, Larson, & Olson, 2003). This teaching and learning event is based on Feurstein's (1980) work on learning modifiability. Wiig et al. (2003) give a powerful illustration of this point: "Simply saying, 'Close the door' does not mediate. But if you say, 'Please close the door because there's a strong draft in the hallway, and I'm afraid the wind might ruin our art projects,' then you have established a reason for closing the door that goes beyond the immediate situation. You have established a relationship between closing the door and preventing a problem (destruction of art projects) and have modeled how to anticipate predictable mistakes" (Larson & McKinley, 2003, p. 345).

The types of activities that are the most helpful for enhancing such teaching strategies were reviewed in greater detail in previous chapters; for convenience, they are summarized here:

1. Thematic approaches enable the student to focus on one content area but from multiple perspectives.

2. Sociodramatic play is an effective way to work on pragmatics (i.e., the student can make requests, use specific terms for specific contexts, and practice working on repairing communication breakdowns).

3. Narratives reinforce verbal specificity, sequencing, language repair, story structure, and cause-effect constructions.

4. Using predictable texts (such as songs, poems, and chants) provides recognizable patterns (which access the student's background knowledge) and language support for listening and comprehension tasks.

5. Visual organizers/aids are very helpful for enabling students to understand word meanings and associations, interpret text titles, analyze stories, understand the cultural features of communication, remember events, and successfully make decisions about answer options (Wiig & Wilson, 2000).

6. Cooperative activities promote listening, negotiation, the asking of questions, language clarification, role-playing, planning, persuasion, and the recording of each of the student's contributions toward the completion of a given assignment.

Applications

Only those students who have an identified language disorder in the primary language should be included in the SLP's caseload. If the student's language difficulty reflects a second-language acquisition pattern rather than a disorder, the student should receive services from other resource personnel, such as an English as a Second Language (ESL) specialist, language development specialist, and/or the classroom teacher.

An Individual Educational Plan (IEP) is the primary tool in special education for organizing and focusing instruction. It is also a vehicle for communicating with parents about their child's progress in a given program. The IEP reflects the SLP's underlying beliefs regarding a number of central issues: the nature of successful instruction, the critical components of the language processes, and the relationship of expectation to performance. Any shifts of focus in theory and practice should be reflected in the IEP plan. The first phase of the IEP consists of matching the student's educational needs with strategies that will enable him or her to perform as successfully as possible in the classroom. The second phase is to decide where and who will assist in implementing the program.

To illustrate these two processes, four scenarios are presented next. These scenarios portray students at four different grade levels (Grades 3, 6, 8, and 12) who have language comprehension/processing difficulties and/or expressive language difficulties that are reflected in the oral and written language areas. In the first phase, described in Boxes 7-1 through 7-4, there are activities that the SLP can carry out to meet the language and learning needs of students in the areas of language arts, reading, and writing. Each box examines areas of concern for a student enrolled in a given grade level—as well as some of the standards for that grade and activities that can be implemented using various activity design strategies. It is important to recognize that other strategies than simply the ones mentioned for each case may also be applicable. When implementing the different activities, it is a good idea for the SLP to have a rationale for using the particular activity. The SLP should also help increase the students' awareness of the strategies used.

The strategies outlined need to be connected to the curricular standards for each grade. Each case uses the Language Arts Standards listed in the California State Department of Education Web site: http://www.cde.ca.gov/index.asp. Other standards that apply to ELL students with various levels of proficiency in English can also be found. Specific standards for each state may be found by consulting the respective state's Department of Education Web site.

The second phase in the implementation process consists of formulating suggestions on how to structure the intervention process to benefit the student. In this phase, the roles of the SLP, the classroom teacher(s), and parents are described. This phase is discussed further in the "Service Delivery" section of this chapter, and is illustrated in Boxes 7-7 through 7-10.

BOX 7-1

A Third-Grade CLD Student with Language Processing/Comprehension Challenges and/or Expressive Language Challenges

The curriculum standards for this grade level require that the student perform in the following ways:

Standards for Comprehension

- Retell, paraphrase, and explain what a speaker has said.

- Connect and relate prior experiences, insights, and ideas to those of a speaker.

- Respond to questions with appropriate elaboration.

- Identify the musical elements of literary language (e.g., rhymes, repeated sounds, instances of onomatopoeia).

Activities

- The SLP can preview a lesson using a visual organizer to highlight key concepts and vocabulary that will be heard during the lesson in the classroom. After the student participates in the classroom lesson, the SLP can use the same visual organizer to help the student review what was learned.

- Planets are one of the science topics in third grade. Have the student ask his or her parents or an older sibling to provide names of planets as well as information on them (if the parents don't remember, ask that they seek the information on the Internet or go with the student to the library). Have the student list the names and information on a piece of paper his or her brings to the therapy room. Every student in the classroom shares what was learned from their research. The SLP writes key ideas on the board. A discussion takes place about the similarities of and differences between the ideas that each student has contributed about the topic.

- Have the student select a poem or passage from a book. Ask the student to clap each time he or she hears a word that rhymes with a previously designated "word of the day." For example, if the word is *bear*, the student will clap if the selection includes words that sound the same even though their spelling might be different. For example, the student should clap when hearing *chair* or *there/their*.

Strategies Used

- Use authentic, purposeful communication interactions to teach language skills.

- Plan activities that use whole texts, themes, events, and experiences.

- Connect the current task to something the child already knows.

- Plan intervention around the goal of achieving effective communication and learning.

Standards for Oral Communication

- Organize ideas either chronologically or around major points of information.

- Provide a beginning, middle, and an end, including concrete details that develop a central idea.

- Use clear and specific vocabulary to communicate ideas and establish the tone.

- Clarify and enhance oral presentations through the use of appropriate props (e.g., objects, pictures, charts).

- Read prose and poetry aloud with fluency, rhythm, and pace, using appropriate intonation and vocal patterns to emphasize important passages of the text.

Activities

- After working on planets, each student selects one planet and explores its description and characteristics. Students then organize this information into a presentation that is delivered first to a small group and then to the entire class. The final presentation includes pictures of each planet. The group works on a chart in which the distance of each planet from the moon and sun is recorded.

- Criteria are developed by the group that are used to create a checklist detailing the characteristics of an effective presentation. The criteria serves to remind each student to structure the presentation so that it has

(Continues)

(Continued)

a beginning, a middle, and an end. Each student makes his or her presentation and the group provides constructive criticism.

- Poems that are read in class are brought to the group and practiced.

Strategies Used

- Connect intervention activities to a larger curriculum context.
- Direct the student/client's attention to salient features of the task.
- Choose cooperative activities that stimulate listening, responding, and discussion.

BOX 7-2

A Sixth-Grade ELL Student with Oral/Written Comprehension Challenges

Standards for Reading

Students read and understand grade-level-appropriate material. They describe and connect the essential ideas, arguments, and perspectives of the text by using their knowledge of text structure, organization, and purpose. For example, the selections in the California State Department of Education's (2004) publication entitled *Recommended Literature, Kindergarten through Grade Twelve* illustrate the quality and complexity of the materials to be read by students. In addition, by Grade 8, students are required to read one million words annually on their own, including a good representation of grade-level-appropriate narrative and expository text (e.g., classic and contemporary literature, magazines, newspapers, online information). In Grade 6, students continue to make progress toward this goal.

Standards: Comprehension and Analysis of Grade-Level-Appropriate Texts

- Connect and clarify main ideas by identifying their relationship to other sources and related topics.
- Clarify an understanding of texts by creating outlines, logical notes, summaries, or reports.
- Follow multiple-step instructions for preparing applications (e.g., for a public library card, bank savings account, sports club, league membership).

Activities

- The teacher provides multiple copies of several titles to students. Students select the book they would like to read; the selection is based on "book talks" given by the teacher. These book talks consist of the teacher giving both a synopsis of the book and a tantalizing piece of information about it that might persuade students to choose that book. Students all read the same text and agree on a time to meet to discuss its content. At the meeting, the teacher begins the discussion by asking open-ended questions about students' personal opinions. Based on the ensuing discussion, the teacher instructs the students to reread the text, and suggests further questions for the students to consider during the second reading. The students report their responses in a literature log that they share with the teacher or, if agreed upon, with other students.

After recording their personal responses, the students are ready to study the story structure elements of literature (e.g., characterization, personalization).

- The SLP can assist students in this literacy event by scaffolding their reading with some of the comprehension activities that were previously mentioned. Once the students understand the text well, the teacher can focus on the language demands of the literature discussion. The students need to (1) express opinions, (2) listen to others' opinions, (3) clarify their thoughts, (4) organize their thoughts logically and clearly, (5) use vocabulary that is sufficiently specific, and (6) record their personal responses (Beaumont, 1992).

- Students are asked to go to their local library and bring an application card. The various applications are read and analyzed using a Venn diagram. Similarities and differences are discussed. The same activity can be completed using the Internet.

- The same topic is read in two different newspapers. The content and organization of each article are then compared and contrasted. Students are encouraged to develop criteria for judging each article in terms of text structure, for example, number of paragraphs, average sentence length, and complexity.

Strategies Used

- Link oral and written language as much as possible in various activities.

- Direct the student/client's attention to salient features of the task.

- Use questioning techniques that lead to problem-solving strategies.

BOX 7-3

An Eighth-Grade CLD Student with Written Comprehension Challenges and Weak Written Expression Skills

Standards for Writing

Students write narrative, expository, persuasive, and descriptive essays of at least 500 to 700 words in each genre. Student writing demonstrates a command of Standard American English and the research, organizational, and drafting strategies outlined in Writing Standard 1.0 of the California Standards for the eighth grade. Although the standards list several activities, the two listed below are selected because they may be more conducive to being immediately applied by the student.

Standard Selected: (1) Write Biographies, Autobiographies, Short Stories, or Narratives

(a)   Relate a clear, coherent incident, event, or situation by using well-chosen details.

(b)   Reveal the significance of, or the writer's attitude about, the subject.

(c)   Employ narrative and descriptive strategies (e.g., relevant dialogue, specific action, physical description, background description, comparison or contrast of characters).

(Continues)

(Continued)

Standard Selected: (2) Write Technical Documents

(a) Identify the sequence of activities needed to design a system, operate a tool, or explain the bylaws of an organization.

(b) Include all the factors and variables that need to be considered.

(c) Use formatting techniques (e.g., headings, differing fonts) to aid comprehension.

Activities

- A group of students prepares a questionnaire to use in interviewing a community worker such as a teacher, postal worker, store manager, nurse, police officer, or restaurant server. After completing the interviews, students share their interviews with the group while being videotaped. Each student transcribes the content of the tape as homework and brings the transcription to class. Each student is asked to narrate their transcription, and end the narrative by stating why the jobs are necessary/important. For helping students with rewrites and edits, consider the SCAN approach (Harris & Graham, 1996): (1) Does it make **s**ense? (2) Is it **c**onnected to my central idea? (3) Is **a**ddition of more detail necessary? and (4) Do I **n**otice errors? Many self-monitoring techniques are described in Westby and Clauser (2005).

- Students brainstorm how to design a playground in a park. What is the equipment needed? What safety features are necessary? What is the material used for each piece of equipment? Where should a playground be located in relation to a park? How many pieces of playground equipment should there be? Which pieces should be installed first and why?

- An architect/designer of playgrounds is invited to listen to the students' report and to contribute information.

    This last activity is a group activity where the SLP takes notes and then all ideas are grouped into categories. The final product is a proposal that includes the appropriate format with headings and subheadings.

Strategies Used

- Cooperative activities increase comprehension, student responses, and general discussion skills.

- The activities demonstrate effective *strategies* (as opposed to teaching *skills*, which are not the same thing).

- The activities model mnemonic devices.

BOX 7-4

A 12th-Grade ELL Student with Language Processing/Comprehension Challenges

One of the greatest challenges for students in the upper grades is to acquire strategies for gaining meaning from the written word, mainly from the readings and textbooks assigned in the various classes. The activities illustrated below are based on using classroom material to gain specific strategies that can be implemented across various subjects.

Standards for Social Studies

Students in Grade 12 pursue a deeper understanding of the institutions of American government. They compare the systems of government in the world today and analyze the history and changing interpretations of the Constitution, Bill of Rights, and current state of the legislative, executive, and judiciary branches of government. An emphasis is placed on analyzing the relationship among federal, state, and local governments, with particular attention paid to important historical documents such as the *Federalist Papers*. These standards represent the culmination of civic literacy as students prepare to vote, participate in community activities, and assume the responsibilities of citizenship.

In addition to studying government in Grade 12, students will also master fundamental economic concepts, applying tools (graphs, statistics, equations) from other subject areas to the understanding of the operations and institutions of economic systems. They will also master basic economic principles of micro- and macroeconomics, international economics, comparative economic systems, measurement, and methods. In helping students who have academic discourse problems, the SLP should refer to the curriculum content covered in class. As in all other activities, the SLP takes on the role of guide or facilitator. In the context of these activities, students may take on the role of teacher and generate questions about a reading passage. This type of interaction is based on the principle of reciprocal teaching in which spoken and written discourse are interwoven. Thus, oral discussions take place in the context of reading. Three text comprehension strategies can be particularly helpful to both ELL students and students with language-learning disabilities: (1) the survey text method, (2) metacognitive strategies, and (3) the method of modifying expository text. The first two strategies are implemented by the student; the third, by the teacher or SLP.

In the survey text method, students can do the following:

1. Analyze features of a chapter—such as the title, subtitles, illustrations, and graphic information.

2. Devise questions to be answered by reading such subsections.

3. Read the introductory and concluding paragraphs, as well as the reading review questions that are provided at the end of the chapter.

4. Predict and then list the ideas that will be covered in the chapter. From this list, the teacher and students generate a statement about the main idea or theme of the chapter.

5. Read the chapter to evaluate predictions made.

To develop the cognitive and metacognitive strategies for text comprehension that are used in the cognitive-academic language-learning approach for second-language students, Chamot and O'Malley (1990) propose that students begin by examining the advanced organization of the text. This includes previewing the main idea and concepts of the material by skimming the text. Intermediate steps include activities on organizational planning, selective attention, and self-monitoring. The activities end with a self-evaluation, which includes judging how well learning has taken place. Some cognitive strategies that can be used include referring students to resource materials such as dictionaries, encyclopedias, textbooks, and the Internet; groupings; note taking; having students create summaries of what they have read and learned; having students do tasks that involve the use of deduction/induction; developing the students' use and understanding of imagery; and incorporating auditory representation tasks—that is, having students verbalize what they understand. Diagramming the story is also helpful.

(Continues)

(*Continued*)
Strategies Used (in addition to the ones listed above)

- Link oral and written language as much as possible in various activities.

- Demonstrate effective *strategies* (as opposed to teaching *skills*, which are not the same thing).

- Use questioning techniques that lead to problem-solving strategies.

Developing Metalinguistic Awareness

In addition to teaching specific strategies that students can apply in accessing the curriculum, the SLP's charge is to enhance students' so-called *metalinguistic awareness.* This is the ability to reflect consciously on the nature of language—and this ability is a part of academic performance and school success. In Chapter 6 we discussed the importance of metalinguistic awareness in the development of the comprehension and expression of written language. Recent research by Catts and Kamhi (2005), Hoskyn (2004), and Torgeson, Otaiba and Grek (2005) indicates that a great proportion of students with reading decoding difficulties have difficulties with the phonological awareness that is one component of metalinguistic awareness.

As they interact with oral and written language, students need to be aware of the following language features:

- Language is symbolic. Words stand for something else.

- Language is arbitrary. The same thing can have different names in various languages. The same sound sequence can have different meanings (e.g., *bark*, which means a dog's sound, or *bark*, which means the covering of a tree). Also, a word may sound the same but have different spellings (e.g., *their, there,* and *they're*).

- Language is segmented. Words have boundaries both aurally and in print.

Because the acoustic stream is not naturally segmented, it is sometimes difficult for children to get the idea of "words." Phonological awareness is part of understanding segmentation.

- Language is held together by grammar. Meaning relationships change as word order changes.

- Language is related to logical thinking. Grammar must precede logical reasoning, and language is necessary for planning, prediction, and reflecting.

Although most studies indicate that metalinguistic awareness does not develop until 4 to 5 years of age, this awareness has been observed in younger children (van Kleeck & Schuele, 1987). Two- and 3-year-olds observe and reflect on language by making conscious word substitutions, playing with sounds (e.g., making rhymes and changing initial consonants), and noticing different language systems (as was discussed in Chapter 2). Bialystok (2001) reviewed various studies that compared monolingual and bilingual children who were speaking various languages while they performed various metalinguistic-based tasks. She concluded that, for the most part, in the majority of studies the bilingual group outperformed the monolingual group (see Chapter 2).

Skills that are associated with reading appear at a more mature level of development. The ability to segment the spoken word into its component sounds is a difficult, late-developing skill for most children. Nevertheless, students are frequently asked to apply knowledge of language to reading tasks that require them to identify words with a given beginning sound, make up sentences with specific words, or compare phonological patterns. Often these "prereading" skills are presented before the larger concepts involved in reading have been addressed—concepts such as print awareness, sense of story, and integration of new knowledge with previous experience. As van Kleeck and Schuele (1987) warned twenty years ago: "Academic difficulties in children may result from assuming that children have a rudimentary awareness of phonemic units and from basing instruction on that assumption" (p. 28). Keeping in mind differences across different languages and cultures, the student's exposure to literacy and to various linguistic experiences needs to be considered in order to avoid the erroneous identification of problems.

Observing students also provides some insights into the level of their metalinguistic awareness. The following examples from Beaumont (1992) illustrate poorly or incompletely developed metalinguistic awareness.

- A bilingual Vietnamese kindergarten student named Xuan (Spring) calls his teacher and points out that his name has a cross in it. (Providing the student with both the symbol and the letter and explaining that the "X" in his name looks like a cross should help him understand the distinction between the two.)

- A first-grade child is asked to copy "I like to play with my doll." In order to guide the child, the teacher provides blank lines for each word: ____ ____ ____ ____ ____ ____ ____. Instead, the child copies *Iliketoplaywithmydoll*. (To assist the student in recognizing word boundaries, the SLP or teacher can provide cards that the student can manipulate and then copy on paper.)

These patterns frequently appear in the work of kindergarten and first-grade children who are just beginning to negotiate the complex world of print. If students are unable to understand word boundaries and make connections between sounds and letters, further in-depth assessment of metalinguistic development may be warranted. In collaborating with teachers on reading instruction, the SLP must consider metalinguistic development and suggest alternative methods of instruction for those students whose skills in that area are not yet well developed.

Specific Activities for Developing Metalinguistic Awareness

Drawing students' attention toward words and their features and uses is an effective way to increase the students' metalinguistic awareness. A particularly successful manner of incorporating word consciousness is to prepare a display center (on a bulletin board or table) that has as its heading the following portion of a poem called "Squeeze a Sneeze" (Morrison, 1977):

> You are using words
>
> And words as you know
>
> Will help you out wherever you go.

A frequently changing display can highlight words in a variety of ways. To increase the students' foreign-language awareness, common objects and action words can be displayed on color-coded word cards that identify each object or action in several languages. Also, small flags from various countries can be displayed across the top of a chart. A familiar object common to all the countries where Spanish is spoken can also be shown, and the word used in the various countries for that object can be listed. For example, *bird* in the Mexican dialect is "pájaro"—but the same word is "pichón" in Puerto Rico. *Camión* (bus) is used in Mexico and in other Hispanic countries, but in Puerto Rico the word is *guagua*.

Finally, newspapers, magazines, posters, and other print media from different countries can be displayed. The students can be asked to use this media to find words in different languages that might have the same meaning.

Discerning word boundaries in a second language can be a very difficult task. It may also be a difficult task for many LLD students, particularly when the task is a written one. Adapting patterned texts by substituting words is a simple way to identify and respond to word boundaries. By working with word cards and a pocket chart device, students receive additional visual and tactile reinforcement because they actually see the words moved around. For example, a class could write a poem that includes a certain pattern (Beaumont, 1992). After looking out the window, students could write

Outside I can see some trees

Outside I can see some trees

No matter what the day

Outside I can see some trees

Outside I can see some trees

This is what we can say.

In a subsequent activity, students could provide words like birds, flowers, and clouds to create another poem:

Outside I can see some birds

Outside I can see some birds

No matter what the day

Outside I can see some birds

Outside I can see some birds

This is what we can say.

In the latter example, the last word in each line was substituted. However, other words within the sentence might also be substituted as in:

We can talk outside

We can talk outside

During school recess

We can talk outside

We can talk outside

Without making any mess.

Subsequently, the word *talk* could be substituted for *walk*, *sit*, *laugh*, etc.

Students who need additional practice with English phonology can use the sound they are trying to master (their emerging sound) to alliterate or repeat sounds and poems in the context of a whole text. Books and games that emphasize alliteration are an enjoyable way for students to make both auditory and visual associations with letters.

This activity may be particularly important for those students whose languages do not have certain sounds, as was discussed in Chapter 6. The unfamiliar sounds may need to be reinforced for those students. For example, the /g/ sound may be a problem for students whose first language is Arabic; /v/ is a problem for students whose first language is Arabic, Chinese, or Spanish; and /z/ might present problems for speakers of Chinese, Khmer, Spanish, or Vietnamese. A large number of alphabet books (that may be adapted to students' ages and abilities) are available in English to SLPs. The following books have varying amounts of text and may contain rhyming words: *ABC's Halloween* (Eubank, 2003), *The Alphabet Ttree* (Lionni, 1996), and *Shiver Me Letters* (Sobel, 2006).

Other alphabet books use short sentences or clauses to tell a story, such as this example from *Alphabet Under Construction* (Fleming, 2002): "Mouse airbrushes the A, buttons the B, carves the C,... " Knight's (2006) *Zoophabet ABC* uses constructions like these: "A—Do Alligators eat apples? B—Do Bears blow bubbles? C—Do Camels like to clean?" Here each letter/sound is presented in a phrase that contains other words beginning with the same sound. Still other alphabet books follow the same principle but are written using categories—such as the insects in *Miss Spider's ABC* (Kirk, 2000): "Ants await, Bumblebees blow balloons, and Caterpillars circle Dragonfly decorations."

Another category of alphabet books are pop-up books such as *Animal ABCs* (Roffey, 2004), which includes the following examples: "A—This <u>A</u>lligator eats apples; B—A big bunch of <u>B</u>ats flies by; C—<u>C</u>ats love to curl up and get cozy." *Alpha Bugs* (Carter, 1994), another pop-up book, includes sentences such as "A is for the agile A-to-Z Alphabet Bug, B is for those boogie-woogie Bubble Bugs, and C is for those not-so-cuddly Cactus Bugs."

In another category of alphabet books the reader is introduced to phonemic sounds such as those in the classic *Dr. Seuss' ABC—An Amazing Alphabet Book* (Dr. Seuss' Enterprises, 1963). For example, "BIG A, little a, what begins with A? Aunt Annie's alligator, A...a...A; BIG B, little b, what begins with B? Barber, baby bubbles, and a bumble bee; BIG C, little c, what begins with C? Camel on the ceiling, C... c...C." Parents who speak another language can be encouraged to make an alphabet book using letters and sounds from their own language. This activity will enhance the child's awareness of the two languages and the languages' similarities and differences.

Alphabet books in Spanish are much more limited in number and variety. Examples include bilingual versions such as Tabor's (1992) *Albertina Anda Arriba—El Abecedario* ("Albertina Walks Up—The Alphabet Book") that gives a short sentence for each letter in addition to a short poem. There is an illustration for each letter with the English translation appearing next to the Spanish text. A more recent bilingual alphabet book by Flor-Ada and Zubizarreta (2001), *Gathering the Sun*, includes poems in Spanish for each letter of the alphabet; each poem is translated into English and the theme of each poem is associated with the life of the farm worker. An earlier alphabet book written by Flor Ada & Escrivá (1990), *Abecedario de Los Animales* ("The ABC of Animals"), includes the letter followed by words that begin with that sound and also includes a short poem in Spanish only. An example follows (with a direct translation in English, for clarity):

La B. La B es la segunda letra.	(B. B is the second letter.)
Con ella dices botón, bata, bate, bota, bote, y burrito barrigón.	(With that letter you say button, robe, bat, boot, can, and pot-bellied little donkey.)
La B es la segunda letra.	(B is the second letter.)
¡Así sigue la lección!	(That's the way the lesson goes!)

Songs and poems that play with sounds are of great interest to children and employ the powerful extralinguistic cues of rhythm and rhyme to emphasize connections between sounds and symbols. If instruction is available in Spanish, the song "La Mar Estaba Serena" (Orozco, 1988) could be used as a pattern, where all vowels are substituted one at one time:

La mar estaba serena, serena estaba la mar

La mar estaba serena, serena estaba la mar

La mar astaba sarana, sarana astaba la mar

La mar astaba sarana, sarana astaba la mar

Le mer estebe serene, serene estebe le mer

Le mer estebe serene, serene estebe le mer.

The exercise could then continue, with the other Spanish vowels /i/, /o/, and /u/ being substituted in the poem.

A similar song in English is "Apples and Bananas" (Cassidy & Cassidy, 1986), which switches vowel sounds:

I like to eat, eat, eat apples and bananas

I like to ate, ate, ate applas and bananas

I like to ote, ote, ote opplos and bononos.

Syllable awareness, so important to Spanish readers, can be developed and reinforced with the use of songs such as "La Pulga de San José" ("At the Flea Market of San José") (Orozco, 1988):

En la pulga de San José, yo compré una guitarra, tarra, tarra, tarra, la guitarra

At the flea market of San José, I bought a guitar, tar, tar, tar, the guitar

En la pulga de San José, yo compré un clarinete, nete, nete, nete, el clarinete

At the flea market of San José, I bought a clarinet, net, net, net, the clarinet

The use of these activities appear to be very effective in helping bilingual language-learning disabled students comprehend and use sound segmentation and establish sound-symbol relationships (personal observation).

Developing Speech Intelligibility

Caution is necessary in planning an intervention program for a phonological disorder. Before deciding that the student has a problem pronouncing a particular sound or sound combination, the SLP should interview the parents and others who know the student to assess whether the pattern is deviant or reflects dialectal differences (Cole & Taylor, 1990; Washington & Craig, 1992; Yavas & Goldstein, 1998). Examples of specific interventions that address language combinations other than English dialects or Spanish-English are scarce. Goldstein (2004b) proposes to treat phonological difficulties by following three steps:(1) work on correcting true error patterns—such as cluster reduction and unstressed-syllable deletion—that have high occurrences in both languages; (2) follow up with treatment of error patterns that are exhibited in both languages with unequal frequency, such as final-consonant deletion in English and trill errors in Spanish; and (3) treat errors that are exhibited in only one language such as final-consonant devoicing in English (p. 278–279).

Goldstein (2004b) recommends that intervention take place in the two languages, if possible, because gains made in English (the most common language of intervention in the absence of enough bilingual SLPs) are necessary to enhance syntactic development in each language. There is no research to direct the SLP in one direction or another; however, treatment in two languages is preferred because not all remediated processes transfer to the other language. As an example, Holm, Dodd, and Ozonne (1997) report that intervention for a Japanese/English-speaking child receiving therapy in English enabled him to pronounce /s/ in both languages, but not consonant clusters. Whereas the child was able to pronounce clusters in English, this ability did not transfer to Japanese. It could have been that cross-linguistic generalization for the /r/ cluster was achieved because /r/ is a Japanese phoneme, but was not achieved for /l/ clusters because /l/ is pronounced as /r/. Auditory training is one way to remediate phonological problems in English-speaking children (Hodson, 2005). I have followed a technique that is based on the above information and that has been helpful with Spanish-speaking children. Box 7-5 illustrates this technique, which makes use the student's curriculum in intervention planning.

Examples of strategies that SLPs can implement when working with CLD students with LLD were reviewed in the preceding sections. In addition to selecting the most relevant strategies for linking the students' communicative and academic needs to the curriculum, it is important to make decisions regarding the language of instruction, therapy delivery, and program options. Even though the option to provide

---

BOX 7-5

Working on Eliminating Phonological Processes: Cluster Reduction and Syllable Reduction in a Spanish/English-Speaking Kindergarten Child

Beginning in kindergarten and, often, even in preschool—there is an increased emphasis on developing phonemic awareness. Selected standards are listed below.

Standards

- Track auditorily each word in a sentence and each syllable in a word.

- Blend vowel-consonant sounds orally to make words or syllables.

Activities

- After writing the consonant cluster of the day or week—for example /kr/ in the initial position of a word—on the board, children listen to words with that sound, while the SLP points to the words one by one on the board. It is best if the selection includes nouns, verbs, names, and adjectives whenever possible (e.g., *crayon-cross-cream-cry-crown-crawl-Christy-crab*).

- Cards are made with three or four words at a time, and students take turns naming the pictures. Different games can be created—like matching, or making a board with the words. Ask the students to draw a picture, but have only one set of crayons to share between two students. They need to request the crayon by saying, for example, "I need a red crayon, please" or "Give me a yellow crayon." After completing the picture, each child talks about the colors he or she used to complete it (e.g., "I used a yellow crayon to make the sun and a blue crayon to do the sky").

- Implement various activities where the words that complete a sentence include a certain sound pattern, in this case, /kr/clusters (e.g., " I feel sad so I cry" or "The king has a crown").

- Select a literature book with a high word count and identify words that begin with /kr/.

  As students look at the book mentioned above, take the opportunity to review some of the activities that the class often focuses on, such as identifying the elements of a book. Instruct students to look at the cover and note the title, author, and illustrations. See if there are words on the cover and pages that they can recognize that contain the cluster sounds they have been practicing.

(Continues)

(Continued)

Strategies

- Connect intervention activities to a larger curriculum context.

- Link oral and written language as much as possible in various activities.

- Plan intervention around the goal of effective communication and learning.

---

intervention in Spanish or any of the student's primary languages may not be viable due to the very limited numbers of SLPs who can provide services in other languages than English, and though today English is the language of instruction in most settings nationwide, it is nevertheless important to keep in mind that providing intervention in the primary language may be in the best interest of the student.

LANGUAGE CHOICE FOR INTERVENTION: FIRST OR SECOND LANGUAGE?

In this section we review the language of intervention. We begin with the language of intervention in the learning environment, followed by the language of intervention in home settings.

The Instructional/Intervention Setting

One of the SLP's most important decisions is to determine the language of intervention to be used in the school setting and to counsel families on how to best enhance and reinforce that language at home. The dilemma of selecting a language of intervention was more of an issue prior to mandates such as Proposition 227, which passed in California in 1997 (and later in other states like Arizona) that called for education in English only. However, it is still important to consider whether speech and language services may be provided in the student's primary language (most commonly

Spanish), in English, or in both languages. As noted by Kohnert (2004), "In the absence of a coherent, convergent literature addressing the issue of language choice, some well-intended professionals have been forced to make their decisions on the basis of anecdotal evidence or bias" (p. 315). The decision to conduct intervention in one or two languages should carry over beyond the confines of the academic setting. Furthermore, a bilingual intervention program should include the collaboration of SLPs, teachers, and families.

There is no evidence that learning in two languages will create an additional cognitive load to a child who is experiencing language-learning difficulties; that is, if the input is offered in "blocks" of time per person. For example, Kohnert and Bates (2002) found that there was no cognitive-load difference when bilingual subjects aged 5 to 25 had to access different lexical items in a condition where the words were presented in blocks of Spanish or English—and then had to perform the task in a mixed condition where words were switched from one language to the other. However, when the subjects needed to use the words, it was more difficult for them when they had to switch from one language to the other. (It was easier for them when they had to answer consistently in one language or the other.) This indicates that there is no detriment to offering input in a random bilingual condition, but the student will respond best when the languages are separated into blocks. This translates into offering the student certain times where only one language is used. In no instance should anyone think that bilingualism causes a language and learning difficulty, an assumption often made by parents and even professionals. A recent study by Kay-Raining Bird et al. (2005) found that children with Down syndrome growing up in a bilingual environment (English-French) performed on various tests in English as well as a matched sample of monolingual English-speaking children with Down syndrome. Therefore, the children's progress in English was equal to the monolingual group even though they were exposed to another language. The comments made above should apply to other languages as well.

Selecting the primary language for intervention is recommended when:

- The first language continues to be the student's dominant language for most aspects of communication (e.g., when using the language, the student demonstrates a larger vocabulary and a wider knowledge of concepts, uses more complex sentences, and demonstrates greater fluency in various contexts).

- The student's background knowledge and prior experiences have been developed and coded linguistically in the first language.

- The first language reflects the cultural environment in which the student was raised.

- The student may potentially lose the ability to communicate with family members who speak only in the first language (e.g., that ability will be lost if the first language is not enhanced) (Wong-Fillmore, 1991).

Other factors must also be considered— among them the student's age, the availability of SLPs who can offer the intervention in the primary language, and last but not least, the student's language preference. More choices are available when the student comes from a Spanish-speaking background in the United States because there are more SLPs who can offer services in that language, and there are more bilingual programs using the English-Spanish combination despite new mandates to focus on English only. Often CLD students have had inconsistent school experiences because of frequent moves, erratic attendance, or changes in the language of instruction from one year to the next. The SLP should determine the languages in which the student has received instruction and the length of time that the student has received instruction in each language. Students with "checkered" school histories need special attention to ensure that their programs are integrated appropriately.

When a choice of languages is available, the language of instruction to be used in the student's classroom should be carefully considered. A bilingual Spanish-English classroom may not necessarily be the answer for the student who is having difficulties in his or her primary language. Such difficulties may occur if the environment is not conducive to learning (i.e., because there is no structure applied to how the languages are used), or if the teacher's proficiency in Spanish is not sufficient and he or she needs to depend on an instructional assistant. Such a classroom setting may not be as suitable as one where instruction is delivered in English only—if and when instruction is delivered using nonlinguistic cues and consistent comprehensible input.

By observing the student in a number of situations and consulting with the classroom teacher and the family, the SLP should determine whether the student will have formal and informal opportunities for peer interaction in both languages. As previously discussed, second-language learners use a variety of strategies for learning. Some children look to peers to help them. They may be concerned primarily with belonging to a social group and may be highly motivated to acquire the second language. Children who adopt observer strategies may not participate actively in verbal exchanges for some time. It is therefore important to observe the type of input that they are receiving as they go through this learning process.

The attitude of school personnel toward the student's primary language is also very important. If the staff ignores or merely tolerates the first language, it will be difficult for the student to sustain the motivation to use that language. If the staff is bilingual, or monolingual but demonstrates respect and encouragement for the primary language, they will support bilingual students in their efforts to learn in their native language. Similarly, the attitudes of parents and other family members, as well as the family's proficiency in each language, are important.

Competence in the student's language can enable an SLP to support the child's first language and to carry on basic conversation. To instruct the student adequately in the primary language, the SLP should be at least a strong intermediate speaker of the language and have near-fluent pronunciation. The Foreign Service Institute uses the International Language Roundtable (ILR) Scale (a scale ranging from Level 1 to Level 5) to describe proficiency level. For more information, visit the ILR on the Web at http://www.govtilr.org/ILRscale2.htm#3. Box 7-6 describes the characteristics of a speaker at Level 3.

BOX 7-6

Characteristics of a Speaker at Level 3 Using the ILR Scale

Using the ILR Scale, a speaker at Level 3 is able to speak the language with sufficient structural accuracy and vocabulary to participate effectively in most formal and informal conversations covering practical, social, and professional topics. Nevertheless, the individual's limitations generally restrict the professional contexts of language use to matters of shared knowledge and/or international convention. Discourse is cohesive. The individual uses the language acceptably, but with some noticeable imperfections; yet, errors virtually never interfere with understanding and rarely disturb the native speaker. The individual can effectively combine structure and vocabulary to convey his or her meaning accurately. The individual speaks readily and fills pauses suitably. In face-to-face conversation with natives speaking the standard dialect at a normal rate of speech, comprehension is quite complete. Although cultural references, proverbs, and the implications of nuances and idiom may not be fully understood, the individual can easily repair the conversation. Pronunciation may be obviously foreign. Individual sounds are accurate, but stress, intonation, and pitch control may be faulty.

Examples of the individual's linguistic capability at this level include the ability to:
- Discuss particular interests and describe specifics about his or her profession with reasonable ease.

- Use the language as part of normal professional duties such as answering objections, clarifying points, justifying decisions, understanding the essence of challenges, stating and defending policy, conducting meetings, and delivering briefings or other extended and elaborate informative monologues.

- Elicit information and informed opinions from native speakers. Structural inaccuracy is rarely the major cause of misunderstanding. Use of structural devices is flexible and elaborate. Without searching for words or phrases, the individual uses the language clearly and relatively naturally to elaborate concepts freely and make ideas easily understandable to native speakers. Errors occur with low frequency and only in highly complex linguistic structures.

No research has been conducted to date that explores the minimum second-language competence necessary for bilingual SLPs who serve ELL students and clients. However, as a minimum level of linguistic competence, Level 3—as it is described for Foreign Service personnel—should be considered.

The decision about which language to choose for intervention is inevitably tied to decisions about service delivery models. The SLP's proficiency in the student's primary language may determine whether the SLP will service the student directly in that language or will function within the consultation model. However, in no instance should school personnel counsel the family to switch to English if the child's family's level of proficiency in that language is not strong—or if the parents do not feel they can adequately communicate with the child because their English is not well developed. Everyone working with a CLD student should remember that a second language develops better when the linguistic foundation of the first language is strong. For sources that support this statement, readers are referred to Gutiérrez-Clellen (1999) and Krashen (1999).

The Home Setting

One important variable to consider when evaluating and planning programs for a CLD student is the student's family's attitude toward the use of each language. The amount of time that the primary language is used may change depending on each parent's proficiency in one or the two languages. But, for the most part, immigrant parents encourage their children to learn English because they view the process of acquiring the new language as a way to better their children's lives. However, even when the primary language is used at home, it may be lost eventually because of marriage (i.e., a spouse no longer speaks the primary language or did not ever speak that language). (See Chapter 2.)

One of the greatest dilemmas of SLPs is counseling families about when and how to best use their languages in the home setting. Although the student's parents' and extended family's language of communication remains a personal matter, the SLP can suggest reasons for maximizing the use of each language in a bilingual home environment. The following sections discuss scenarios in which (1) both parents are bilingual, (2) only one parent is bilingual, (3) neither parent speaks English, and (4) the parents have only a receptive knowledge of English.

Both Parents Are Bilingual

Parents should be encouraged to express themselves on various topics in the language of their choice. For example, some bilingual parents may feel more at ease explaining events, scolding, or comforting in one language than in the other. A communication breakdown may occur if parents feel pressed to change their language use so that it conforms to the mainstream culture. As a result, children may lose their native language, and the parents will not necessarily acquire the competence to express themselves fully in the second language. To maximize the use of each language, it may be beneficial to communicate in one or the other language when addressing specific topics. For example, English may be used to discuss school and job matters, whereas Spanish, Vietnamese, Mandarin, etc., may be used to express personal feelings. The primary language may be used in a home setting, whereas English may be used for activities outside the home. Ultimately it is the family who must make the choice about how to use each language.

Only One Parent Is Bilingual

The way each language is used may affect family dynamics, especially if the children attend schools where the majority of students are English speaking. Eventually, as they spend more time in school or with English-speaking peers, the children may speak English more fluently than Spanish, Vietnamese, Mandarin, etc. If only one parent speaks English, the children may turn to that parent when they have a problem or need to discuss an issue. However, the other parent who is not fluent in English may therefore lose the ability to communicate with the family. It is important that the bilingual parent maintain a balance by encouraging the children to speak Spanish, Vietnamese, Mandarin, etc., at home as much as possible to allow the participation of the monolingual parent. At the same time, the parent who does not speak English should be encouraged to learn more English to increase his or her receptive—and eventually expressive—language skills. In this manner, the children can maintain their first language and its culture, and the entire family can understand the parent who is not as fluent in English.

Neither Parent Speaks English

It is not advisable for a family to learn to communicate in English at the expense of their primary language. Switching to a language in which the family's skills are weaker may cause a loss of communication between parents and children. Rodríguez (1982) noted that his parents' compliance with a suggestion to switch to English to facilitate his adjustment to school resulted in such a loss of communication. The parents' English was never proficient enough to enable them to express more complex ideas. Similarly, Rodriguez's Spanish could never develop because of a lack of practice in the language. Cummins (2000) indicated that, when they use their native language naturally, parents increase their children's pride in their own culture. In his early works, Cummins (1981) cited cases in which parents had switched to the majority language to help their children with language and learning problems. Those children whose parents maintained their native language eventually performed better than did those whose parents tried to use the second language (Bhatnagar, 1980; Chesarek, 1981). The parents who only used the second language were unable to express more complex ideas and were not good language models for their children. This finding corroborates the theory of "common underlying proficiency" (Cummins, 1981). Two languages have common underlying characteristics, such as the ability to express similar concepts and functions, even though the surface structures (words and word order) are different. In other words, skills are transferable across languages.

Parents Have a Receptive Knowledge of English Only

If the children speak English and the parents answer in the home/primary language, they reinforce in Spanish, Vietnamese, Mandarin, etc., what the children have said—which will enable the children to preserve and expand their understanding of their home language. When the children have more natural opportunities to use their primary language, their expressive abilities will develop faster and more completely. As an example, one child who had been exposed to French since birth could understand the language, but would answer using English only. After attending a three-hour immersion program in French for three weeks at age 6, she began using more complete and longer sentences in the French language. Thus, when given the time, opportunity, and motivation, children who have a good understanding of one language and a passive understanding of a second language can develop expressive language in the second language more quickly. This process may take longer for students with language-learning disabilities. However, eventually these students may develop a greater command of their home language.

More than twenty years ago, Cummins (1984) made the following suggestions, which are applicable even today: (1) "Never advise minority parents to switch to English at home. This may lower the quality of interaction between parents and children," and (2) "Communicate to minority children that bilingualism is a special achievement to be valued and developed" (p. 267). It may be difficult for educators to follow these suggestions, but doing so not only will help preserve the identity of the persons and their communication with their families, but will also emphasize the value of bilingualism.

PREFERRED SERVICE DELIVERY MODELS

In previous sections we discussed the role played by families in the enhancement of their children's language skills in the home environment. In this section we will discuss various models for fostering the learning of ELL students with language-learning disabilities.

School-Based Programs

The language used during intervention will depend on the SLP's proficiency in the student's primary language as well as on whether the student is enrolled in a bilingual program that is being implemented in a given district. As previously mentioned, bilingual programs are rare today due to regulations that demand that English be used as the primary language of instruction.

When a bilingual SLP is available, instruction in the primary language may take place during the specific intervention session (even if there is no bilingual language instruction in the regular classroom) in order to facilitate the development of concepts and to communicate with the student's family. SLPs who are not proficient in the student's language can follow up the session by providing other direct services to the student in English or consultation services to the teachers. Instruction may be provided in either a self-contained classroom or on an "in-class–pull-out" basis. When the SLP does not speak the students' language, working with a bilingual trained assistant may also be an option. In a consultative model, the SLP provides suggestions to the regular and/or special education teacher.

Family Support

Working with parents and significant others of the student's personal community should be an important goal for SLPs, whether or not they are fluent in the student's primary language. Parents need to know that they too are teachers of their children. They need to know that using their primary language at home is not detrimental to their children's linguistic and educational progress. Rather than focus on the language itself, they need to assist their children in expanding the variety of uses for the language, depending on their children's school needs. To develop their children's understanding of story structure, not only can parents read with their children, but they can also watch TV with them and discuss what they see. For example, they can comment on the positive or negative aspects of commercials for products or programs. Another approach is to discuss activities that they do together as a family, such as shopping, visiting the post office or bank, or going to the park. In fact, parents should expose their children to as many activities as possible in order to familiarize them with varying types of discourse exchanges.

Reading books and magazines expands the children's exposure to written language. Visiting the library and taking out books is an activity that will engage both parents and children. If the parents' literacy is limited in English and even in their primary language, looking at wordless books—or at pictures in books—and talking about them is an option. If students are older and have some reading ability, they can read to their parents. In turn, parents can ask their children to explain the meaning of what they are reading. The participation of other family members, such as older siblings or extended family members, is also very helpful.

Parents should show interest in what their children have done in school by asking questions about their activities. A set time should be allocated for the children to complete their homework, or for a parent and siblings to complete a joint project or to play a game with them. For example, the family can make special decorations for the home for different holidays, or play a universal game like lotto or checkers. Also, the family could prepare a special meal together by planning the menu, shopping for the ingredients, sharing in the cooking, and setting up the table. Parents can also help other parents by creating networks that are facilitated by bilingual personnel or an interpreter.

The role of the SLP is more difficult when the student has a phonological disorder. However, the SLP can work with the student by making an analysis of sounds that are common between the two languages, determining where most errors occur, and having the student practice those. (Refer to the suggestions offered by Goldstein, 2004b, in the phonology section of this chapter.) Subsequently, the SLP can teach those sounds that do not exist in the student's phonological repertoire. It may be necessary to seek the assistance of an aide, community

member, or relative in engaging the student to both produce target sounds and practice in the primary language. Under no circumstances should that person be asked to work with a student without adequate preparation, guidance, or supervision.

In summary, SLPs and school staff should recommend strategies that will empower the parents and the family of CLD students who have language-learning disabilities. Thus, clinicians and universities should collaborate on projects to document the success of various intervention strategies. For example, one or two classes within a district could be designated as models for the implementation of specific programs. Sufficient time and funds must be allocated for these programs, however. There should be a commitment from school administrators, staff, parents, and community to carry out such projects with consultation from university faculty.

Applications

Box 7-7 to Box 7-10 describe the implementation of intervention programs for various grade levels and various curricular goals. However, program implementation may vary depending on the student's strengths and on the severity of the student's difficulties. Although several of the scenarios may occur because some bilingual programs may still be in place—especially in the younger grades—the suggestions in the boxes focus primarily on two situations: (1) the SLP is monolingual or may be bilingual but not in the student's language, or (2) the SLP is bilingual. In addition, the suggestions may vary depending on the parents' and family's linguistic and literacy skills in each language. The scenarios described below are provided to illustrate certain situations, but adaptations will need to be made for each case.

A Third-Grade CLD Student with Language Processing/Comprehension Challenges and/or Expressive Language Challenges

If the SLP is English speaking or not bilingual in the student's language:

- Provide small-group instruction once or twice a week in the therapy room, and another time in the classroom depending on the student's needs.

- Consult with the classroom teacher and model strategies for the entire group; if necessary, do this a couple of times a month.

- Provide tutoring services for the student after school.

A school liaison or interpreter assists in ensuring that parents can follow up. Parents may assist by helping the student practice following instructions, responding to requests, and engaging in conversations. Telling stories, looking at books, and going to the library is helpful, and the activities mentioned earlier in the chapter can also be used. Using English is not as important as enhancing communication. If parents are asked to assist with a science project (e.g., the student is seeking information on planets), the information may be provided in their own language. The student may be able to express some of the information shared at home with the help of a bilingual assistant or interpreter.

If the SLP is bilingual:

- Use the strategy mentioned above with regard to collaborating with the classroom teacher. However, small-group instruction will be in the student's primary language.

- Use the ideas mentioned above with regard to parents, except that the SLP can communicate directly with the family. If the family is literate, a journal can be sent home that describes the activities that were completed at school.

A Sixth-Grade CLD Student with Oral/Written Comprehension Challenges

If the SLP is English speaking or not bilingual in the student's language:

- Work with the student in small groups both in the therapy room and in the classroom.

- Offer to demonstrate some lessons to the entire class and/or participate in small group activities within the classroom that will be beneficial to the LLD student.

- Communicate with parents via a bilingual school liaison or interpreter. Even if parents are not literate in either language, the student can read to the family and parents may ask questions about what is read— even if parents' knowledge of English is limited. Older siblings, friends, and relatives who are more proficient in English can assist in the process.

- Parents can assist by watching a TV program and talking about what might come next, or by making comments about who or what they like about the program.

(Continues)

(Continued)

If the SLP is bilingual:

- Provide small-group instruction once or twice a week in the native language to reinforce concepts and vocabulary and enhance the student's ability to organize ideas.

The other suggestions offered earlier also apply. Because the SLP shares the language of the family, closer contact can be maintained with the family. The importance of nurturing the native language needs to be communicated so that the student may progress as much as possible in both languages. In addition, greater proficiency in the native language will reinforce the student's self-esteem. When the time comes to work on a foreign language, the transition will be smoother. Often students who speak Spanish cease to use this language for various reasons, and are not exposed to the language again in any formal context until they take classes in Spanish at the high-school level.

BOX 7-9

An Eighth-Grade CLD Student with Written Comprehension Challenges and Weak Written Expression Skills

If the SLP is English-speaking or not bilingual in the student's language:

- The service delivery model for the older student will be different. Usually, older students are very conscious of being "pulled out"; therefore the best way to serve these students is during a special period designated as Resource or Special Skills class. Collaboration with the resource specialist/reading specialist is important.

- The delivery model could be one where the SLP takes charge of a group of students who are working on different aspects of the same project, such as constructing interviews, or transcribing a presentation. During this time, the SLP works on developing metacognitive skills: "What have we done? Why have we done it? Where do we go from here …?"

- The SLP works both as the direct service provider who participates with the student in a small group, and as a consultant who visits with teachers in order to ensure that the student is receiving the appropriate accommodations in the classroom.

- The role of the parents is to offer the student support by providing time and a place to do homework—and by encouraging the student to try his or her best. Parents should follow up with school staff on the student's progress. The assistance of a bilingual school liaison or interpreter will be important.

If the SLP is bilingual:

- Service delivery would be similar to the one outlined above. The advantage for the student is that the SLP, with his or her knowledge of the native language, may provide a bridge by enhancing the student's comprehension of the academic content and by emphasizing analogies and differences between the reading/spelling of different words across the two languages. Research has demonstrated that by making bilingual students aware of similarities and differences between their two languages, they become more aware of the linguistic characteristics of a second language. (See Gutiérrez-Clellen, 1999, for further details.)

- The bilingual SLP can also point out similarities and differences in text formats such as narratives, expository text, or poems. Recipes written in different languages can be discussed or demonstrated.

- As the bilingual SLP communicates directly with the family, he or she can involve the student in the process.

BOX 7-10

A 12th-Grade ELL Student with Language Processing/Comprehension Challenges

If the SLP is English speaking or not bilingual in the student's language:
- The same suggestions made above and in previous sections for students attending upper middle school and high school will apply. As mentioned earlier, older students are more conscious about being "pulled out"; therefore, the best way to serve these students is during a special period designated as a Resource or Special Skills class. Collaboration with the resource specialist/reading specialist is important.

- The delivery model could be one where the SLP takes charge of a group of students who are working on different aspects of the same project (for example, a social studies project). During this time, the SLP has students continue to work on tasks such as analyzing the layout of a chapter, finding the chapter headings, and having discussions about what may be included in each section of the chapter.

- Tapping into the student's prior knowledge is important for helping the student link what he or she knows with what is written in a text.

- As would also be true for eighth-graders, the role of the parents is to offer the student support by providing a time and a place to do homework—and by encouraging the student to try his or her best. Also, realistic plans should be made (for after graduation) by matching the student's interests and skills to available educational programs or work settings. Involving the parent in the process may be very helpful; this can be accomplished with the assistance of a counselor. If necessary, a bilingual school liaison or interpreter should be involved as well.

If the SLP is bilingual:
- Service delivery would be similar to the suggestions listed in Box 7-9. The advantage for the student is that the SLP, with his or her knowledge of the native language, may provide a bridge between the student's current program content, by emphasizing analogies and differences between the reading/spelling of different words across the two languages (see Gutiérrez-Clellen, 1999).

- The bilingual SLP can also point out similarities and differences in text formats such as narratives, expository text, or poems. Recipes in different languages can be discussed or demonstrated.

- While making plans for after the student's graduation, the bilingual SLP can communicate directly with the family and involve the student in the process.

SUMMARY

This chapter offered suggestions for the implementation of intervention strategies that are based on "best practices"—or "evidence-based practices," as the term is used today. A large portion of the chapter was devoted to the delineation of those strategies in conjunction with the demands of the student's specific curriculum. Another section of the chapter was devoted to the discussion of language choice for intervention in educational and home settings. SLPs encounter daily dilemmas regarding the best approaches for counseling parents and families both on language choice and on the ways parents can enhance their children's language and communication abilities and academic performance—even when the parents do not speak English well. More longitudinal studies are needed to document the best teaching strategies to use for ELL students without disabilities that could be applied to those who are LLD. Difficulty in follow-up is one the greatest barriers. Students, particularly ELL students, move from school to school and district to district. Practices vary from setting to setting, and the very same strategies that were successful in one classroom may not necessarily be used in the next one. More coordination in the implementation of effective strategies within schools, districts, and regions would alleviate this problem.

OUR CLIENTS

Eric, Ana, Jack, Grace, and Leonardo

Detailed reports on Eric, Ana, and Jack were included in Chapter 6. School programs and interventions for each of these three students—and suggestions for their parents—are presented next.

Eric

Eric's parents have reviewed various options with the preschool SLP, who has recommended a biweekly 90-minute special program that will develop Eric's language and communication skills. Eric's regular preschool program will continue for the rest of each week, as usual. All intervention will need to be in English, because there are no bilingual Vietnamese-speaking SLPs or interpreters available. In addition, it was felt that Eric had some basis in the English language upon which to build his language skills. However, it was recommended that in no instance should educators encourage Eric's parents to switch to English. For most of his life, Eric has heard Vietnamese and interacted in Vietnamese with his family, and this is the language of communication he and his family feel most comfortable with. What Eric will learn in one language will transfer to the other language—but only if and when both languages continue to be nurtured. Eric will not learn English faster if he practices it at home. Moreover, as Eric progresses, he will have the benefit of being bilingual.

Suggested Speech and Language Goals

- Being able to respond to "who," "what," and "where," questions during play and while being read a story (being able to point to and/or verbalize the answer)

- Being able to follow two-step directions (for example, "put the man in the car and push the truck")

- Being able to demonstrate increasing comprehension and use of some basic concepts such as prepositions, quantifiers, comparatives, and superlatives ("under," "over"; "one," "two," "three"; "more," "most," "the rest," etc.)

- Being able to expand his utterances and rephrase those that may not be clearly stated.

Eric's parents should participate in a parent support program that can address any concerns they may have. The parent support program can also provide suggestions for further activities at home.

Suggestions for Home

- Eric's parents should continue interacting in Vietnamese with him. Using Vietnamese will not prevent Eric from acquiring more communication skills or arrest his language development in English. If his parents wish to interact with him English, they may try doing so at specific times. (Consistency in language use—i.e., keeping the language linked to a specific person or persons and/or situation—has been found to be one of the best strategies for bringing up children bilingually.)

- Eric's parents should provide a predictable schedule. It is useful to create some pictures and icons that show what Eric has already finished and what is coming up next.

- Eric's parents should praise him for what he does well and be consistent in their expectations.

- When Eric responds with a short phrase, his parents should try to expand on what he said.

- During play, Eric's parents should continue commenting on what he and they are doing, and ask him to follow what they are doing. This will enhance his ability to reciprocate actions.

- Eric's parents should ask him to help them around the house as a way to provide him the opportunity to practice his ability to follow directions. For example, before supper, they could ask him to give them "two little spoons [instead of big ones] and one fork." While folding the laundry, they could ask Eric to: "give us the two red socks and the green shirt."

- His parents should play games with him—like lotto or other board games where he can practice taking turns.

Ana

Suggested School Program

Because Ana is so far behind in basic reading, a special class (a smaller group of students) is recommended for part of her school day to address areas of phonological processing, reading decoding, reading fluency, and comprehension. Topics that relate to the regular curriculum could be discussed in small groups using videos and books that contain high-interest/low-interest vocabulary. Using visual organizers, checking for comprehension and integration of comprehension into speaking, and writing (as much as possible)—will assist in enhancing her oral and written skills. The suggested language of intervention is English because it has been the language of instruction since she began school.

Ana should be integrated into her regular classroom for subjects where reading and writing can be integrated into hands-on activities such as science and art. The SLP can review and discuss key words and concepts that will be the focus of her science class.

Suggestions for Home

- Her parents should continue to follow up on Ana's progress in school.

- To enhance Ana's practice in verbalizing ideas, her parents should encourage dialogue about what she sees on TV shows and/or the news.

- Her parents should continue going to the library and continue reading to Ana in Spanish. They should listen to her read in English. They should ask her to explain what she has read using her own words.

- Ana's parents should encourage the use of Spanish as a way to promote her bilingual skills. Her bilingualism is an asset that should be maintained as much as possible in order to promote her and her community's appreciation for the Spanish language and culture.

(Continues)

(Continued)

Jack

Suggested School Program

The best program for Jack will be one where he can receive more individual attention.

- Services in a Resource room can provide both academic support and support from Jack's other teachers as they follow up on his progress. This is a class where Jack can learn various strategies for listening, taking notes, reading a book chapter with comprehension, writing an essay, giving effective oral presentations, and asking clarification questions. Using the curriculum from some of his classes would be one of the most effective ways to teach him those strategies.

- The team could work on some of the standards that are key to success in improving performance on any subject. (The following examples are taken from the seventh-grade California Standards for English Language Arts. The interested reader can find them on the Web at: http://www.cde.ca.gov/ci/rl/cf/index.asp.)

  - Understand and analyze the differences in structure and purpose between various categories of informational materials (e.g., textbooks, newspapers, instructional manuals, signs).

  - Use strategies of note taking, outlining, and summarizing to impose structure on composition drafts.

  - Deliver focused, coherent presentations that convey ideas clearly and relate to the background and interests of the audience. Students evaluate the content of oral communication.

- The SLP should ensure that teachers are made aware of Jack's learning needs. Adapting lectures and activities is a helpful way to enhance his learning.

- Jack should be encouraged to maximize computer use in order to do research for projects and write essays both at school and at home.

- The SLP should have Jack keep a daily log in which he will keep track of his homework assignments and check that he has completed them.

Suggestions for Jack's Grandmother

- She should insist that Jack complete his homework before he is allowed to talk on the phone with friends. (She could reward him by enabling him to talk on the phone for as many minutes as he has spent completing his homework.)

- She could encourage Jack to read with her on topics of common interest.

- She could consult the local library in order to obtain titles that would be of interest to Jack.

- She could enhance Jack's expressive skills by discussing with him the main ideas of TV programs or movies.

FURTHER READINGS

Farr. B., & Quintanar-Sarellana, R. (2005). Effective instructional strategies for students learning a second language or with other language differences. In E. Trumbull & B. Farr (Eds.), *Language and learning: What teachers need to know* (pp. 215–267). Norwood, MA: Christopher Gordon.

Herrell, A. (2000). *Fifty strategies for teaching English-language learners*. Upper Saddle River, NJ: Merrill.

Wiig, E. H., Larson, V., & Olson, J. (2005). *S-Maps: Rubrics for curriculum-based assessment and intervention*. Eau Claire, WI: Thinking Publications.

CHAPTER 8

CLD/ADULT POPULATIONS: ASSESSMENT AND INTERVENTION ISSUES

"With the increasing number of older Americans and the number of bilingual and bicultural individuals living in the United States and in many parts of the world, it is time that we also focus on the CLD adult populations." (Author)

CHAPTER OUTLINE

Note: In this chapter, the terms "client" and "patient" will be used interchangeably, as will the terms "SLP" and "Clinician."

INTRODUCTION

Speech and language services delivered to older populations are different from services provided to younger populations for many reasons. Adults have more life experiences and usually more formal education. They have specialized knowledge, and this population may represent a wider range of ages—anywhere from the early 20s to 90+. Most speech and language impairments occurring within that age span result from acquired neurological disorders caused by accidents such as traumatic brain injury. Impairments occurring at more advanced ages also often result from decreased hearing, stroke, memory difficulties, or other illnesses that are more prevalent in older populations (65 and over). Services rendered to this population are primarily available in hospitals, rehabilitation centers, and clinics—instead of at school-based locations.

CHARACTERISTICS OF OLDER CLD POPULATIONS

In this section, major characteristics of older CLD populations will be discussed; these include population percentages, education and employment, and health issues.

Percentages of Older Adults

In 2000, one in eight Americans were 65 years old or older. The over-65 population in the United States was 12% (as compared with 15% for European countries and as much as 19% for Italy and Japan). The approximate numbers were 30 million white, 2.7 million black, 1.5 million Hispanic, 615,000 Asian-American and Pacific Islander, and 134,000 Native American, Eskimo, and Aleut. By 2025, the number of Americans 65 years old or older will increase to one in six individuals (U.S. Census Bureau, 2000). The number of older Hispanics, Asian-Americans, and Pacific Islanders will triple within the next 50 years, whereas the number of blacks, Native Americans, and Alaskan Natives will increase by only 50%. By 2050, the total percentage of the population 65 and over will decrease to 61.3% for whites, and

increase from 5.7% to 17.5% for Hispanics. The black population will increase from 8.4% to 12%, while the Asian-American/Pacific Islander population will increase from 2.7% to 7.8%. Native Americans and Alaskan Natives will increase from 1.1% to 2.7%. Projections for the various older CLD groups in the United States from 2000 to 2050 are presented in Figure 8-1 (Federal Interagency Forum on Aging-Related Statistics, 2006).

Education and Employment

The education level of older Americans has improved in the last fifty years. In 1950, only 17% of Americans graduated from high school and only 3% obtained a bachelor's degree. By 2003, a significantly greater number had received a high school diploma (72%), but only 17% held a bachelor's degree. Fifty-two percent of older blacks and 36% of older Hispanics had received a high school diploma.

The percentage of older people living in poverty declined from 35% in 1959 to 10% in 2002. However, in 2001, the median net worth of older white households ($205,000) was five times larger than for older black households ($41,000). Another salient finding is that today

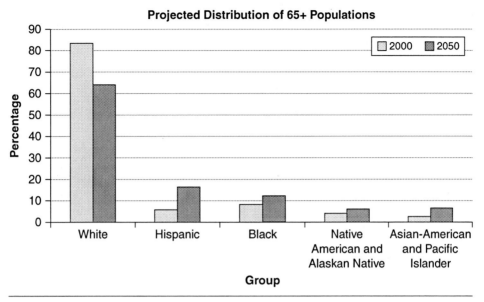

FIGURE 8-1 *Projected Distribution of 65+ Populations (2003–2050).* (Adapted from Federal Interagency Forum on Aging-Related Statistics, 2006.)

women aged 55–60 work more than ever before. In 2003, about three-fifths of women aged 55–61, almost two-fifths of women aged 62–64, and more than one-fifth of women aged 65–69 were in the labor force.

An important implication for the health care system is that Americans live longer then ever before. Specifically, by 2030, the average 65-year-old could expect to live almost 12 more years, and the average 85-year-old could expect to live an additional 4 years. It is significant that one in five persons will be 65 or older in about 25 years, and that the proportion of people aged 85+ will remain stable for the next thirty years. In 2030, populations aged 65+ and 85+ will have doubled in number from what they were in 1975. The percentages of elderly persons aged 65+ and 80+ are presented in Table 8-1. The reader who is interested in additional statistics regarding the age, income, and health of the world's older population is referred to Kinsella and Velkoff (2001).

Health Issues

In 2002, nearly one-half of all older men and nearly one-third of older women reported trouble hearing without a hearing aid. This

TABLE 8-1 Percentage of Elderly Americans (Aged 65+ and 85+): 1975–2030

Ages	1975	2000	2015	2030
65+	10.5%	12.6%	14.7%	20%
85+	2.1%	3.3%	3.8%	5.3%
80+ as a percentage of 65+	20.4%	26.8%	25.8%	26.4%

Source: Adapted from Kinsella and Velkoff, 2001.

finding has significant implications for the assessment of this population and for the availability of an adequate number of hearing devices that could facilitate the communication skills of the elderly. Vision problems, even with glasses or contact lenses, affected 16% of older men and 19% of older women. The prevalence of overweight and obese older adults has also increased dramatically and this has been the subject of numerous health articles and alerts. Mjoseth (2004) reports that between 1999–2002, 69% of Americans aged 65 and over were overweight or obese. Furthermore, she states that "in the last two decades, the increases among those aged 65–74 have been especially striking. Between 1976–1980 and 1999–2002, the percentage of people aged 65–74 who were overweight or obese rose from 57% to 73%; the percentage who were obese doubled from 18% to 36%" (p. 2). This information has important implications for SLPs working with older populations because being overweight or obese has health consequences that can enhance conditions such as stroke, diabetes, and other ailments.

The American Speech-Language-Hearing Association (ASHA, 2005b) published a series of documents that list the prevalence and incidences of relevant medical conditions in various populations. A summary is provided in Figures 8-2 through 8-5. For further details the reader is referred to Castrogiovanni (2004), who compiled information on this subject from various sources. The reader can also directly access the ASHA information on the Web at the following ASHA Web site: http://www.asha.org/about/leadership-projects/multicultural/epi.htm. Figures 8-2 through 8-5 report the prevalence of four medical conditions among CLD populations in the United States. Figure 8-2 provides data on cardiovascular diseases, Figure 8-3 provides data on stroke, Figure 8-4 provides data on hypertension, and Figure 8-5 provides data on obesity.

The reader will note that data on the epidemiology of various cultural groups remain incomplete or limited in some cases. For example,

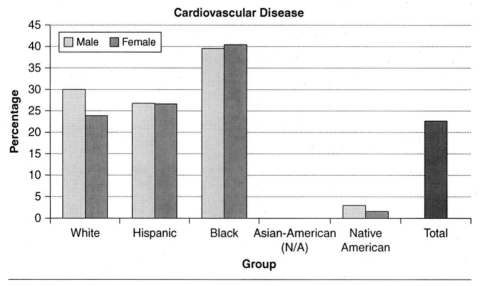

FIGURE 8-2   *Cardiovascular Disease among CLD Populations.* (Adapted from Castrogiovanni, 2004, and ASHA, 2005b.)

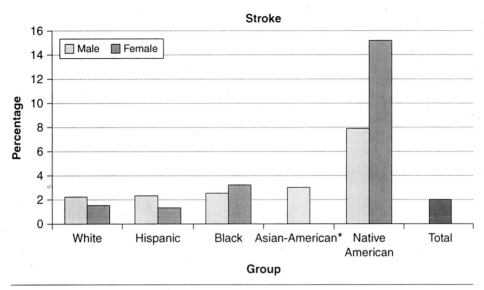

FIGURE 8-3 *Stroke among CLD Populations.* (Adapted from Castrogiovanni, 2004, and ASHA, 2005b.)

*Data are only available for Japanese males.

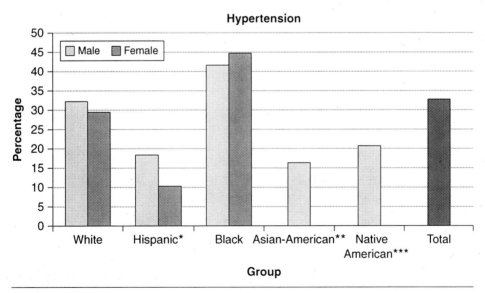

FIGURE 8-4 *Hypertension among CLD Populations.* (Adapted from Castrogiovanni, 2004, and ASHA, 2005b.)

*Data available on only Mexican-American and Puerto Rican (males and females).

**Data available on only Chinese-American, Filipino-American, and Japanese-American males.

***Data available on males only.

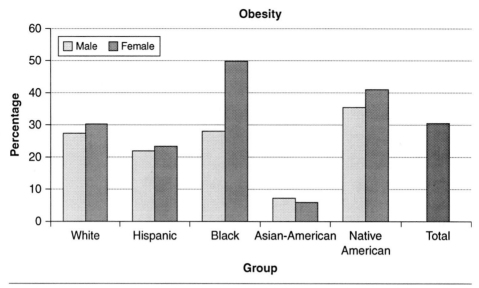

FIGURE 8-5   *Obesity among CLD Populations.* (Adapted from Castrogiovanni, 2004, and ASHA, 2005b.)

information on Hispanics is sometimes based on Mexican-American populations, or on only a few other Hispanic groups such as Cuban-Americans or Puerto Ricans. Data on Asian-Americans are either omitted or based on only one group (Japanese) or a few others. For example, an analysis of the data in the figures indicates that there is no information on cardiovascular disease for Asian-American populations.

African-American men and women are the ones who are most prone to cardiovascular disease (males 39.6% and females 40.5%). Cardiovascular incidence among the white population is 30% for men and 24% for females. Hispanics (both males and females) are also prone to cardiovascular disease, but to a somewhat lesser degree: the percentage for males is 28.8%, and for females, 26.6% (data are for only Mexican-Americans). For an illustration of cardiovascular disease among CLD populations see Figure 8-2.

The highest incidence of stroke (Figure 8-3) is for female and male Native Americans (15.2% and 7.9%, respectively). Data on stroke

for Asian-Americans are available for Japanese males exclusively, and stands at about 2.4%. Incidence of stroke is similar among whites and Hispanics for both males and females.

Hypertension (Figure 8-4) is more prevalent among African-American females (45%), and stands at 42% for males. The second-highest incidence is for whites, with 32.2% for males and 29.5% for females. The data on hypertension for Hispanics are only available for Cuban-Americans, Mexican-Americans, and Puerto Ricans; the combined percentage for these groups stands at 18.4% for males and 10.3% for females. Data on hypertension among Asian-Americans are limited to Chinese-, Filipino-, and Japanese-American males only and stands at 16.3%.

Obesity (Figure 8-5) in every group is higher for females than for males. The highest percentages are for African-American females (49.7%), as compared with only 28.1% for males in that group. Asian-American groups have the smallest percentages of obesity among females and males (7.1% and 5.8%, respectively).

Stroke, head trauma, various infections and/or chemical toxicity may result in acquired neurological disabilities. The incidence of stroke in the United States is approximately 600,000 (Center for Health Statistics, 2005), and about 25% of these cases are fatal. As noted in Chapter 1, the incidence of stroke is higher in the African-American population than in the white population. Today, stroke occurs at equal rates among women and men. Alchemic strokes are more prevalent in people older than 65, whereas hemorrhagic stroke is more common among younger people. Stroke is the third-leading cause of death (following heart disease and cancer).

Adamovich (2005) reports that head trauma among children and older adults is the leading cause of death and long-term disability in the United States. Motor vehicle accidents account for the largest percentage of traumatic brain injuries (TBI) among the younger population, whereas falls are the leading cause of TBI in the elderly population (75+) (Thurman & Guerrero, 1999). For example, statistics collected over a three-year period from 1996 to 1999 in California on almost 30,000 cases of TBIs that required hospitalizations indicated that that the majority of those who died were persons 65 and older (Center for Disease Control and Prevention, 2003). Falls were caused primarily because of osteoarthritis, Parkinson's disease, and the intake of drug combinations that produce dizziness or drowsiness in older persons.

ACQUIRED NEUROLOGICAL DISABILITIES: A REVIEW

It is impossible to describe in great detail all the variations of acquired neurological disabilities in a text of this scope. In this chapter, therefore, a short review of (1) cerebral vascular disease, (2) traumatic brain injury, and (3) selected progressive neurogenic diseases (Alzheimer's and Parkinson's) will be provided as a frame of reference for discussing these disabilities as they apply to the older CLD populations. For more in-depth information on these topics the reader is referred to Brookshire (2002), Chapey (2001), Hegde (2006), La Pointe (2005), and Murray and Clark (2006). Textbooks with some limited information on neurological language disorders that focus primarily on CLD populations are currently available. Some books that contain more information on this subject include the classic text written in the 1970s by Albert and Obler (1978) in which the authors describe the general patterns of recovery of bilingual individuals with various types of aphasia, and more recent works edited by Wallace (1997a), Paradis (2001), and de Bot & Makoni (2005).

The edited text by Wallace is a helpful resource for SLPs working with monolingual and bilingual CLD clients. It includes a review of the characteristics of the largest cultures currently represented in the United States (African-American, Hispanic, Asian-American, Native American, and Pacific Islander). Wallace's text is a good complement to the information included in Chapter 4 of this book. Wallace's text also includes case studies of clients with diseases such as aphasia, TBI, motor-speech disorders, Alzheimer's disease, and dysphasia. The edited text by Paradis (2001) describes the patterns of recovery of monolingual non-English-speaking clients who have sustained a cerebral lesion causing aphasia. The various languages featured by Paradis include African-American, Catalan, Czech, Greek, Hebrew, and Spanish.

The edited text by de Bot & Makoni (2005) includes several chapters that address issues regarding language and aging in multicultural societies. To understand declines in physical skills and social functioning, the authors advocate for further study of the way that communication and aging relate to several cultural linguistic groups. They argue that "physical decline has effects on basic skills such as memory, speed of processing, and attention that will affect language skills and language use. Language proficiency is seen as a skilled behavior and this implies that without regular 'training,' skills will decline…. [Further,] to maintain a complex skill, it needs to be activated regularly. This is what renders elderspeak harmful: if elderly people are spoken to in a restricted register, they will not have a chance to use language in all its complexity and may gradually lose the more advanced of the language skills" (p. 135). Communication patterns between elderly patients and the caregivers who come in contact with them in many different types of facilities have not been studied in multilingual subjects. There needs to be more research into this subject, and such research should take place in collaboration with the community and with medical establishments.

Another pressing issue is preparing both monolingual and bilingual SLPs to work with the ever-increasing CLD adult populations in their caseloads. Several resources are available to help professionals develop cultural sensitivity in their interactions with these populations. Among specific sources that refer to older populations is a document from the Administration on Aging called *Achieving Cultural Competence* (2001). A recent issue of ASHA's *Perspectives on Communication Disorders and Sciences in CLD Populations* (Salas-Provance, 2005) is also devoted to this topic. As the editor, Salas-Provance, indicates in her introduction, "All four articles emphasize the importance of getting to know our adult clients, keeping in mind that they are individ-

uals who lived full lives before their disability. It is our job to reconnect them, as much as possible, to their full and rich lives with family and friends" (p. 1).

Classification of Cerebral Vascular Accidents

The anatomical and physiological causes of cerebral vascular accidents (CVAs) or strokes determine their classification (Chusid, 1982; Mlcoch & Metter, 2001; Stein, 1986). They can be classified as either ischemic or hemorrhagic.

Ischemic CVAs, which are the most common, can be further classified as thrombotic or embolic. These CVAs result from partial or complete occlusion of a cerebral vessel. The most common ischemic CVA is thrombotic in nature and occurs when a blood clot obstructs a blood vessel feeding into the brain. The clot may result from atherosclerotic plaques (cholesterol and calcium deposits), inflammation of the vessel walls, or damage following a head injury. In an ischemic CVA that is embolic in nature, a fragment of clot or plaque travels from its site or origin to the brain, where it occludes the vessel.

There are two types of hemorrhagic CVAs, depending on their location in the brain. Intracerebral hemorrhagic CVAs originate from a vessel within the brain and are caused by excessive blood pressure, weakening of the vessel wall, injury, inflammation, or congenital defects. The subarachnoid type results from an aneurysm or malformation of the arterial walls that leads to bleeding in the subarachnoid space surrounding the brain. All CVAs have one feature in common—they interrupt the blood supply to the brain, leading to damage to the nervous tissue. The damage can involve cortical and subcortical areas, the lower brain stem cerebellar areas, and peripheral nerve areas. Numerous types of speech and language disorders can result. In general, the more severe the interruption of the blood supply, the more significant the resultant deficits. Stroke-like syndromes can also be caused by brain tumors, chronic subdural hematoma, infections of the brain, and multiple sclerosis and head trauma, among other events.

Recent technological advances, such as the increased use and improvement of computed tomography (CT) and magnetic and functional resonance imaging (MRI and fMRI), have been helpful in localizing the site of different lesions in the brain. Localization of a lesion alone does not necessarily make it possible to determine the appropriate assessment or treatment for a client, however. The results should be supplemented by a description of behaviors associated with the stroke, head trauma, or any acquired neurological deviation. A localization-alist model often lends itself to a better association between brain-behavior relationships, especially with the accessibility of imaging techniques to establish this connection in cases of CVA.

Traumatic Brain Injury

Classifying the symptoms associated with head trauma is complex, as one of the problems is that symptoms vary from moment to moment. Ylvisaker, Szekeres, and Feeney (2001) comment that disabilities that follow TBI are very variable regarding the impact on language and on general cognitive processing. They propose considering both the primary and secondary impacts of TBI in order to define the degree of involvement of any lesion. The primary impact may result in various kinds of damage—such as the abrupt movement of the brain within the skull, or fractures. However, the site of the lesion is not as important as "the differential tissue movements within the skull, both brain-skull and Brain-brain movements" (p. 747). Secondary

damage may include hemorrhage, cerebral edema, intracranial pressure and other symptoms. Ultimately, a classification system is helpful in the selection of appropriate treatment measures. For example, Hagen (1984) developed a classification system that delineates three different phases of neurological communicative-cognitive dysfunction. First, there is a global suppression of all communicative and cognitive functions. In the phases that follow one can still note persisting symptoms with some impairments. Finally, a permanent and irreversible neurological impairment can be identified, along with an associated neurobehavioral and communicative impairment. The majority of clients will go through these three phases, although not all of them do. As a result, clients may have various cognitive impairments along with secondary language problems; have a minimal number of cognitive impairments, but have a specific language impairment; or have attentional, retentional problems but have no problems with short-term memory or no specific language problems (Schwartz-Cowley & Stepanic, 1989).

Some of the most widely used scales that measure TBI clients' levels of cognitive and behavioral activity include the *Rancho Los Amigos Level of Cognitive Functioning* (Hagen, 1981) and the *Glasgow Outcome Scales* (Jennett & Bond, 1975). These measures can also be applied to CLD populations and are briefly described later in this chapter.

Progressive Neurogenic Diseases

The prevalence of gradual neurogenic damage and dementia, such as that associated with Alzheimer's, Huntington's, or Parkinson's disease, increases with age. Some families adjust rather well, perhaps too well, to the gradual onset of a neurogenic illness such as Alzheimer's, because the onset may be so gradual that there is no sense of urgency to seek professional help. Often, this disease is not diagnosed or treated until the psychosocial impact begins to obviously influence family life. In some CLD families, attitudes toward the disease may cause a further delay in a family's seeking appropriate care. All too often families interpret a possible neurogenic disorder to be the result of "old age," just as if old age made mental deterioration inevitable. Pope (2005), in her review of Alzheimer's disease (AD) in CLD populations, concluded that the disease has not been studied adequately. Most of the studies on AD do not make differentiations among persons who come from various linguistic or cultural groups, and many studies focus on testing and screening instead of on issues related to communication.

ASSESSMENT ISSUES

Despite the many advances in technology that have facilitated the detection of lesions caused by CVAs and other traumas that affect the neurological system, the role of the SLP remains paramount in the assessment and intervention process. In addition to understanding the medical aspects of the disease, the SLP should be familiar with the client's cultural and social background as well as with the controversies surrounding the recovery of bilingual clients' linguistic skills. If the SLP and client do not share the same languages, collaboration with an interpreter/translator (I/T) will be essential for achieving a fair assessment. Ideally, an evaluation of the language ability of a bilingual client with an acquired neurological impairment should include three components: (1) assessment of communicative and cognitive skills, (2) socio-

cultural appraisal, and (3) the results of radiological and technological tests.

The formal diagnosis of a problem in a client who has sustained a stroke or traumatic brain injury, or is suffering from a progressive neurological illness, should include an assessment of the client's phonological, linguistic, suprasegmental, and cognitive skills. Sociocultural issues (discussed in detail in Chapter 4) must be considered as well.

When the SLP does not speak the patient's language it is necessary to collaborate with a well-trained interpreter/translator (I/T) even though the patient may not need to respond verbally. It is important that the patient understands the directions for every task, including pure-tone testing, to assess hearing and oral-motor abilities. The oral-motor abilities assessment may include an evaluation of the physical parameters of the oral peripheral mechanism. This evaluates the use of all oral structures including lips and tongue, and is used to determine adequacy of velar pharyngeal closure and efficient swallowing. It is also important to question the spouse, a relative, a friend, or the client (when possible) to obtain a careful language history of the client prior to the neurological event. In addition, obtaining educational and occupational histories is important because expectations about a client need to remain as objective and realistic as possible. For example, it would not be surprising if the written skills of a client are weaker in English than in the client's native language if the client learned to read and write in the native language. Knowing the client's favorite activities and foods can also be helpful in the treatment of various linguistic and physical problems.

The ratio of nonnative English-speaking clients to bilingual SLPs fluent in their clients' language continues to be low. Alternative strategies, such as seeking the collaboration of a bilingual consulting SLP or an I/T, must therefore be adopted. Even if the SLP is monolingual or partially bilingual in a non-English language (but not in the client's language), he or she should not work with the client alone without the consultation of a bilingual professional or I/T fluent and trained in the client's language. Doing so may be a disservice to the client and, at times, may even be detrimental to treatment. It is therefore imperative that the SLP objectively recognize his or her own linguistic capabilities and limitations in a second language.

The process of collaborating with I/Ts in the communicative disorders field was discussed in Chapter 6. Langdon and Cheng (2002) also provide some guidelines for how to work effectively with an I/T in a variety of settings—including hospitals and rehabilitation centers.

Assessment Tools Appropriate for CLD Clients

Various communicative areas can be assessed using screenings or bedside tests for aphasia, and by using more thorough assessments. However, the number of tests that are specifically suitable for CLD clients is very limited (Roberts, 2001). Two tests that are recommended by Roberts include the *Reliable Assessment of Neurobehavioral Organization* (RANBO) (Wallace, 1997b), and *The Functional Assessment of Communication Skills* (FACS) (Frattali et al., 1995). The RANBO is available in both Spanish and English.

The RANBO enables the SLP to obtain information about the entire spectrum of communication, including cognitive communication, speech and language, and dysphagia. The battery includes 10 subtests that are listed in Figure 8-6.

1 Profile of Emerging Responsiveness from Coma (PERC)
2 Profile of Emerging Cognition, Communication, and Language (PECCL)
3 Profile of Emerging Pragmatic Skills (PEPS)
4 Profile of Emerging Oral Motor-Sensory Skills (PEOMSS)
5 Profile of Emerging Oral and Speech Praxis (PEOSP)
6 Profile of Emerging Motor Speech (PEMS)
7 Profile of Emerging Limb Praxis (PELP)
8 Profile of Emerging Motor Potential for Assistive Communication (PEMPAC)
9 Profile of Emerging Proficiency with Assistive Communication (PEPAC)
10 Profile of Emerging Swallowing Skills (PESS)

FIGURE 8-6 *Subtests of the RANBO.* (Adapted from Wallace, 1997b.)

The test includes adaptations that can be made when assessing clients who speak African-American Vernacular English (AAVE), Hawaiian pidgin dialect, and Appalachian English. In addition, the scoring guidelines included in the manual take into account the influence of 28 languages on the rating of the various English-language subtests. Formal and informal adaptations of the test are also available. Normative data are still being collected for the various subtests (G. L. Wallace, personal communication, May 8, 2006).

The FACS measures functional disability and assesses performance of all functions that are fundamental for successful communication. There are items that can be performed by individuals regardless of age, gender, socioeconomic status, education, vocational background, or cultural background (Frattali et al., 1995).

The conceptual framework of the FACS includes four domains: (1) Social Communication; (2) Communication of Basic Needs; (3) Reading, Writing, and Basic Concepts; and (4) Daily Living. Each item measures seven levels of performance that are rated as "Does" (7) to "Does Not" (1). Intermediate

---

TABLE 8-2   Examples of Items for Each of the Four Domains Tapped by the Functional Assessment of Communication Skills (FACS) Test[*]

Domain	Example
Social Communication (Total: 21 questions)	8—Follows simple verbal directions (e.g., "Get the mail") 11—Understands nonliteral meaning and inference (e.g., "He has a heavy heart," or other culturally appropriate idioms)
Communication of Basic Needs (Total: 7 questions)	22—Recognizes familiar faces 28—Responds in an emergency (e.g., calls 911)
Reading, Writing, Number Concepts (Total: 10 questions)	35—Writes messages (e.g., "Call your mother") 37—Makes basic money transactions (e.g., pays for items at the grocery store, recognizes when given the wrong change)
Daily Planning (Total: 5 questions)	38—Knows what time it is (e.g., tells time) 42—Uses a calendar for time-related activities (e.g., scheduling, planning)

Source: Adapted from Frattali, Thompson, Holland, Wohl, and Ferketic, 1995.
[*]The different subject areas of the FACS have been condensed in this table. The numbers next to the examples refer to specific numbered questions in the FACS.

---

qualifiers include "Does with Minimal Assistance" (6) and "Does with Moderate to Maximal Assistance" (3). The assessment features a total of 43 items. Examples of items for each assessment domain are provided in Table 8-2.

For a more comprehensive assessment, the SLP may use one of several language adaptations from the Boston Aphasia Test (Googlass & Kaplan, 1983) in 60 different languages. Each language version includes specific vocabulary and pictures that are linguistically and culturally appropriate. Each version also includes norms for monolingual speakers of that language. Paradis and Libben (1987) reported that bilingual individuals who speak any of the 60 languages and/or have taken 400 or more hours of language training—should score 100% on most of the items. However, some studies contradict these findings. Manuel-Dupont, Ardila, Rosselli, and Puente (1992) found that this was not true for 14 Spanish/English well-educated individuals, indicating that norms for bilingual individuals taking the test should be considered. Roberts (2001) has compiled a detailed list of BAT tests

available in a number of languages (e.g., Chinese, Dutch, English, Finnish, French, German, Italian, Japanese, Korean, Punjabi, Spanish, and Thai).

For Alzheimer's patients, administration of the *Alzheimer's Quick Test (AQT) Assessment of Temporal-Parietal Function* (Wiig, Nielsen, Minthon, Warkentin, 2002) is an effective tool for determining whether further neuropsychiatric testing is necessary. This test asks the client to name a specific number of color and form combinations as rapidly as possible. The time that this takes for the patient—together with the number of errors—determines whether further neurological testing is necessary to assess the patient for a possible degenerative disease. This criterion-referenced test has been administered to individuals who speak one of many non-English Germanic languages, and is valid for literate speakers (educated at an eighth-grade level or above)—regardless of the individual's advanced level of education. The test has not yet been validated on individuals who have been exposed to two languages, although norm-referenced criteria are available for West

African speakers of Krio (Nielsen & Wiig, 2006), bilingual Spanish-English speakers residing in the U.S.-Mexico border regions (Radford & Wiig, 2005), and Arabic speakers (Al-Halees, Nielsen, & Wiig, 2007). A Spanish adaptation of the AQT is also available (Bruna et al., 2007).

The Importance of a Comprehensive Case/ Language History

Although the FACS includes a case history and other tests might do the same, it is important to have as much information as possible about the client's language history and onset of neurological disease. The above tests may supply some of the overall linguistic/communicative information needed to evaluate, refer, or plan a treatment for the client. Figure 8-7 contains a list of areas that should be evaluated with regard to the languages spoken by the client. The client's exposure to and experience with each language should also be considered. As always, it is important for the SLP to gather a careful history. A sample client questionnaire is presented in Figure 8-7.

Background information on a CLD patient who is evaluated because of a neurological disease should be collected systematically. This information should include several areas:

- Date of birth (Note: Use the correct date format. Speakers of other languages may write 9/12 instead of 12/9, because in many cultures, the day precedes the month.)

- Languages spoken at home; age of patient when the first and second language were acquired; domains in which each language is used

- Age of patient when reading and writing skills were acquired in the first and second language; handedness

- Educational background, occupational history, and medical history

Oral and Written Language Communication/Cognitive Skills

Even though some of the previously mentioned tests (the RANBO and the FACS, especially) include the assessment areas listed below, the SLP should ensure that all of the following information is obtained:

- Language Comprehension/Processing
  - Ability to follow simple and complex oral and written directions
  - Ability to engage in conversation
  - Ability to answer factual, cause-and-effect, and inferential questions (oral and written) based on paragraphs that include a variety of topics

- Language Expression—Evaluating Form, Content, and Use
  - Presence of apraxia/dysarthria
  - Fluency (word-finding problems, circumlocution, grammar and sentence complexity, and pragmatic skills)
  - Ability to explain sequences of events; expression of solutions (e.g., "what would you do if … ")
  - Written expression

- Cognitive Skills
  - Attention; visual and auditory discrimination
  - Memory-sentence repetition; recall of information
  - Orientation (time, place, biographical history, awareness of impairment)

Sociocultural Appraisal

The contact between the SLP and the client constitutes a specific communicative event.

Name: _____

DOB: _____   Age: _____

Occupation: _____

Language Use and Preferences:

Language(s): _____   Country of origin: _____

How long has the adult resided in the United States? _____

Has the adult resided in countries where other languages were spoken? Yes_____No_____

Describe the adult's experiences with other languages: _____

_____

What is the main language used at home (i.e., home language)? _____

Language(s) of interactions between the adult and:

Spouse_____Siblings_____Children_____Parents_____

Other family members/friends _____

Language preference for listening to the radio or watching TV?

❑ Home language   ❑ English   ❑ No preference

Language preference for reading and writing?

❑ Home language   ❑ English   ❑ No preference

Rate the adult's proficiency in English:

❑ Very low   ❑ Low average   ❑ Above average   ❑ Very high

Education and Occupation:

Did the adult attend school in his or her country of origin (if country is other than the United States)?

❑ Yes   If yes, how many years? _____   ❑ No

Did the adult attend school in the United States?

❑ Yes   If yes, how many years?_____   ❑ No

Highest level of education: _____

List jobs held in the past five years: _____

Health Information: Any problems? (circle response)

Prior to the accident			*After the accident*		
Listening	Y	N	Listening	Y	N
Hearing	Y	N	Hearing	Y	N
Recalling what is said	Y	N	Recalling what is said	Y	N
Following directions	Y	N	Following directions	Y	N
Speaking clearly	Y	N	Speaking clearly	Y	N
Expressing ideas clearly	Y	N	Expressing ideas clearly	Y	N
Swallowing	Y	N	Swallowing	Y	N
Walking	Y	N	Walking	Y	N
Using hands	Y	N	Using hands	Y	N
Writing	Y	N	Writing	Y	N
Reading	Y	N	Reading	Y	N

Handedness   ❑ Right   ❑ Left

Previous significant problems?   Y   N

Describe any problems: _____

Does the client have any food/dietary preferences?   Y   N

If yes, please describe: _____

List the adult's favorite activities and hobbies: _____

_____

Additional comments: _____

FIGURE 8-7   *Questionnaire for Older CLD Clients.* (Adapted with permission from *Interpreters and Translators in Communication Disorders: A Practitioner's Handbook,* by H. W. Langdon, 2002, pp. 33–34. Eau Claire, WI: Thinking Publications.)

The interaction is bound by the cultural background of the SLP and the client. As noted in Chapter 4, many CLD clients may have difficulty relating to a clinician. Some clients feel alienated by the clinician-client situation, and the language barrier further escalates this feeling. Thus, the clinician must be aware of possible conflicts that arise from the client's cultural and communicative norms that were present prior to the onset of his or her trauma or illness. The expectations of the family, as well as the family's trust in the delivery of services, must be considered. The family's educational background, degree of acculturation, and level of bonding to ill family members are important variables as well. Some families have great respect for therapists, clinicians, and physicians as individuals, yet do not adhere to a prescribed treatment plan. They feel the elderly family member "has had a difficult life," and that it is the family's turn to take care of the client. The philosophy of "helping clients help themselves"—a philosophy upon which rehabilitation professionals' efforts to instill a sense of independence in the client are based—often conflicts with what the CLD family and client desires. Nevertheless, out of respect for medical professionals, the family may not clearly communicate their desires. The rehabilitation team may find out too late that their efforts were essentially in vain.

The culture, religion, and traditional beliefs of CLD parents may also affect treatment. For example, the church or religious parish in many countries continues to influence various facets of life, particularly in the more rural or remote areas of a given country. The belief in "higher" forces that intervene in the cause and healing of a disease is quite prevalent. As noted in Chapter 4, the American mainstream relies on medical technology to define the causes of illness and to treat medical problems. In several third-world countries, the lack of public services and medical technologies can result in very different attitudes. Therefore, SLPs must acknowledge those differences in beliefs and attitudes by suggesting a service delivery model from a mutually acceptable perspective.

The role of the SLP should be to listen to the client and offer explanations for the client's condition that have been confirmed by physicians and other specialists, while at the same time respecting the beliefs of the client.

Results of Radiological and Technological Tests

The information obtained by computed tomography (CT) scans, magnetic resonance imagery (MRI), single-photon, emission-computed tomography (SPECT), and positron-emission tomography (PET), are valuable for clarifying the reasons that clients sometimes present such peculiar linguistic profiles.

CT scans are radiological techniques in which sections, or "slices," of a client's cerebral tissue are irradiated with a beam. A computer calculates average differences in density as the beam moves through the tissue, and these density differences are then plotted on a screen or photographic plates to show the intracerebral structures, including damaged tissue. Bourgeois (2005) reports that CT scans are more valuable than other techniques for assessing cognitively impaired and agitated clients because it is faster and cheaper.

MRI, a more sophisticated procedure, involves the use of a large electromagnet that induces a magnetic field throughout the tissue in the brain. All atoms in the body have nuclei that react as if they were spinning. They possess some physical characteristics, such as a magnetic movement of their own. The magnetism in the atomic nuclei is random, however, because the atoms and molecules are mostly randomly oriented in bodily tissue. The powerful electromagnet of the MRI forces the atoms (hydrogen for the most part) to align themselves with the magnetic field that it induces. In the process they absorb energy and are excited. Through rapid oscillating absorptions and a release of energy—from the hydrogen atoms, as well as from the water content in all the body's tissue—it is possible to detect small differences in intracerebral density. Lesions can be identified more accurately with this method than with the CT scanner. Because of their greater sensitivity, MRIs are used for differential diagnoses of clients suspected of having Alzheimer's. For example, Alzheimer's can be differentiated from other types of dementia because in AD there is more medial temporal-lobe atrophy and less preservation of hippocampal volume. Other techniques, such as functional MRI (fMRI), assess blood flow during the performance of a task. An intravenous injection of a contrast agent such as gadolinium allows examiners to detect changes in blood flow measured by the MRI.

Other techniques, such as SPECT, are used to measure the biochemical status of cells, including blood flow, synaptic density, and tumor metabolism. The PET technique is used to measure the glucose and record the gamma rays produced when the isotope decays (Kennedy, 2000).

These technological advances provide clinicians with unprecedented and exciting tools for conducting research—and often for clarifying and differentiating the recovery of monolingual and bilingual clients. However, Bourgeois (2005) indicates that despite the advancements in radiological and technological procedures, "many definitive diagnoses are still not possible until postmortem examination of the brain" (p. 201).

RECOVERY PATTERNS OF CLD ADULTS WITH ACQUIRED NEUROLOGICAL DISORDERS

In order to implement effective intervention techniques, it is important to understand the possible recovery mechanisms that a bilingual person may experience. Researchers have provided various insights into the possible underlying mechanisms of language recovery following strokes or traumatic brain injury. Some of these theories were developed as far back as the late 1800s. They still have considerable applicability for categorizing many stages of recovery; however, they are based on single-case histories and it may therefore be difficult to make generalizations from them.

Early Theories

In 1882, Ribot hypothesized that a bilingual with an acquired language deficit recovers the first language first because it is most resistant to damage. To illustrate this hypothesis, Dreifuss (1961) reported the case of a 34-year-old bilingual poet who had emigrated from Germany to the United States at the age of 10 and had had no exposure to German since then. Migraine headaches resulted in the loss of his second language (English), while his first language (German) remained intact. Eventually, English was recovered, but not to the same level of proficiency as German.

Pitres (1985) proposed that the most familiar or most recently learned language returned first. Consistent with this theory, Halpern (1941) reported the case of a 24-year-old German who had gone to Israel at age 20 and had been hit by a bullet. It damaged the left temporal region, resulting in sensory aphasia. In recovering, his comprehension and expression of Hebrew preceded his comprehension and expression of German in both the oral and written modalities. Both languages gradually recovered, but he regained Hebrew at a faster rate than German.

A theory proposed by Minkowski (1963) was based on the premise that the emotional importance of a language may influence its recovery. In his review of the Russian literature, he presented cases where multilingual aphasics from central Asia who spoke Turkmenian, Kazakh, or Georgian were inducted into the Russian army, where they learned to speak Russian. After suffering brain injury, the clients were admitted to hospitals at which there were only Russian speakers, and the clients' Russian skills recovered first. In this case Russian, rather than the soldier's native language, became the "emotionally charged" language. It is possible that for these soldiers, Russian symbolized the primary communication vehicle used to plan the country's defense as well as the protection of their own lives. Although these earlier studies were clearly not stringent in their methodologies, they are useful for illustrating the complexity of bilingual aphasia syndromes.

Some early researchers proposed still other theoretical neurological mechanisms of language recovery. Goldstein (1948), for example, suggested that the recovery of only one language results from an inhibition of the switching mechanism. He hypothesized that, under certain conditions, the recovery of one language may inhibit the recovery of the other. He reported the case of an English-Swedish bilingual woman who switched from English to Swedish when she was making emotional statements. She could not translate from either language on command, however, and she could not perform all language functions voluntarily. Thus, "the switching ability" could operate only under certain conditions. Cases such as this one are relatively rare.

Minkowski (1963) proposed a model that involved two switches. According to this theory, an "output" switch that operates under voluntary control inhibits one language, while allowing the production of the other. An "input" switch alerts or sets the language processing system to filter in or out the different incoming languages.

More Recent Theories

When Paradis (1977) retrospectively analyzed recovery in 138 multilingual aphasics, he organized the paths of recovery into five general patterns. The first three refer to the recovery patterns of bilingual clients, whereas the last two refer to the recovery patterns of trilingual or multilingual aphasics. The types of recovery are still referenced in the current literature (Paradis, 1995; Pearce, 2005; Roberts, 2001). In

the literature, these patterns of recovery may be listed in slightly different ways, (i.e., the concept of impairment may be separated from the concept of recovery), but they remain equivalent. In the following sections, five different recovery patterns are described.

Synergistic and Differential Recovery

In a synergistic recovery, both languages are impaired, and they eventually recover—although not necessarily at the same time. In a differential recovery, the languages are not equally impaired and therefore recover at different rates. The synergistic and differential patterns are by far the most common, as 95% to 98% of bilingual aphasic clients follow the course of language restitution. Of the 138 cases reviewed by Paradis (1977), 87 were synergistic and 56 were differential. Of those 138 individuals, 6 were speakers of Spanish and a language other than English. The recovery patterns may be different for bilingual clients from countries other than the U.S., however—countries where the combined influences of culture and cross-linguistic similarities or differences and individual language histories are more varied.

Antagonistic Recovery

Also referred to as regressive recovery, an antagonistic recovery involves the return of one language at the apparent expense of a previously recovered language. One language may gradually improve, but begins to fade upon the emergence of the second language.

Successive Recovery

When one language returns only after another has been completely restored, the recovery is successive. The second language does not reemerge until the client has achieved relative fluency in the first one.

Mixed Recovery

In one type of mixed recovery, the languages are intermingled in all language processes (i.e., comprehension, expression, reading, and writing). A person may be able to read better in one language and speak better in another. In another variety of mixed recovery, also referred to as reciprocal antagonism, successive restitution is followed by antagonistic recovery for a person speaking three languages. For example, two languages recover successfully to a relatively fluent degree. After a few months, the patient's third language emerges, detrimentally affecting the most dominant, fluent language recovered up to that point.

Selective Recovery

When one of the languages never recovers and remains impaired, even when the other language(s) have returned, the recovery is selective. The recovery patterns depend on several factors that include the nature and structure of the two languages and the type of lesion. In addition, age, premorbid IQ, and level of education play a role in the process of recovery. For the most part, these clients recover the language that was most familiar to them before their impairment. If a given grammatical form is frequent in a given language, the less vulnerable it will be (Paradis, 2001). However, the SLP needs to keep in mind that one type of grammatical error in one language may not be manifested in the other language, due to the differing structures of the languages. Even thirty years after Paradis' work we are not quite sure what to expect in patients who have suffered various lesions and have spoken two or more languages during

their lives. Pearce (2005) summarized this dilemma by stating: "These diverse and at times conflicting observations imply that in certain patients impairment or recovery is differential, and in others it is parallel. Clearly, further studies are needed to define mechanisms associated with differential effects: types of aphasia, size and site of the lesion, etiology, educational level, proficiency, and age of language acquisition that determine the subsequent disintegration when the brain is injured. It appears that multiple languages can in some subjects be represented, at least partially, in different brain areas" (p.131).

TREATMENT

Most SLPs agree that the success of therapeutic intervention for clients suffering from acquired neurological problems depends on three primary factors: (1) the quality of service delivered, (2) the client's neurological deficits, and (3) the client's support network. As Bollinger (1983) stated, however, "There are few areas of communicative intervention in which the clinician's personal feelings influence treatment as much as they do in the management of the aphasic individual.... [The] intervention process is closely related to the clinician's philosophy of aphasia treatment, the amount and type of clinical experience, and ability to observe and modify behavior in various contexts" (p. ix). Moreover, because of a lack of bilingual personnel, the bilingual SLP or consultant to the case may function as the spokesperson for the entire treatment team.

The bilingual SLP can apply the same treatment principles to bilingual clients as are applied to English-speaking monolingual clients, provided that sociocultural and sociolinguistic factors are taken into account. Including family members in the intervention process is always crucial. In this manner, the SLP can be more certain that a planned program will be followed once the client is dismissed from the hospital. The process of rehabilitation should include strategies that teach and facilitate—to the highest degree possible—processes for reestablishing both communicative competence and the patient's productive reentry into his or her former daily routines. As for children and adolescents, the focus of treatment has shifted from form to functional aspects of communication. Overall, "the principles for unilingual treatment apply to bilinguals: goals should be realistic, meaningful to the patient, and tailored to the individual patient's deficits" (Roberts, 2001, p. 222). Comparisons of traditional treatment and functional communication treatment are outlined in Table 8-3.

Ulatowska and Bond (1983) suggested more than 20 years ago that "traditional sentence-level activities should be incorporated along with discourse-level tasks" (p. 33), and this is still relevant today. Therefore, it is necessary to consider pragmatic activities such as (1) initiating and sustaining conversation, (2) using contextual information to understand and produce messages as a situation may

---

TABLE 8-3 A Comparison of Traditional and Functional Communication Treatment Approaches

Traditional Communication Treatment	Functional Communication Treatment
1. Major focus on language	1. Major focus on functionality
2. SLP more often plays the role of stimulator/facilitator and initiates and directs linguistically based exchanges (Sarno et al., 1970; Schuell et al., 1964).	2. SLP more often alternates between playing the role of listener and speaker (dyadic exchange), and creates situations requiring equal participation from the patient (Chapey, 2001; Davis & Wilcox, 1981).
3. Goals are to improve to successful criterion level the comprehension of language (spoken, written) via stimulation of input modalities (Marshall, 2001).	3. Goal is to maximize comprehension of information exchanges by enriching the context of natural conversation, which is accompanied by writing and gestures (Chapey, 2001; Wilcox, 1983).
4. Frequently uses cloze and other convergent/confrontative approaches to increase available vocabulary.	4. Encourages divergent utterances of circumlocutions stimulated by general situations, cues, and interrogative probes, accepting related, holophrastic, and prosodic productions when natural settings are unavailable (Chapey, 1981; Marshall, 2001; Martin, 1981).
5. Most treatment is conducted in individual clinical settings using pictorial and/or printed stimuli; reduced emphasis on personal relevancy of lexicon or grammar.	5. Treatment is conducted in settings as natural as possible—including groups. When contrived situations are employed, they simulate real-life scenes/content and stress functional communicative content. Family members are actively involved (Chapey, 2001; Elman, 1999; Holland, 1999).
6. Treatment is based upon analysis of the individual client's profile of language strengths and deficits obtained from results of formal language tests. SLP selects preferred input/output modalities for language reception/production (Porch, 1981).	6. Treatment is based upon formal language test results, but also stresses the use of functional measures of communicative ability (CADL, FACS, discourse analysis, observation of client's communicative performance in real-life settings) (Chapey, 2001; Frattali et al., 1995; Holland, 1983).

Source: Adapted from Arámbula, 1992.

require, and (3) clarifying or asking for clarification.

Although pragmatic competence may be relatively intact in certain aphasic clients, therapy may be required to develop communicative rather than purely linguistic competence. This may be achieved by, for example, using the model for promoting aphasic communicative effectiveness developed more than 20 years ago by Davis and Wilcox (1981), and which was further elaborated by the "Life Participation Approach to Aphasia" (LPAA) described by Chapey et al. (2001). This approach focuses on aspects of communication (such as the exchange of new information, equal participation by the SLP and client, and free choice in selecting a channel for conveying a specific piece of information), rather than on linguistic accuracy. These strategies have assisted patients in achieving their degrees of linguistic competence.

The similarities and differences between the languages spoken by the individual, as well as the proficiency and use of each of the languages premorbidly—must also be considered in the process. The recovery of a formerly Spanish/French-speaking bilingual client with a given type of lesion may be different from that of a client who spoke Spanish and a Slavic language, or a Germanic language—even if all the clients have similar bilingual language histories and had similar types of proficiency in each language. Given the paucity of studies on the specific recovery paths of bilingual individuals, outcomes for bilinguals are difficult to predict. However, it may not be unusual for the client to use words from the two languages in a code-switching mode (as is frequent in the case of bilingual individuals)— and the code-switching may be more prevalent at the word or sentence level. Some research on code-switching patterns in aphasics is documented in works by Marty and Grosjean

(1998); Muñoz, Marquart, and Copeland (1999), and Springer, Miller, and Bürk (1998).

Selecting the Appropriate Language(s) for Intervention

Following the principles of bilingual language use, the choice of language for intervention will depend on the client's language proficiency in each language after trauma. The path of recovery may follow any of the five recovery patterns described earlier. The choice of language should match the pattern of use by the patient prior to the trauma. Two principal scenarios apply:

1. If the patient recovers in only one language (at least initially), therapy should be offered in that language until the other language or languages recover. At times, the language may not be the majority language, and the collaboration of an interpreter may be necessary.

2. If the patient recovers simultaneously in the two languages, therapy can be offered in one language, and then be followed by carry-over at home to the other language.

Another alternative recommended by Roberts (2001) is to offer treatment in each language during blocks of sessions in case the SLP is bilingual and competent in the patient's languages. For example, if the patient recovers in English and French, offer therapy in English first for a few sessions, followed by therapy in French. There may be a conflict with regard to deciding which language(s) should be used during treatment, because bilingual SLPs who can offer services in the client's language may not be accessible. However, every effort should be made to meet the patient's needs in at least one language.

Ultimately, the language that is appropriate for intervention depends on three important factors: (1) the client's premorbid language history, (2) the client's relative strengths and weaknesses in each language, and (3) environmental factors at the time of the client's discharge from the hospital (e.g., the family constellation, ability to sustain a job).

Materials

With the ever-advancing field of technology, computers are becoming important tools in the intervention process. Although the availability of software in languages other than English or Spanish is limited (and limited to some degree even in Spanish), several software packages allow the SLP to meet the unique needs of a patient. Even then, the SLP should be aware of the limitations of computer programs when planning intervention. The goal of the treatment of patients with various communication disorders is to enhance patients' comprehension and expressive language skills. However, the applications of software programs are limited to the specific practice of linguistic grammatical forms or sentences, which may not convert to real-life situations. Nevertheless, certain programs can be very helpful for offering patients ways to improve their communication skills. One of the most helpful programs is the Computer-Aided Visual Communication System, or C-VIC (Steele, Weinrich, Wertz, Kleczewska, & Carlson, 1989), that has been commercialized as Lingraphica® (Lingraphicare of America, 15 Spring St., 2nd floor, Princeton, NJ 08542). This program incorporates animation and digitized speech (Katz, 2001). Some preliminary data indicate that the program has been effective in the treatment of aphasic patients when used in combination with more traditional methods (Aftonomos, Steels, & Wertz, 1997).

The computerized reading and writing programs have greater applicability for treating patients with acquired neurological disorders. For example, Aphasia Tutor (Parrot Software, Inc., P.O. Box 250755, West Bloomfield, MI 48825) and Bungalow (Bungalow Software, Inc., 2905 Wakefield Dr., Blacksburg, VA 24060) both provide exercises in reading comprehension that begin with letter recognition and then move to more complex language. They are also available in Spanish. Several other materials from the Parrot Software Company are available in Spanish as well. For example, programs are available with exercises that follow event sequences (*Secuencia de Eventos*) and enhance categorization (*Razonar y Discriminar Categorías*), sentence completion (*Completar Frases*), and cause-and-effect (*Causa y Efecto*) language relationship skills. The majority of programs require some level of literacy and may need to be modified for patients who have lost their reading skills or whose reading skills were limited premorbidly.

Materials that are designed specifically for adults with various neurological disorders and that are available in languages other than English are scarce. This is true even for materials published in Spanish. One exception is the Spanish adaptation of Tomlin's workbooks (2006a, 2006b).

Materials that were available about 10 years ago are not currently available. Examples include the *Manual Terapéutico para el Adulto con Dificultades del Habla y Lenguaje* (Kilpatrick, Jones, & Reller, 1982), which was written in Spanish but was not translated into English, and *El Habla después de una Embolia* (Stryker, 1985), which had both English and Spanish texts. The bilingual versions of materials are useful for clinicians who may have a practical command of Spanish; they can refer to the English text and follow along as an I/T or family member assists the patient.

The majority of these materials continue to focus on language form. Some computer programs, however, now address the functional aspects of language; they assist patients in following specific directions, requesting specific foods items both at home and at a restaurant, and describing their health status. It is crucial that the SLP adopt a pragmatic-functional approach to therapy that will best meet the real-life needs of the patient.

SUMMARY

In this chapter we reviewed some important factors that should be considered by SLPs working with CLD adult populations with various acquired neurological disorders. First, the number of adults 65 years old and older in the U.S. and the world is increasing exponentially. Ideally, the languages spoken by the SLPs should match those of the patient so that the best possible speech and language services can be provided. However, the likelihood that there will be a match between the language(s) of the monolingual or bilingual SLP and the languages of the patient is remote. Therefore, an SLP working with a CLD adult must possess the specific skills necessary for producing a client assessment and treatment plan that best addresses the client's communication needs. The following suggestions for the SLP are recommended:

- Assess your patient by implementing as holistic an approach as possible—given the time and constraint of the situation.

- Consider your patient's bi/multilingual language history. Obtain as much information on the patient's history and use of each language as possible.

- Be prepared to work with a trained bilingual interpreter, and attempt to follow the best possible practices for partnering with this individual—always keeping in mind the best interests of your client. If you do not have access to trained interpreters of the languages that are most common in your patient caseload, work closely with the directors or supervisors at your work site who may have access to those individuals.

- Involve the family as much as possible and to the degree that is appropriate to the situation.

- Be as practical as possible when implementing therapy goals (they should match the patient's current language skills). Plan realistic goals to match (as much as possible) the premorbid skills and functional needs of the patient in each of the languages.

- Respect the wishes and requests of the patient. Some patients may not acquire independence again and may prefer to spend time on activities different from those planned by the SLP or the family.

In summary, speaking the language of patients is not as important as understanding the culture, beliefs, and attitudes of the ethnic group to which the patient belongs—while at the same time allowing for possible individual variations. SLPs, in conjunction with their colleagues in related professions, need to foster further research into both the best assessment practices to use with the older CLD populations and the best language(s) to use for intervention. Also, documentation of best practices in the treatment of CLD patients' various communication disorders needs to continue. As stated in Langdon and Cheng (1992), "The relatively few SLPs who are involved in working with this segment of the population have the opportunity to do significant and important research and to develop useful diagnostic and treatment materials" (pp. 403–404). After 15 years, this sentiment is still valid.

OUR CLIENTS

Eric, Ana, Jack, Grace, and Leonardo

The cases of our older clients Grace and Leonardo were discussed in earlier chapters—but not in Chapters 5 through 7 because those chapters discussed issues related to younger populations. The next sections will highlight the best strategies for assessing and treating Grace's and Leonardo's unique situations. Using a commentary format (rather than a report format) is the most appropriate and useful way to outline the cases of these two clients.

Grace

Background Information   Grace is a 60-year-old multilingual businesswoman, originally from Shanghai, China, who sustained a stroke in the right hemisphere of her brain while visiting the United States. Her business was in the clothing industry. She speaks Mandarin, Cantonese, English, and French. She completed her business degree in China, but spent five years in the United States when she was first developing her business. The languages she speaks most frequently are Mandarin and English. She communicates in Cantonese with her relatives, and speaks French when she visits Canada and France for business transactions. Prior to her stroke, she could converse on several topics in all the languages she knew. However, she felt most at ease reading and writing in Chinese and English. She was very proficient at reading and writing everyday English, but her strongest area was business English.

Grace learned the languages she speaks in various contexts. There is no information on how she first acquired English, but it is possible she attended a bilingual Chinese-English school and learned English through additional programs. Because Grace is well educated and lived in the United States for five years, she is most likely familiar with the various health care establishments. She may, however, not be able to advocate for herself because her speech and mobility skills are limited at this time. She will need a friend or relative to assist her in mediating her medical transactions. Luckily, Grace has several friends who were able to assist her when she had her accident. Grace has appeared, for the most part, to be able to resume the life she had prior to the stroke.

Assessment   The *Boston Aphasia Test* (BAT) was used in English, Chinese, and French. To assess all of Grace's languages, two trained interpreters (Cantonese/Mandarin-English and French-English) were hired to assist with the evaluation. Table 8-4 summarizes Grace's assessment results for the four languages that she had command of prior to her accident.

TABLE 8-4   Grace's Linguistic Profile for Four Languages

Area	English	Mandarin	Cantonese	French
Word discrimination	60%	70%	60%	20%
Commands	70%	70%	70%	20%
Response naming	70%	80%	70%	20%
Confrontation naming	40%	50%	65%	10%
Reading sentences	50%	70%	70%	10%

A language sample indicated that Grace was able to understand Mandarin, Cantonese, and English quite well—but not French. She could use sentences to express herself in the three languages but there was some code-switching between Mandarin and Cantonese and even some between Cantonese or Mandarin and English—especially when she wanted to express more complex ideas. Her recovery pattern reflected a mixed recovery; Mandarin, Cantonese, and English recovered fairly well, but not French, the language of least competence and use.

Treatment   Due to the lack of availability of a bilingual Chinese/Mandarin- and English-speaking SLP, all treatment was provided in English. Because Grace's friends were primarily Mandarin speaking, and the one she was staying with was her business partner, Grace and the friend were asked to follow up at home with practice in Mandarin of language activities similar to those that had been practiced in the hospital. Grace continued having therapy as an outpatient once she was dismissed from the hospital.

Goals for Therapy

1. Review important vocabulary that Grace needs in order to conduct her clothing business successfully. Review names and terminology: types of clothing, their make, sizes, etc. Review vocabulary associated with paperwork that needs to be filled to complete various transactions. Grace's business partner, who is bilingual Mandarin-Chinese, was asked to participate in the sessions to assist in planning typical scenarios that may occur in the daily life of their business.

2. Improve reading skills in both English and Mandarin-Chinese. Because Grace has right-hand weakness, she practiced dictating her letters and correspondence into a computer instead of typing the messages independently. Computer programs such as iListen™ and iDictate™ may be appropriate for further rehabilitation.

Grace made great progress after four weeks of rehabilitation. However, she was easily fatigued and could not speak very fluently. Some word-finding problems were still apparent, resulting in pauses and hesitations and also code-switching. A reassessment of her French skills after this period revealed some improvement, but not to the level of her former ability. Grace was saddened by this fact, but she was happy that she could go back to the business on a part-time basis in the U.S. with a prospect of returning full time to China within the following six months.

Reflections: What Is So Special about Grace's Case?

1. Grace could communicate in more than one language prior to her stroke. Therefore, the assessment and treatment needed to take this fact into account.

2. To be comprehensive, her assessment needed to be conducted in all the languages before the languages of intervention could be selected. Well-trained interpreters needed to be hired before a more comprehensive evaluation could be conducted. In this case, Mandarin, Cantonese, and English were recovered at about the same levels, but not French.

3. Treatment goals were specifically tailored to enhance those areas that were most essential for enabling her return to her former occupation. Her friends were able to help her practice at home.

4. Grace is fortunate to be familiar with the medical establishment because she has lived in the United States before and has traveled back and forth from China for business purposes. It is unknown if she has insurance coverage in China, but, most likely, she does have some personal coverage and her company may be able to reimburse her expenses (at least some of them).

5. She has friends who can help her follow up with her recovery. After completing the case, we found out that she is a widow and that her children live in different parts of the world—so they could not be of great assistance to her.

Leonardo

Background Information   Leonardo is a 45-year-old fieldworker from Guatemala who suffered a traumatic brain injury following a dispute with a neighbor. Leonardo is an illegal immigrant who has been traveling back

(Continued)

and forth between the U.S. and Guatemala for more than 20 years. He works as a crop picker in several states, including Washington, Ohio, Michigan, California, and Oregon. He completed seven grades in Guatemala but was able to get his GED while in the U.S. after attending night classes. His family lives in Cobán, Guatemala, and he has some friends in the U.S. that he has met over time. He is able to communicate in English, but even after his years in the U.S., he is still much more fluent in Spanish. Prior to his accident, he could read newspapers in both English and Spanish, but concentrated primarily on sports and local news. Leonardo prefers watching the Spanish TV channels and his favorite music is Latin.

Leonardo's family and relatives depend on the money he sends them every month. During a recent party, he got into a fight with someone over money that he had borrowed, but had not returned on time. Two heavier persons attacked him and hit his head with a baseball bat. He remained unconscious in the hospital for more than a week. At this time, he can walk, but he cannot process what is said to him. He is disoriented, he cannot keep track of time, and he forgets daily routines. After spending two weeks in a rehabilitation center he was dismissed because he can walk independently and his orientation is improving. Currently he is staying with some friends who own a restaurant.

Leonardo will need the assistance of a bilingual friend to help him navigate through the medical establishment, since he is significantly impaired at this time. Hopefully, it will be someone who has some knowledge of the medical services available and who speaks English fluently. Otherwise, he would need to rely on bilingual social workers to guide him and to ensure that he has appropriate language interpreting services in case his friend does not understand the intricacies of the health system. His illegal status should not be a deterrent in receiving the appropriate medical services, however. Because Leonardo's friend has located a charity foundation that will pay for his treatment, he can be seen at the local rehabilitation hospital. In addition, he has been very lucky to find a bilingual SLP in Spanish and English even though the therapist's Spanish is from Puerto Rico and uses slightly different vocabulary words and pronunciation. This, however, does not interfere with communication.

Assessment   Leonardo sustained a 3 × 2-cm lesion over the left midtemporal lobe; this was evident from his CT scan. Yet his language deficits involved receptive and expressive areas, with English, his second language, being more severely impaired than Spanish. Leonardo's test results are presented in Table 8-5. As can be noted, Leonardo initially was moderately to severely impaired receptively and expressively in English, but relatively less impaired in Spanish. His recovery was characteristic of synergistic improvement in which both languages return at the same time, but the originally dominant language (Spanish) maintains its dominance over the second (English).

TABLE 8-5   Leonardo's Linguistic Profile

Area	Spanish	English
Word discrimination	70%	30%
Body part identification	60%	30%
Commands	60%	20%
Paragraph level	40%	10%
Responsive naming	70%	40%
Confrontation	50%	20%
Oral reading	80%	40%
Sentence reading	60%	40%

Treatment   Because Leonardo's language skills in Spanish were not as affected as his skills in English were, all initial intervention took place in Spanish. A home program was developed in Spanish to allow maximal communication with friends. At first, activities centered on everyday events, including routines such as getting dressed, having meals, and getting into and out of his wheelchair. Many visual cues and repetitions were provided as well. The complexity of output gradually improved until Leonardo could describe pictures in books and magazines and could read headlines, titles, and short sentences. Materials were taken from his home on topics of interest to him, such as sports and some local news. His attention and concentration improved slowly, but he continued to get fatigued very easily. Eventually, when Leonardo was able to communicate his basic needs and feelings in Spanish, the SLP began to introduce English every other session (as recommended in the literature) in order to enhance both languages in the best possible environment. The therapy was designed to enhance his communication skills because Leonardo was very popular in his community—and being able to interact with the community was therefore very important to him. The charity that assisted him found a lawyer who worked pro bono and who began transactions to facilitate the immigration of his family. Leonardo had not seen his children for a long time. One of them had become a bilingual science teacher in Guatemala who won a scholarship to complete a master's degree in science education in the United States. Because Leonardo could not resume full-time occupation in the fields anymore, he asked his friend to train him to become a waiter in his Mexican restaurant. He shadowed his friend for two months, serving water and bread to clients as a transition to becoming a waiter.

Once Leonardo began making progress, his therapist concentrated on enhancing his speech and language skills so that he could communicate with customers. Leonardo was also taught how to use the computer to take orders. Even though it took more than six months to retrain him, he was very glad to be able to enter into another profession. The prospect of having his family coming to live with him enhanced his progress.

Reflections: What Is So Special about Leonardo's Case?

1. Leonardo is a success story. Even though he did not fully recover his written skills in Spanish or English, he was able to gain sufficient speech, language, and communication skills to retrain into another occupation.

2. Leonardo was very lucky. Not all persons in his situation find a charitable foundation that will take over the medical expenses.

3. Even though Leonardo did not know the ins and outs of the medical profession, he knew how to appreciate all the help he received from his friends, the community, and his therapist. A follow-up visit to the restaurant by the bilingual SLP a year after his accident indicated that Leonardo's speech and communication in both languages had continued to improve. His boss and restaurant clients were very pleased with his service. His family was on its way to the U.S. within the following three months.

FURTHER READINGS

De Bot, K., & Makoni, S. (2005). *Language and aging in multilingual contexts*. Clevedon, UK: Multilingual Matters.

Paradis, M. (2001). *Aspects of bilingual aphasia*. Tarrytown, NY: Elsevier.

Wallace, G. I. (1997). *Multilingual neurogenics: A resource for speech-language pathologists providing services to neurologically impaired adults from culturally and linguistically diverse backgrounds*. San Antonio: The Psychological Corporation.

EPILOGUE

I am writing these couple of pages as I complete the second revision of this book. After working in this topic almost continuously for the last 15 months, I realize that there are many resources available that address the needs of the growing culturally and linguistically diverse (CLD) populations currently represented in every state of the nation. However, there are still many gaps in resources, education, and research, which makes it very challenging to work effectively with those who are not successfully acquiring English language skills or who have not learned the language sufficiently due to social or personal reasons.

How to differentiate a language difference from a language disorder continues to be the most common question posed by not only speech-language pathologists (SLPs) but other professionals who come into contact with individuals who are not sufficiently able to learn effectively or who cannot communicate as well as expected. The reason for this situation cannot be discovered by using "a simple test." The process of ascertaining whether an individual indeed has a language disorder requires rigorous work, almost like that undertaken by a detective. We have seen that many factors may interfere with an individual's language development. Thus, the answer cannot be given in just a few minutes. We need to collect information, observe the individual in his or her familiar surroundings, converse with persons who know that individual well, and interpret our findings while taking those variables into account. Also, it is important to assess the individual's proficiency in the two languages (L1 and L2) where appropriate. The SLP does not need to be bilingual but he or she absolutely must understand the process of bilingualism. Collaborating with a well-trained interpreter/translator is therefore very important.

If I had a magic wand, my first wish would be to ensure that students are receiving the best possible teaching in the world. However, this is not always possible because of pressure put on the teacher, and because of political and social factors. I strongly believe that some CLD students have had less than effective experiences in the classroom. My second wish would be to make every possible effort to educate our communities about the value of speaking another language. As a professional, I have heard colleagues say on numerous occasions that they have discouraged parents from speaking their native language because the child had a language disorder. Research on normally developing students, as well as some emergent research on students with language disabilities, indicates that being exposed to another language will not deter the child from making progress in language development. Dissuading children from embracing an additional language feels to me like destroying a potentially beautiful tree by choosing not to add it to a garden.

Future efforts should concentrate on the effectiveness of the programs offered to CLD students with various disabilities. Instead of duplicating information that has already been disseminated over the years, more effort should be made to document various strategies that have demonstrably assisted students in going forward. Longitudinal studies are difficult to conduct but merit some attention. Collaboration between universities and schools would yield important data. Regarding older CLD populations, it is very important that more attention be given to that segment of our society. Further research relating to this population needs to be conducted. This should include research on assessment practices, the best course and best language(s) of intervention, and the design of materials that focus on functional language development and that can be used in the home by the patient's family. The very few bilingual clinicians who work with this special population have a great opportunity to make significant contributions toward assisting CLD clients who have various language impairments, and an equally great opportunity to educate the clients' families as to the most effective ways to enhance their loved ones' communication and independence.

From now on my efforts will be put forth in the direction that I have outlined.

Henriette W. Langdon,
April 7, 2007.

REFERENCES

Acosta, D. (2005, September 13). Millenium goals—Cuba: Educational focus shifts from quantity to quality. *Interpress Services News Agency*. Retrieved September 16, 2005, from http://www.ipsnews.net/search.shtml

Adamovich, B. L. (2005). Traumatic brain injury. In L. LaPointe (Ed.), *Aphasia and neurological-related disorders* (3rd ed., pp. 225–236). New York: Thieme.

Administration on Aging. (2001). *Achieving cultural competence*. Retrieved April 11, 2007 from http://www.aoa.gov/prof/adddiv/cultural/CC-guidebook.pdf

Aftonomos, L. B., Steele, R. D., & Wertz, R. T. (1997, August). Promoting recovery in chronic aphasia with an interactive technology. *Archives of Physical Medicine, 78*, 841–846.

Al-Halees, Y., Nielsen, N. P., & Wiig, E. H. (2007). *AQT cognitive-screening criteria for Middle-Eastern speakers of Arabic*. Working paper, University of Jordan, Amman, Jordan.

Albert, M., & Obler, L. (1978). *The bilingual brain*. New York: Academic Press.

Ambert, A. (1986). Identifying language disorders in Spanish speakers. In A. C. Willig & H. F. Greenberg (Eds.), *Bilingualism and learning disabilities* (pp.15–33). New York: American Library.

Ambert. A., & Meléndez, S. (1985). *Bilingual education: A sourcebook*. New York: Garland.

American Educational Research Association, American Psychological Association, and National Council on Measurement in Education. (1985). *Standards for educational and psychological testing*. Washington, DC: American Psychological Association.

American Speech-Language-Hearing Association. (1985). Clinical management of communicatively handicapped minority language populations. *ASHA, 7*(6).

American Speech-Language-Hearing Association. (1988, March). Bilingual speech language pathologists and audiologists definition. *ASHA, 31*, 64.

American Speech-Language-Hearing Association. (2001). Roles and responsibilities of speech-language pathologists with regard to reading and writing in children and adolescents. Position statement, executive summary of guidelines, technical report. *ASHA Supplement, 21*, 17–27.

American Speech-Language-Hearing Association. (2003). *2003 Omnibus survey: Caseload report SLP*. Rockville, MD: Author.

American Speech-Language-Hearing Association. (2005a). *Background information and standards and implementation for the Certificate of Clinical Competence in Speech-Language Pathology*. Rockville, MD: Author.

American Speech-Language-Hearing Association. (2005b). *Epidemiology of communication disorders*. Retrieved April 12, 2007, from http://www.asha.org/about/leadership-projects/multicultural/epi.htm

American Speech-Language-Hearing Association. (2005c). *Evidence-based practice in communication disorders: An introduction*. Rockville, MD: Author.

Anderson, N., & Battle, D. (1993). Cultural diversity in the development of language. In D. Battle (Ed.), *Communication disorders in multicultural populations* (pp.158–185). Boston: Andover Medical Publishers.

Anderson, R. (2004). First-language loss in Spanish-speaking children: Patterns of loss and implications for clinical practice. In B. Goldstein (Ed.), *Bilingual language development and disorders in Spanish-English speakers* (pp.187–212). Baltimore: Brookes.

Aprenda: La Prueba de Logros en Español (Tercera Edición) [Aprenda3]. (2004). San Antonio, TX: Harcourt Assessment.

Arámbula, G. (1992). Acquired neurological disabilities in Hispanic adults. In H. W. Langdon with L. Cheng (Eds.), *Hispanic children and adults with communication disorders: Assessment and intervention* (pp. 373–407). Gaithersburg, MD: Aspen.

Asher. J. (1979). *Learning another language through actions: The complete teachers' guidebook*. Los Gatos, CA: Skyoak Productions.

August, A., & Hakuta, K. (1998). *Educating language-minority children*. Washington, DC: National Academy Press.

Bailey G., & Thomas. E. (1998). Some aspects of African-American vernacular English phonology. In S. Mufwene, J. Rickford, G. Batley, & J. Baugh (Eds.), *African-American English: History and use* (pp. 85–109). London: Routledge.

Bain, B., & Yu, A. (1978). Toward an integration of Piaget and Vygotsky: A cross-cultural replication (France, Germany, Canada) concerning cognitive consequences of bilinguality. In M. Paradis (Ed.), *Aspects of bilingualism*. Columbia, SC: Hornbeam Press.

Baker, C. (2000). *A parents' and teachers' guide to bilingualism*. Clevedon, UK: Multilingual Matters.

Baker, C. (2006). *Foundations of bilingualism and bilingual education*. Clevedon, UK: Multilingual Matters.

Baker, C., & Prys Jones, S. (1998). *Encyclopedia of bilingual education and bilingualism*. Clevedon, UK: Multilingual Matters.

Baker, K., & de Kanter, A. (Eds.). (1983). *Bilingual education: A reappraisal of federal policy*. Lexington, MA: Lexington Books.

Ballard, W. S., Tighe, P. L., & Dalton, E. F. (Eds.). (1979, 1982, 1984, 1991, 2005). *Idea Language Proficiency Test* [IPT]. Brea, CA: Ballard & Tighe.

Barik, H., & Swain, M. (1978). Evaluation of a French immersion program: The Ottawa study through grade five. *Canadian Journal of Behavioral Sciences, 10*, 192–201.

Bashir, A. S., Kuban, K. C., Kleinman, S., & Scavuzzo, A. (1984). Issues in language disorders: Considerations of cause, maintenance, and change. *ASHA Reports, 12*, 92–106.

Bashir. A. S., & Scavuzzo, A. (1992). Children with language disorders: Natural history of academic success. *Journal of Learning Disabilities, 25*(1), 53–65.

Bates, E. (1976). *Language and context: The acquisition of pragmatics*. New York: Academy Press.

Beaumont, C. (1992). Language intervention strategies for Hispanic LLD students. In H. Langdon with L. Cheng (Eds.), *Hispanic children and adults with communication disorders: Assessment and intervention* (pp. 201–272). Gaithersburg, MD: Aspen.

Bedore, L. M., & Leonard, L. B. (2001). Grammatical morphology deficits in Spanish-speaking children with specific language impairment. *Journal of Speech and Hearing Research, 44*, 905–924.

Ben-Zeev, S. (1977). The influence of bilingualism on cognitive development and cognitive strategy. *Child Development, 46*, 1009–1018.

Beringer, M. (1977). *Ber-Sil Level I and Level II*. Ranchos Palos Verdes, CA: Ber-Sil.

Berman. P. B., McLaughlin. B., McLeod. B., Minicussi, C., Nelson, B., & Woodsworth, K. (1995). *School reform and student diversity: Case studies of exemplary practices for LEP students*. Berkeley, CA: National Center for Research on Cultural Diversity and Second Language and B.W. Associates.

Bhatnagar, J. (1980). Linguistic behaviour and adjustment of immigrant children in French and English schools in Montreal. *InternationalReview of Applied Psychology, 29*, 141–159.

Bialystok, E. (Ed.). (1991). *Language processing in bilingual children*. New York: Cambridge University Press.

Bialystok, E. (2001). *Bilingualism in development: Language, literacy, and cognition*. New York: Cambridge University Press.

Birdwhistell, R. L. (1970). *Introduction to kinesis*. Philadelphia: University of Pennsylvania Press.

Bloom L., & Lahey, M. (1978). *Language development and language disorders*. New York: Cambridge University Press.

Bollinger, R. L. (1983). Foreword. *Topics in Language Disorders, 3*, ix–xi.

Bonder, B., Martin, L., & Miracle, A. (2001). *Culture in clinical care*. Thorofare, NJ: Slack.

Bosh, L., & Sebastián-Gallés, N. (2001). Early language differentiation in bilingual infants. In J. Cenoz & F. Genessee (Eds.), *Trends in bilingual acquisition* (pp. 231–256). Amsterdam: John Benjamins.

Bourgeois, M. S. (2005). Dementia. In L. La Pointe (Ed.), *Aphasia and neurological-related disorders* (3rd ed., pp. 19–21). New York: Thieme.

Bowers, L., Huising, R., & LoGiudice, C. (2005). *Test of Problem Solving: Elementary (TOPS 3)* (2nd ed.). Moline, IL: Linguisystems.

Bowers, L., Huising, R., & LoGiudice, C. (2007). *Test of Problem Solving: Adolescent (TOPS 2)* (2nd ed.). Moline, IL: Linguisystems.

Brigance, A. (1983). *Brigance Diagnostic Assessment of Basic Skills* [Spanish version]. North Billerica, MA: Curriculum Associates.

Brisk, M. (2005). *Bilingual Education: From compensatory to quality schooling* (2nd ed.). Mahwah: NJ: Lawrence Erlbaum Associates.

Brooks, M. (1986). Culture in the classroom. In J. Valdés (Ed.), *Culture bound* (pp.123–129). New York University: Cambridge University Press.

Brookshire, R. H. (2002). *Introduction to neurogenic communication disorders*. St. Louis, MO: Mosby.

Brownell, R. (2001a). *Expressive One-Word Picture Vocabulary Test* [Spanish-English ed.]. Novato, CA: Academic Therapy Publications.

Brownell, R. (2001b). *Receptive One-Word Picture Vocabulary Test* [Spanish-English ed.]. Novato, CA: Academic Therapy Publications.

Bruna, O., Puyuelo, M., Wiig, E. H., Cullell, N., Villalta, V., Dergham, A., & Nieves, G. (2007, August). *Early detection of cognitive and language disorders in Alzheimer's disease: Adaptation of Alzheimer's Quick Test to Spanish populations.* Oral presentation to the 27th World Congress of the International Association of Logopedics and Phoniatrics, Copenhagen, Denmark.

Bungalow Software. 2905 Wakefield Dr., Blacksburg, VA 24060-8184 [Tel: 1-508-526-0305]. Web site: http://www.BungalowSoftware.com

Burt, M., Dulay, H., & Hernández-Chávez, E. (1980). *Bilingual Syntax Measure* [BSM] [Levels I and II]. San Antonio, TX: The Psychological Corporation.

Butler, K. G., Nelson, N. W., Wallach, G. P., Fujiki, M., and Brinton, B. (Eds.). (2005). Language disorders and learning disabilities: A look across 25 years. *Topics in Language Disorders, 25*(4).

Butler, K. G., & Silliman, E. R. (Eds.). (2003). *Speaking, reading, and writing in children with language-learning disabilities: New paradigms in research and practice.* Mahwah, NJ: Lawrence Erlbaum Associates.

California Education Language Development Test [CELDT]. (2001). New York: McGraw-Hill.

California State Department of Education. (1986). *Case studies in bilingual education second-year report (1984–1985).* Sacramento: Bilingual Education Office.

California State Department of Education. (2004). *Recommended literature, kindergarten through grade twelve.* Retrieved March 16, 2007 from http://www.cde.ca.gov/ci/rl/ll/documents/newstitles2004.doc

California State Department of Education. (2007). *Curriculum frameworks.* Retrieved March 13, 2007, from http://www.cde.ca.gov/be/st/fr

Camarota, S. A. (2001, January). Immigrants in the United States–2000: A snapshot of America's foreign-born population. Washington, DC: Center for Immigration Studies.

Campbell, G. (1995). *Compendium of the world's languages.* New York: Routledge.

Campbell, G. (1998). *Handbook of scripts alphabets.* New York: Routledge.

Carr, S. E., Roberts, R., Dufour, A., & Steyn, D. (Eds.). (1997). *The critical link: Interpreters in the community.* Philadelphia: John Benjamins.

Carrow, E. (1973). *Test of Auditory Comprehension of Language* [TACL] [English and Spanish]. Allen, TX: DLM Teaching Resources.

Carrow, E. (1974). *Austin Spanish Articulation Test.* Allen, TX: DLM Teaching Resources.

Carter, D. (1994). *Alpha bugs.* New York: Simon & Schuster.

Carter, T., & Chatfield, M. (1986). Effective bilingual schools: Implications for policy and practice. *American Journal of Education, 95,* 200–232.

Cassidy, J., & Cassidy, N. (1986). *Apples and bananas* [Song]. Palo Alto: Klutz Press.

Castrogiovanni, A. (2004). [Note to reader: The information in this book that was compiled by Castrogiovanni in 2004 for the American Speech-Language-Hearing Association can be accessed at the ASHA Web site listed in an earlier reference. See American Speech-Language-Hearing Association, 2005b.]

Catts, H. W., & Kamhi, A. G. (2005). *Language and reading disabilities* (2nd ed.). Boston: Allyn & Bacon.

Center for Disease Control and Prevention. (2003). *Public health and aging: Nonfatal fall-related traumatic brain injury among older adults–California, 1996–1999*. Atlanta: Author.

Chamberlain, P., & Medeiros-Landurand, P. (1991). Practical considerations for the assessment of LEP students with special needs. In E. B. Hamayan & J. S. Damico (Eds.), *Limiting bias in the assessment of bilingual students* (pp. 111–156). Austin, TX: Pro-Ed.

Chamot, A., & O'Malley, J. (1990). Adaptation of the Cognitive Academic Language Learning Approach (CALLA) to special education. In A. L. Carrasquillo & R. E. Baecher (Eds.), *Teaching the bilingual special education student* (pp. 218–223). Norwood, NJ: Ablex.

Chamot, A., & O'Malley, J. (1994). *The CALLA handbook: Implementing the cognitive academic language-learning approach*. Reading, MA: Addison Wesley.

Chan, S., & Lee, E. (2004). Families with Asian roots. In E. Lynch & M. Hanson (Eds.), *Developing cross-cultural competence: A guide for working with children and their families* (3rd ed., pp. 219–298). Baltimore: Brookes.

Chapey, R. (Ed.). (1981). *Language intervention strategies in adult aphasia*. Baltimore: Williams & Wilkins.

Chapey, R. (Ed.). (2001). *Language intervention strategies in aphasia and related neurogenic communication disorders* (4th ed.). Philadelphia: Lippincott Williams & Wilkins.

Chapey, R., Duchan, J. F., Elman, R. J., Garcia, L. J., Kagan, A., & Lyon, J. G., et al. (2001). Life participation approach to aphasia: A statement of values for the future. In R. Chapey (Ed.), *Language intervention strategies in aphasia and related neurogenic communication disorders* (4th ed., pp. 235–245). Philadelphia: Lippincott Williams & Wilkins.

Chen, G. M, & Starosta, W. J. (1998). *Foundations of intercultural communication*. Boston: Allyn & Bacon.

Cheng, L. (1991). *Assessing Asian language performance: Guidance for evaluation of limited-English-proficient students* (2nd ed.). Oceanside, CA: Academic Communication Associates.

Cheng, L (1993). Deafness: An Asian/Pacific Islander perspective. In K. M. Christensen & G. L. Delgado (Eds.), *Multicultural issues in deafness* (pp. 113–126). White Plains, NY: Longman.

Cheng, L. (1996). Beyond bilingualism: Language acquisition and disorders—A global perspective. *Topics in Language Disorders, 16*(4), 9–21.

Cherry, B., & Giger, J. N. (1999). African-Americans. In J. N. Giger & R. E. Davidhizar (Eds.), *Transcultural nursing: Assessment and intervention* (3rd ed.). St. Louis, MO: Mosby.

Chesarek, S. (1981, March). *Cognitive consequences of home or school education in a limited second language: A case study in the Crow Indian community*. Paper presented at the Language Proficiency Assessment Symposium, Airlie House, VA.

Children's Defense Fund. (2001). *School-age child care: Keeping children safe and helping them learn while their families work*. Retrieved on May 22, 2007 from http://www.childrensdefense.org/site/DocServer/keyfacts2003schoolagecare.pdf?docID=593

Choi, S. (1999). Acquisition of Korean. In O. Taylor & L. Leonard (Eds.), *Language acquisition across North America: Cross-cultural and cross-linguistic perspectives* (pp. 291–334). San Diego, CA: Singular Publishers.

Chu, T. L. (1990, April). *Working with Vietnamese parents.* Paper presented at the Harbor Regional Center Conference, Towards Competence in Intercultural Interaction, Torrance, CA.

Chusid, J. G. (1982). *Correlative neuroanatomy and functional neurology.* Los Altos, CA: Lange Medical Publications.

Coe, G., & McConnell, J. L. (2004). The children of Cuba. *Young Children, 59*(5), 44–48.

Cole, P., & Taylor, O. (1990). Performance of working class African-American children on three tests of articulation. *Language, Speech, and Hearing Services in Schools, 21,* 171–176.

Collier, V. (1987). Age and rate of acquisition of second language for academic purposes. *TESOL Quarterly, 21,* 739–764.

Condon, J. C. (1986). "…So near the United States." In J. M. Valdés (Ed.), *Culture bound* (pp. 85–93). New York: Cambridge University Press.

Condon, J., & Yousef, F. (1975). *An introduction to intercultural communication.* Indianapolis, IN: Bobbs-Merrill.

Confusion Is Rife about Drug Plan as Sign-Up Nears. (2005, November 13). *New York Times.*

Cook, V., & Bassetti, B. (2005). *Second-language writing systems.* Clevedon, UK: Multilingual Matters.

Cossu, G., Shankweiler, D., Liberman, I. Y., Katz, L., & Tola, G. (1988). Awareness of phonological segments and reading ability in Italian children. *Applied Psycholinguistics, 9,* 1–16.

Crawford, J. (1989). *Bilingual education: History, politics, theory, and practice.* Trenton, NJ: Crane.

Crawford, J. (2004). *Educating English-language learners: Language diversity in the classroom.* Los Angeles: Bilingual Educational Services.

Critchlow, D. E. (1974). *Dos amigos verbal language scales.* Novato, CA: Academic Therapy Publications.

Crockett, J. B. (2004). The science of schooling for students with learning disabilities: Recommendations for service delivery linking practice and research. In B. Wong (Ed.), *Learning about learning disabilities* (3rd ed., pp. 451–484). Boston: Elsevier.

Crystal, J. (1997). *The Cambridge encyclopedia of language* (2nd ed.). New York: Cambridge University Press.

Cummins, J. (1981). The role of primary language development in promoting educational success for language minority students. In Office of Bilingual Bicultural Education, California State Department of Education (Ed.), *Schooling and language minority students: A theoretical framework* (pp. 3–49). Los Angeles: Evaluation, Dissemination, and Assessment Center, California State University.

Cummins, J. (1984). *Bilingualism and special education.* Clevedon, UK: Multilingual Matters.

Cummins, J. (1989). *Empowering minority students.* San Francisco: California Association for Bilingual Educators.

Cummins, J. (2000). *Language, power, and pedagogy: Bilingual children in the crossfire.* Clevedon, UK: Multilingual Matters.

Davis, G., & Wilcox, M. (1981). Incorporating parameters of natural conversation in aphasia treatment. In R. Chapey (Ed.), *Language intervention strategies in adult aphasia.* Baltimore: Williams & Wilkins.

De Avila, E., & Duncan, S. E. (2005). *Language assessment scales* [LAS] [Levels I and II, Spanish]. Monterey, CA: McGraw-Hill.

De Bot, K., & Makoni, S. (2005). *Language and aging in multilingual contexts.* Clevedon, UK: Multilingual Matters.

Delgado-Gaitán, C. (1992). School matters in the Mexican American home—Socializing children for education. *American Educational Research Journal 29*, 495–513.

Delgado-Gaitán, C., & Trueba, T. (1991) *Crossing cultural borders.* New York: Falmer Press.

Delpit, T. (1998). What should teachers do? Ebonics and culturally responsive instruction. In T. Perry & L. Delpit (Eds.), *The real Ebonics debate: Power, language, and the education of African-American children.* Boston: Beacon Press.

Diaz, R. (2000). *Latina parent educational participation: A pro-active approach.* Unpublished doctoral dissertation, UCLA, Los Angeles, CA.

Díaz-Rico, L., & Weed, K. (2005). *The cross-cultural, language, and academic development handbook. A complete K–12 reference guide* (2nd ed.). Boston: Allyn & Bacon.

Dopke, S. (2000). Generation of and retraction from cross-linguistically motivated structures in bilingual first-language acquisition. *Bilingualism: Language and Cognition, 3,* 209–226.

Dore, J. (1975). Holophrases, speech acts, and language universals. *Journal of Child Language, 2,* 21–40.

Dr. Seuss Enterprises. (1963, 1996). *Dr. Seuss's ABC: An amazing alphabet book!* New York: Random House.

Dreifuss, F. (1961). Observations of aphasia in a polyglot poet. *Acta Psychiatrica Scandinavia, 36,* 91–97.

Duffy, G. (2002). The case for direct explanation of strategies. In C. C. Block & M. Pressley (Eds.), *Comprehension instruction: Research-based best practices.* New York: Guilford Press.

Dulay, H., & Burt, M. K. (1973). Should we teach children syntax? *Language learning, 23,* 245–258.

Dulay, H., & Burt, M. K. (1974). Natural sequences in child second-language acquisition. *Language learning, 24,* 37–53.

Dunn, L. M., Padilla, E. R., Lugo, D. E., & Dunn, L. M. (1986). *Test de Vocabulario en Imágenes Peabody.* Circle Pines, MN: American Guidance Service.

Dunoff M., Coles, F., McLaughlin, D., & Reynolds, D. (1977, 1978). *Evaluation of the impact of ESEA Title VII Spanish-English bilingual education program* (Vols. 1–3). Palo Alto, CA: American Institutes of Research.

Echevarría, J., & Graves, A. (2003). *Sheltered content instruction: Teaching English-language learners with diverse abilities* (2nd ed.). Boston: Allyn & Bacon.

Echevarría J., Vogt, M., & Short, D. (2004). *Making content comprehensible for English learners: The SIOP model* (2nd ed.). Boston: Pearson.

Edwards, V. (2004). *Multilingualism in the English-speaking world*. Malden, MA: Blackwell.

Ehren, B. J. (2005). Looking for evidence-based practice in reading comprehension-instruction. *Topics in Language Disorders, 25*(4), 310–321.

Ehren, B. J. (2006, January). *Literacy—SLPs' unique contributions*. Presentation to the San Mateo County Speech-Language-Hearing Association, San Mateo, CA.

Ehren, T., & Whitmire, K. A. (2005). Leadership opportunities in the context of responsiveness to intervention activities. *Topics of Language Disorders, 25*, 168–179.

Ekstrand, L. (1978). *Bilingual and bicultural adaptation*. Unpublished doctoral dissertation, University of Stockholm, Sweden.

Elman, R. (Ed.). (1999). *Group treatment of neurogenic communication disorders*. Woburn, MA: Butterworth-Heinemann.

Eubank, P. (2003). *ABCs Halloween*. Nashville, TN: Ideal Children's Books.

Everatt, J., Smythe, I., Ocampo, D., & Veii, K. (2002). Dyslexia assessment of the biscriptal reader. *Topics in Language Disorders, 22*(5), 32–45.

Fadiman, A. (1997). *The spirit catches you and you fall down*. New York: Farrar, Strauss and Giroux.

Farr, B., & Quintanar-Sarellana, R. (2005). Effective instructional strategies for students learning a second language or with other language differences. In E. Trumbull & B. Farr (Eds.), *Language and learning: What teachers need to know* (pp. 215–267). Norwood, MA: Christopher Gordon.

Farr, B., & Richardson Bruna, K. (2005). Second-language acquisition and development. In E. Trumbull & B. Farr (Eds.), *Language and learning: What teachers need to know* (pp. 113–158). Norwood, MA: Christopher Gordon.

Federal Interagency Forum on Aging-Related Statistics. (2006). *Older Americans: Update*. Retrieved April 14, 2007, from http://www.agingstats.gov

Feurstein. R. (1980). *Instrumental enrichment: An intervention program for cognitive modifiability*. Baltimore: University Park Press.

Fishman, J. (1972). *The sociology of language*. Rowley, MA: Newbury House.

Flege, J., Frieda, E., & Nozawa, T. (1997). Amount of native-language (L1) use affects the pronunciation of an L2. *Journal of Phonetics, 25*, 169–186.

Fleming, D. (2002). *Alphabet under construction*, New York: Henry Holt and Co.

Fletcher, T., Dejud, C., Klingler, C., & López-Mariscal I. (2003). The changing paradigm of special education in Mexico: Voices from the field. *Bilingual Research Journal, 27*, 409–430.

Flor Ada, A., & Escrivá, V. (1990). *Abecedario de animales*. Madrid: Espasa-Calpe.

Flor Ada, A., & Zubizarreta, S. (2001). *Gathering the sun: An alphabet in Spanish and English*. New York: HarperCollins.

Foreign Service Institute. (n.d.). *International Language Roundtable (ILR) Scale*. Retrieved March 1, 2006, from http://www.govtilr.org/ILRscale2.htm#3

Fortin, J., & Crago, M. (1999). French-language acquisition in North America. In O. Taylor & L. Leonard (Eds.), *Language acquisition across North America: Cross-cultural and cross-linguistic perspectives* (pp. 209–242). San Diego, CA: Singular.

Fradd, S. H., & Tikunoff, W. J. (1987). *Bilingual education and bilingual special education: A guide for administrators*. Austin, TX: Pro-Ed.

Francis, N., & Reyhner, J. (Eds.). (2002). *Language and literacy teaching for indigenous teaching: A bilingual approach*. Clevedon. UK: Multilingual Matters.

Frankenberg, E., Lee, C., & Orfield, G. (2003). *A multiracial society with segregated schools: Are we losing the dream?* Cambridge, MA: The Civil Rights Project, Harvard University.

Frattali, C., Thompson, C., Holland, A., Wohl, C., & Ferketic, M. (1995). *Functional Assessment of Communication Skills in Adults* [FACS]. Rockville, MD: ASHA.

Fujiki M., & Brinton, B. (2005). Foreword. *Topics in Language Disorders, 25*(4), 337.

Galambos, J., & Hakuta, K. (1988). Subject-specific and task-specific characteristics of metalinguistic awareness in bilingual children. *Applied Psycholinguistics, 9*, 141–152.

Gallegos, A., & Gallegos, R., (1988). The interaction between families of culturally diverse handicapped children and the school. In S. García & R. C. Chávez (Eds.), *Ethnolinguistic issues in education* (pp. 125–132). Lubbock: College of Education, Texas Tech University.

Gardner, R. (1985). *Social psychology and second-language learning*. London: Edward Arnold.

Gay, G. (2000). *Culturally responsive teaching: Theory, research, and practice*. New York: Teachers College Press.

Genesee, F. (2003). Rethinking bilingual acquisition. In J. Dewaele, A. Housen, & L. Wei (Eds.), *Bilingualism: Beyond basic principles* (pp. 204–229). Clevedon, UK: Multilingual Matters.

Genesee, F., Nicoladis, E., & Paradis, J. (1995). Language differentiation in early bilingual development. *Journal of Child Language 22*, 611–631.

Genesee, F., Paradis, J., & Crago, M. (2004). *Dual language development and disorders: A handbook on bilingualism and second-language learning*. Baltimore: Brookes.

Genesee, F., Tucker, G., & Lambert, W. (1976). Communication skills of bilingual children. *Child Development, 46*, 1010–1014.

Geva, E., & Wade-Wolley, J. (2003). Issues in the assessment of reading disability in second-language children. In I. Smythe, J. Everatt, & R. Salter (Eds.), *International book of dyslexia* (2nd ed.). London: John Wiley & Sons.

Gile, D. (1995). *Basic concepts and models for interpreter and translator training*. Philadelphia: John Benjamins.

Giles, H., & Makoni, S. (2005). *Perceptions of age stereotypes, filial norms, communication behaviors, and communication satisfaction: Young, middle-aged, and older U.S. and African adult targets*. Manuscript submitted for publication.

Gillam, R., Peña, E., & Miller, L. (1999). Dynamic assessment of narrative and expository discourse. *Topics in Language Disorders, 20*, 33–47.

Goldenberg. C. (1993). Instructional conversations: Promoting comprehension through discussion. *The Reading Teacher, 46*(4), 316–326.

Goldenberg. C., & Gallimore G. (1995). Immigrant Latino parents' values and beliefs about their children's education: Continuities and discontinuities across cultures and generations. *Advances in Motivation and Achievement, 9*, 183–228.

Goldenberg, C., Gallimore, R., Reese, L., & Garnier, H. (2001). Cause or effect? A longitudinal study of immigrant Latino parents' aspirations and expectations, and their children's school performance. *American Educational Research Journal, 38*, 547–582.

Goldenberg, D., & Sullivan, R. (1994). *Making change happen in a language-minority school: A search for coherence*. Washington, DC: Center for Applied Linguistics.

Goldstein, B. (2000). *Cultural and linguistic diversity resource guide for speech-language pathologists*. San Diego, CA: Singular.

Goldstein, B. (Ed.). (2004a). *Bilingual language development and disorders in Spanish-English speakers* (pp. 259–285). Baltimore: Brookes.

Goldstein, B. (2004b). Phonological development and disorders. In B. Goldstein (Ed.), *Bilingual language development and disorders in Spanish-English speakers*. (pp. 259–285). Baltimore: Brookes.

Goldstein, K. (1948). Disturbances of language in polyglot individuals with aphasia. In K. Goldstein (Ed.), *Language and language disturbances*. New York: Grune & Stratton.

Goldstein, B., & Iglesias, A. (2006). *Contextual probes of articulation competence (Spanish) (CPAC-S)*. Greenville, SC: Super Duper.

Goodenough, F. (1926). Racial differences in the intelligence of school children. *Journal of Experimental Psychology, 9*, 388–397.

Goodglass, H., & Kaplan, E. (1983). *Boston diagnostic aphasia exam*. Philadelphia: Lean & Febiger.

Goodz, N., Legarré, M., & Bilodeau, L. (1990). *Language acquisition in bilingual families*. Poster session presented at the 7th Annual Conference of the American Association for Applied Linguistics, Vancouver, Canada.

Gordon, C. (1997). The effect of cancer pain on quality of life in different ethnic groups: A literature review. *Nurse Practitioner Forum, 8*(1), 5–13.

Gorman, B. K., & Gillam, R. B. (2003). Phonological awareness in Spanish: A tutorial for speech-language pathologists. *Communication Disorders Quarterly, 25*(1), 13–22.

Gottardo, A. (2002). The relationship between language and reading skills in bilingual Spanish-English speakers. *Topics in Language Disorders, 22*(5), 46–70.

Graham, L., & Bellert, A. (2004). Difficulties in reading comprehension for students with learning disabilities. In B. Wong (Ed.), *Learning about learning disabilities* (3rd ed., pp. 251–279). New York: Elsevier.

Graham, L., Harris, K. R., & Mac Arthur, C. (2004). Writing instruction. In B. Wong (Ed.), *Learning about learning disabilities* (3rd ed., pp. 281–313). New York: Elsevier.

Greene, J., & Forster, G. (2003). *Public high school graduation and college readiness: Rates in the United States* (Executive Summary No. 3). Education working paper presented at the Center for Civic Innovation, Manhattan Institute for Policy Research, New York, NY.

Greenfield, P. (1984). A theory of the teacher in the learning activities of everyday life. In B. Rogott & J. Lave (Eds.), *Everyday cognition: Its development in a social context*. Cambridge, MA: Harvard University Press.

Greenfield, P., & Smith, J. (1976). *The structure of communication in early language development*. New York: Academic Press.

Gromme, D. (1999). *An introduction to cognitive psychology: Processes and disorders*. London: Psychology Press Ltd.

Grosjean, F. (1982). *Life with two languages*. Cambridge, MA: Harvard University Press.

Grosjean, F. (2001). The bilingual's language models. In J. Nicol. (Ed.), *One mind, two languages: Bilingual language processing* (pp. 1–22). Williston, VT: Blackwell.

Guendelman, S., (1983). Developing responsiveness to the health needs of Hispanic children and families. *Social Work in Health Care, 8,* 1–15.

Gutiérrez-Clellen, V. (1999). Language choice in intervention with bilingual children. *American Journal of Speech-Language Pathology, 8,* 291–302.

Gutiérrez-Clellen, V. (2004). Narrative development and disorders in bilingual children. In B. Goldstein (Ed.), *Bilingual language development and disorders in Spanish-English speakers* (pp. 235–256). Baltimore: Brookes.

Gutiérrez-Clellen, V., & Erickson. A. (2003). *Codeswitching in bilingual SLI children.* Poster session presented at the 4th International Symposium on Bilingualism, Arizona State University, Tempe, AZ.

Gutiérrez-Clellen, V., & Kreiter, J. (2003). Understanding child bilingual acquisition using parent and teacher reports. *Applied Psycholinguistics, 24,* 267–298.

Gutiérrez-Clellen, V., Peña, E., Conboy, B., & Pasechnic, P. (1996). *Dynamic assessment of language: Research issues and clinical applications across cultures.* Paper presented at California Association of Mediated Learning Conference, San Diego, CA.

Gutiérrez-Clellen, V., & Quinn, R. (1993). Assessing narratives in diverse cultural/linguistic populations. Clinical implications. *Language, Speech, and Hearing Services in Schools, 24,* 2–9.

Hagen, C. (1981). Language disorders secondary to closed head injury. *Topics in Language Disorders, 1,* 73–87.

Hagen, C. (1984). Language disorders in head trauma. In A. Holland (Ed.), *Language disorders in adults* (pp. 247–281). San Diego, CA: College Hill Press.

Hakuta, K., & Díaz, R. (1985). The relationship between degree of bilingualism and cognitive ability: A critical discussion and some new longitudinal data. In K. Nelson (Ed.), *Children's language* (Vol. 5). Hillsdale, NJ: Lawrence Erlbaum Associates.

Hall, E. (1977). *Beyond culture.* Garden City, NY: Anchor Books.

Halpern, L. (1941). Beitrag zur Restitution der Aphasic bei Polyglotten im Himblick auf das Habräische. *Schweitzer Archiv für Neurologie und Psychiatrie, 47,* 15–156.

Hamman, S., & Square, L. (1996). Levels of processing effects in word-completion priming. A neuropsychological study. *Journal of Experimental Psychology: Learning, Memory, and Cognition, 22,* 933–947.

Hamman, S., & Square, L. (1997). Intact perceptual memory in the absence of conscious memory. *Behavioral Neuroscience, 111,* 850–854.

Hammer, C., Miccio, A., & Rodriguez, B. (2004). Bilingual language acquisition and the child socialization process. In B. Goldstein (Ed.), *Bilingual language development and disorders in Spanish-English speakers* (pp. 21–50). Baltimore: Brookes.

Hammill, D. (1998). *Detroit Test of Learning Aptitude* [DTLA-4]. Austin, TX: Pro-Ed.

Hanson, M. (2004). Families with Anglo-American roots. In E. Lynch & M. Hanson (Eds.), *Developing cross-cultural competence: A guide for working with children and their families* (3rd ed., pp. 81–108). Baltimore: Brookes.

Harris K., & Graham, S. (1996). Constructivism and students with special needs: Issues in the classroom. *Learning Disabilities: Research and Practice, 11,* 133–137.

Harris K., Graham, S., & Mason L. (2003). Self-regulated strategy development in the classroom: Part of a balanced approach to writing instruction for students with disabilities. *Focus on Exceptional Children, 25*(7), 1–16.

Hayes., J. R. (1996). A new framework for understanding cognition and affect in writing. In C. M. Levy & S. Ransdell (Eds.), *The science of writing* (pp. 1–27). Mahwah, NJ: Lawrence Erlbaum Associates.

Heath, S. B. (1986). Sociocultural contexts of language development. In California State Department of Education (Ed.), *Beyond language: Social and cultural factors in schooling language minority students* (pp. 143–186). Los Angeles: Evaluation, Dissemination, and Assessment Center, California State University.

Hegde, N. M. (2006). *Coursebook on aphasia and other neurogenic language disorders.* Clifton Park, NY: Thomson Delmar Learning.

Herrell, A. (2000). *Fifty strategies for teaching English-language learners.* Upper Saddle River, NJ: Merrill.

Herrera, S., & Murry, K. (2005). *Mastering ESL and bilingual methods: Differentiated instruction for culturally and linguistically diverse (CLD) students.* Boston: Pearson.

Hodson, B. (1986). *Assessment of Phonological Processes—Spanish.* San Diego, CA: Los Amigos Research Associates.

Hodson, B. (2005). *Enhancing phonological and metaphonological skills of children with highly unintelligible speech* [VHS/DVD and manual]. Rockville, MD: ASHA.

Holland, A. (1983). Nonbiased assessment and treatment of adults who have neurological speech and language problems. *Topics in Language Disorders, 3*(3), 67–75.

Holland, A. (1999). *Counseling adults with neurogenic communication disorders* [Videotape]. Rockville, MD: ASHA.

Holm, A., Dodd, H., & Ozonne, A. (1997). Efficacy of intervention for a bilingual child making articulation and phonological errors. *International Journal of Bilingualism, 1,* 55–69.

Hopstock, P., & Stephenson, T. (2003). *Native languages of LEP students.* Washington, DC: U.S. Department of Education, National Clearinghouse for English Language Acquisition and Language Instruction Educational Programs.

Hoskyn, M. (2004). Language processes and reading disabilities. In B. Wong (Ed.), *Learning about learning disabilities* (3rd ed., pp. 93–131). Boston: Elsevier.

Hresko, W. P., Reid, D. K., & Hammill, D. D. (1982). *Prueba del Desarrollo Inicial del Lenguaje.* Austin, TX: Pro-Ed.

Hummert, M., Shaner, J., Garstka, T., & Henry, C. (1998). Communication with older adults. The influence of age stereotypes. Context and communicator age. *Human Communication Research, 25*(1), 124–151.

Hwa-Froelich, D., & Westby, C. (2003a). Considerations when working with interpreters. *Communication Disorders Quarterly, 24,* 78–85.

Hwa-Froelich, D., & Westby, C. (2003b). A Vietnamese Head-Start interpreter: A case study. *Communication Disorders Quarterly, 24,* 86–98.

Hyter, Y. (1996). Ties that bind: The sounds of African-American English. *ASHA Special Interest Division 14 Newsletter, 2,* 3–6.

Individuals with Disabilities Education Improvement Act of 2004. Pub. L. No. 108–446 (2004).

Jackson-Maldonado, D., Bates, E., & Thal, D. J. (2003). *Mac Artur Inventario del Desarrollo de Habilidades Comunicativas.* Baltimore: Brookes.

James, P. (1974). *The James Language Dominance Test* [Spanish-English]. Allen, TX: DLM Teaching Resources.

Jennett, B., & Bond, M. (1975). Assessment of outcome after severe brain damage: A practical scale. *Lancet, 1*, 480–484.

Jiménez, J. W., & García, C. R. H. (1995). Effects of word linguistic properties on phonological awareness in Spanish children. *Journal of Educational Psychology, 87*, 23–40.

Joe, J., & Malach, R. (2004). Families with American Indian roots. In E. Lynch & M. Hanson. (Eds.), *Developing cross-cultural competence: A guide for working with children and their families* (3rd ed., pp. 99–131). Baltimore: Brookes.

Johnson, C. (2006). Getting started in evidence-based practice for childhood speech-language disorders. *American Journal of Speech-Language Pathology, 15*, 20–35.

Johnson, D. J., & Myklebust, H. (1967). *Learning disabilities: Educational principles and practices*. New York: Grune & Stratton.

Justice, L., & Kaderavek, J. (2004). Embedded-explicit emergent literacy intervention: Background and description of approach. *Language, Speech, and Hearing Services in Schools, 35*, 201–211.

Kagan, S. (1986). Cooperative learning and sociocultural factors in schooling. In California State University (Eds.), *Beyond language: Social and cultural factors in schooling language minority students* (pp. 231–298). Los Angeles: Evaluation, Dissemination, and Assessment Center, California State University.

Katz, R. C. (2001). Computer application in aphasia treatment. In R. Chapey (Ed.), *Language intervention strategies in aphasia and related neurogenic communication disorders* (4th ed., pp. 718–741). Philadelphia: Lippincott Williams & Wilkins.

Katzner, K. (2002). *The languages of the world*. London: Routledge.

Kay-Raining Bird, E., Cleave, P., Trudeau, N., Thordardottir, E., Sutton, A., & Thorpe, A. (2005). The language abilities of bilingual children with Down syndrome. *American Journal of Speech-Language Pathology, 14*, 187–199.

Kayser, H. (1989, November). *Communicative strategies of Anglo and Hispanic clinicians with Hispanic preschoolers*. Paper presented at the American Speech-Language-Hearing Association Annual Convention, St. Louis, MO.

Kayser, H. (1990). Social communicative behaviors of language-disordered Mexican-American students. *Child Language Teaching and Therapy, 6*, 255–269.

Kennedy, A., (2000). Positron-emission tomography in dementia. In J. O'Brien, D. Ames, & A. Burns (Eds.), *Dementia* (2nd ed., pp. 163–177). London: Edward Arnold.

Kilpatrick, K, Jones, C. L, & Reller, J. (1982). *Manual terapéutico para el adulto con dificultades del habla y lenguaje—Tomo I* (I. Bahler & B. K. Gatto, Trans.). Akron. OH: Visiting Nurse Services.

Kindler, A. (2002). *Survey of the states' limited-English-proficient students and available educational programs and services: 2000–2001 summary report*. Washington, DC: National Clearinghouse for English Language Acquisition and Language Instruction Educational Programs.

Kinsella, K., & Velkoff, V. A. (2001). *An aging world*. National Institute on Aging, Washington, DC: U.S. Department of Commerce.

Kirk, D. (2000). *Miss spider's ABC*. New York: Calloway & Kirk.

Kirk, S., & van Isser, A. (1980). *Prueba Illinois de Habilidades Psicolingüísticas*. Tucson, AZ: University of Arizona, Special Education Department.

Kitano, H. (1989). A model for counseling Asian-Americans. In P. B. Pedersen, J. G. Draguns, W. J. Lonner, & J. E. Trimble (Eds.), *Counseling across cultures* (pp. 130–151). Honolulu: University of Hawaii Press.

Knight, K. (2006). *Zoophabet: ABC*. Franklin, TN: Dalmatian Press.

Kochman, T. E. (1981). *Black and white styles in conflict*. Chicago: University of Chicago Press.

Kohnert, K. (2004). Processing skills in early sequential bilinguals. In B. Goldstein (Ed.), *Bilingual language development and disorders in Spanish-English speakers* (pp. 53–76). Baltimore: Brookes.

Kohnert, K., & Bates, E. (2002). Balancing bilinguals: Lexical comprehension and cognitive processing in children learning Spanish and English. *Journal of Speech, Language, and Hearing Research, 45*, 347–359.

Kohnert, K., & Derr, A. (2004). Language intervention with bilingual children. In B. Goldstein (Ed.), *Bilingual language development and disorders in Spanish-English speakers* (pp. 311–338). Baltimore: Brookes.

Kolchin, O. (1995). *American slavery 1619–1877*. Harmondsworth, UK: Penguin.

Krashen, S. (1981). Bilingual education and second-language acquisition theory. In Office of Bilingual Bicultural Education, California State Department of Education (Ed.), *Schooling and language minority students: A theoretical framework* (pp.51–79). Los Angeles: Evaluation, Dissemination, and Assessment Center, California State University.

Krashen, S. (1982). *Second-language acquisition and second-language learning*. Oxford, UK-Oxford, UK: Pergamon Press.

Krashen, S. (1999). *Condemned without a trial: Bogus arguments against bilingual education*. Portsmouth, NH: Heineman.

Krashen, S., & Biber, D. (1988). *On course: Bilingual education's success in California*. Sacramento: California Association for Bilingual Education.

Kucer, S., & Silva, C. (1989, Winter). The new California English-language-arts framework: A step in the right direction. *California Association of Supervisors of Curriculum Development Journal*, 14–15.

Kuhlman, N. (2005). The language assessment conundrum: What tests claim to assess and what teachers need to know. *The ELL Outlook,4*(2). Electronic newsletter, retrieved July, 2005, from http://www.coursecrafters.com/ELL-Outlook/2005/mar_apr/ELLOutlookITIArticle1.htm

Langdon, H. W. (1977). *Determining a language disorder in a bilingual Spanish-English population*. Unpublished doctoral dissertation, Boston University, Boston, MA.

Langdon. H. W. (1983). Assessment and intervention strategies for the bilingual-language-disorder student. *Exceptional Children, 50*, 37–56.

Langdon H. W. (1989). Language disorder or language difference? Assessing the language skills of Hispanic students. *Exceptional Children, 56*, 160–167.

Langdon, H. W. (1992a). Language communication and sociocultural patterns in Hispanic families. In H. W. Langdon with L. R. Cheng (Eds.), *Hispanic children and adults with communication disorders: Assessment and intervention* (pp. 99–131). Gaithersburg, MD: Aspen.

Langdon, H. W. (1992b). Speech and language assessment of LEP/bilingual Hispanic students. In H. W. Langdon with L. R. Cheng (Eds.), *Hispanic children and adults with communication disorders: Assessment and intervention* (pp. 201–266). Gaithersburg, MD: Aspen.

Langdon, H. W. (2002). *Interpreters and translators in communication disorders: A practitioner's handbook.* Eau Claire, WI: Thinking Publications.

Langdon H. W. (2003). *Working with interpreters to serve bilingual children and families* [Video]. Rockville, MD: ASHA.

Langdon, H. W., & Cheng. L. R. (1992). Defining bilingual education in the United States. In H. W. Langdon with L. R. Cheng (Eds.), *Hispanic children and adults with communication disorders: Assessment and intervention* (pp.168–200). Gaithersburg, MD: Aspen.

Langdon, H. W., with L. R. Cheng (Eds.). (1992). *Hispanic children and adults with communication disorders: Assessment and intervention.* Gaithersburg, MD: Aspen.

Langdon, H. W., & Cheng, L. R (2002). *Collaborating with interpreters and translators: A guide for communication disorders professionals.* Eau Claire, WI: Thinking Publications.

Langdon, H. W., & Merino, B. (1992). Acquisition and development of a second language in the Spanish speaker. In H. W. Langdon with L. R. Cheng (Eds.), *Hispanic children and adults with communication disorders: Assessment and intervention* (pp. 132–167). Gaithersburg, MD: Aspen.

La Pointe, L. (Ed.). (2005). *Aphasia and neurological-related disorders* (3rd ed.). New York: Thieme.

Larson, V. L., & McKinley, N. L. (2003). *Communication solutions for older students: Assessment and intervention strategies.* Eau Claire, WI: Thinking Publications.

Leigh, J. W., & Green, J. W. (1982). The structure of the black community: The knowledge base for social services. In J. W. Green (Ed.), *Cultural awareness in the human services* (pp. 94–121). Englewood Cliffs, NJ: Prentice-Hall.

Lenneberg, E. (1967). *Biological foundations of language.* New York: Wiley.

Leopold, W. (1970). *Speech development of a bilingual child* (Vols. 1–4). New York: AMS Press.

Lessow-Hurley, J. (2005). *The foundations of dual-language instruction* (4th ed.). Boston: Pearson.

Linares-Orama, N. (1977). Evaluation of syntax in three-year-old Spanish-speaking Puerto Rican children. *Journal of Speech and Hearing Research, 20,* 350–357.

Lingraphicare of America—Lingraphica®. 15 Spring St., 2nd floor, Princeton, NJ 08542 [Tel: 888-274-2741]. Web site: http://www.aphasia.com/contact.html

Lionni, L. (1996). *The alphabet tree.* New York: Random House.

Lipman, P. (1998). *Race, class, and power in school restructuring.* Albany: State University of New York Press. *Logramos.* (2nd ed.). (2006). Itasca, IL: Riverside.

Loop, C. (2002). *Which tests are commonly used to determine English and/or Spanish language proficiency?* Washington, DC: National Clearinghouse for English Language Acquisition and Language Instruction Educational Programs.

Luckmann, J. (2000). *Transcultural communication in health care.* Clifton Park, NY: Thompson Delmar Learning.

Lustig, M., & Koester, J. (1999). *Intercultural competence: Interpersonal communication-across cultures* (3rd ed.). New York: Longman.

Lynch, E. W. (2004). Developing cross-cultural competence. In E. W. Lynch & M. J. Hanson, (Eds.), *Developing cross-cultural competence: A guide for working with children and their families* (3rd ed., pp. 41–77). Baltimore: Brookes.

Lynch, E. W., & Hanson, M. J. (2004). *Developing cross-cultural competence: A guide for working with children and their families* (3rd ed.). Baltimore: Brookes.

Lyon, G. R. (1998, April 28). *Overview of reading and literacy initiatives. Statement to the Committee on Language and Human Resources.* Washington DC: U.S. Senate.

Madding, C. C. (1995). The stuttering syndrome: Feelings and attitudes of stutterers and non-stutterers among four cultural groups. *Dissertation Abstracts International, 56* (12), 4959A.

Maestas, A. G., & Erickson, J. E. (1989, November). *Mexican immigrant parents and the education of their handicapped children: Factors that influence parent involvement.* Paper presented at the American Speech-Language-Hearing Association Annual Convention, St. Louis, MO.

Mandlawitz, M., (2006). *What every teacher should know about IDEA 2004.* Boston: Pearson.

Manuel-Dupont, S., Ardila, A., Rosselli, M., & Puente, A. E. (1992). Bilingualism. In A. E. Puente & R. J. McCaffrey (Eds.), *Handbook of neuropsychological assessment* (pp. 193–210). New York: Plenum Press.

Manuel–Dupont, S., & Yoakum. S. (1997). Training interpreter paraprofessionals to assist in the language assessment of English-language learners in Utah. *Journal of Children's Communication Development, 18*(1), 91–102.

Mares, S. (1980). *Pruebas de Expresión Oral y Percepción de la Lengua Española* [PEOPLE]. Downey, CA: Los Angeles County Office of Education.

Marshall, R. C. (2001). Management in Wernicke's aphasia: A context-based approach. In R. Chapey (Ed.), *Language intervention strategies in aphasia and related neurogenic communication disorders* (4th ed., pp. 435–456). Philadelphia: Lippincott Williams & Wilkins.

Martin, A. D. (1981). An examination of Wepman's thought-centered therapy. In R. Chapey (Ed.), *Language intervention strategies in adult aphasia.* Baltimore: Williams & Wilkins.

Marty, S., & Grosjean, F.(1998). Aphasie, bilinguisme et modes de communication. *Aphasie und Verwandte, 12*(1), 8–28.

Mason, M. A., Smith, B. F., & Hinshaw, M. M. (1976). *Medida Española de Articulación* [MEDA]. San Ysidro, CA: San Ysidro School District.

Mattes, L. (1995). *Spanish Articulation Measures* [SAM]. Oceanside, CA: Academic Communication Associates.

Mayer, M. (1969). *Frog, where are you?* New York: Dial Books for Young Readers.

Mayer, M., & Mayer, M. (1975). *One frog too many.* New York: Dial Books for Young Readers.

McKinnon, J. (2003). *The Black population in the United States(March 2002).* Washington, DC: U.S. Census Bureau.

McLaughlin, J. (2003). *Schooling in Mexico: A brief guide for U.S. educators. ERIC Digest,* ED 470987. Retrieved April 14, 2005, from http://www.ericdigests.org.2003-4/mexico.html

McLaughlin, M., & Allen, M. B. (2002). *Guided comprehension: A teaching model for grades 3–8*. Newark, DE: International Reading Association.

Mehrabian, A. (1972). *Nonverbal communication*. Chicago: University of Chicago Press.

Melgar de González, M. (1980). *Cómo detectar al niño con problemas del habla*. Mexico City (D. F.), Mexico: Trillas.

Meyerson, M. (1983). Genetic counseling for families of Chicano children with birth defects. In D. R. Omark & J. G. Erickson (Eds.), *The bilingual exceptional child* (pp. 285–298). San Diego, CA: College Hill Press.

Meyerson, M. (1990). Cultural considerations in the treatment of Latinos with craniofacial malformations. *The Cleft Palate Journal, 27*, 279–288.

Miller, D. L. (1979). *Mother's perception of Indian child development*. Unpublished research report. San Francisco: Institute for Scientific Analysis.

Miller, L., Gillam, R., & Peña, E. (2001). *Dynamic assessment and intervention: Improving children's narrative abilities*. Austin, TX: Pro-Ed.

Miller, R. (1984). *The primary schools in Mexico*. Los Gatos, CA: Paradox Press.

Minkowski, M. (1963). *On aphasia in polyglots: Problems in dynamic neurology*. Jerusalem: Hebrew University [Press].

Mjoseth, J. (2004). *Federal forum reports Americans aging well, but gaps remain* [News release]. Retrieved August 30, 2005, from http://www.agnagstats.gov/charbook2004/pr.html

Mlcoch, A., & Metter, E. J. (2001). Medical aspects of stroke rehabilitation. In R. Chapey (Ed.), *Language intervention strategies in aphasia and related neurogenic communication disorders* (4th ed., pp. 37–54). Philadelphia: Lippincott Williams & Wilkins.

Moll, L. (1988). Some key issues in teaching Latino students. *Language Arts, 65*(5), 465–472.

Morine-Dershimer, G. (1985). *Talking, listening, and learning in elementary classrooms*. New York: Longman.

Morrison, B. (1977). *Squeeze a sneeze*. Boston: Houghton Mifflin.

Muñoz, M. L., Marquart, T., & Copeland, G. (1999). A comparison of the code-switching patterns of aphasic and neurologically normal bilingual speakers of English and Spanish. *Brain and Language, 66*, 249–274.

Muñoz-Sandoval, A., Cummins, J., Alvarado, C., & Ruef, M. (1998). *Bilingual Verbal Ability Test* [BVAT]. Itasca, IL: Riverside.

Murray, L., & Clark, H. M. (2006). *Neurogenic disorders of language*. Clifton Park, NY: Thomson Delmar Learning.

Myers-Scotton, V. (1992). Comparing code-switching and borrowing. *Journal of Multilingual and Multicultural Development, 13*, 19–39.

Myers-Scotton, V. (2002). *Contact linguistics*. Cambridge, UK: Cambridge University Press.

National Center for Health Statistics. (2005). *Health, United States 2005 with chartbook on trends in the health of Americans*. Hyattsville, MD: Author.

National Clearinghouse for English Language Acquisition and Language Instruction Educational Programs. (2002). *Survey of the states' limited-English-proficient students and available educational programs and services: 2000–2001 summary report*. Washington, DC: U.S. Department of Education.

National Clearinghouse for English Language Acquisition and Language Instruction Educational Programs. (2003). *The growing numbers of limited-English-proficient students (1992/1993–2002/2003)*. Washington DC: U.S. Department of Education.

National Institute for Literacy. (2007). Data last retrieved April 14, 2007, from http://www.nifl.gov/nifl/contact.html

National Virtual Translation Center. (2006). Data last retrieved March 31, 2007, from http://www.nvtc.gov

Negroni-Rodríguez, L., & Morales, J. (2001). Individual and family assessment skills with Latino-Hispanic Americans. In R. Fong and S. Furuto (Eds.), *Cultural competence practice: Skills, interventions, and evaluations* (pp. 132–146). Boston: Allyn & Bacon.

Nelson-Barber, S., & Dull, V. (1998). Don't act like a teacher. Images of effective instruction in a Yu'ik Eskimo classroom. In J. Lipka, (Ed.), with G. V. Mohatt & The Ciulistet Group. *Transforming the culture of schools: Yup'ik Eskimo examples* (pp. 91–105). Mahwah, NJ: Lawrence Erlbaum Associates.

Nettle, D. (1999). *Linguistic Diversity*. Oxford, UK: Oxford University Press.

Nicoladis, E., & Secco, G. (2000). The role of a child's productive vocabulary in the language choice of a bilingual family. *First Language, 58*, 3–28.

Nielsen, N. P., & Wiig, E. H. (2006). Alzheimer's Quick Test screening criteria for West African speakers of Krio. *Age & Ageing, 35*, 503–507.

Nieto, S. (2004). Affirming diversity: The sociopolitical context of multicultural education (4th ed). Boston: Pearson. No Child Left Behind Act of 2001. Pub. L. No. 107–110, 115 Stat. 1425 (2001).

Office of Minority Health. (2000). *Hispanics in the United States: An insight into group characteristics*. Washington, DC: Author.

Ogbu, J. (1987). Variability in minority responses to schooling: Non-immigrants vs. immigrants. In G. Spindler & L. Spindler (Eds.), *Interpretive ethnography of education at home and abroad* (pp. 255–278). New Jersey: Lawrence Erlbaum Associates.

Ogunwole, S. O. (2002). *The American Indian and Alaska Native population*. Washington DC: U.S. Census Bureau.

Oller, D., & Eilers, R. E. (2002). *Language and literacy in bilingual children*. Clevedon, UK: Multilingual Matters.

Orozco, J. L. (1988). *La pulga de San José (San José's flea market)* [Recorded by J. L. Orozco]. On *La lírica infantil, Vol. I* [CD]. Berkeley, CA: Arcoiris Records.

Ovando. C. (2003). Bilingual education in the United States: Historical development and current issues. *Bilingual Research Journal, 27*(1), 1–2.

Pang, V. O., & Cheng, L. (1998). *Struggling to be heard: The unmet needs of Asian/Pacific-American children*. Albany: State University of New York Press.

Paradis, J. (2001). Do bilingual two-year olds have separate phonological systems? *International Journal of Bilingualism, 5*, 19–38.

Paradis, J. (2005). Grammatical morphology in ESL: Similarities with SLI. *Language, Speech, and Hearing Services in Schools, 36*, 172–187.

Paradis, J., & Genesee, F. (1996). Syntactic acquisition in bilingual children: Autonomous or interdependent. *Studies in Second-Language Acquisition, 18*, 1–25.

Paradis, M. (1977). Bilingualism and aphasia. In H. Whitaker & H. A. Whitaker (Eds.), *Studies in neurolinguistics* (Vol. 3). New York: Academic Press.

Paradis, M. (1987). *Bilingual aphasia test*. Hillsdale, NJ: Lawrence and Erlbaum.

Paradis, M. (1995). *Aspects of bilingual aphasia*. Tarrytown, NY: Elsevier.

Paradis, M. (Ed.). (2001). *Manifestations of aphasia symptoms in different languages*. New York: Pergamon.

Paradis, M., & Libben, G. (1987). *The assessment of bilingual aphasia*. Hillsdale, NJ: Lawrence Erlbaum Associates.

Parrot Software. P.O. Box 250755, West Bloomfield, MI 48825 [Tel: 800-PARROT-1]. Web site: http://www.parrotsoftware.com/contact/contact.htm

Patterson, J., & Pearson, B. (2004). Bilingual lexical development: Influences, contexts, and processes. In B. Goldstein (Ed.), *Bilingual language development and disorders in Spanish-English speakers* (pp. 77–104). Baltimore: Brookes.

Paul, R. (2001). *Language disorders from infancy through adolescence: Assessment and intervention* (3rd ed.). New York: Mosby.

Paul, R. (2006). *Language disorders from infancy through adolescence: Assessment and interaction* (4th ed.). New York: Mosby.

Peal, E., & Lambert, W. E. (1962). The relation of bilingualism to intelligence. *Psychological Monographs, 76*(27, Whole No. 546).

Pearce, J. M. (2005). A note on aphasia in bilingual patients: Pitres' and Ribot's laws. *European Neurology, 54*, 127–131.

Pearson B., Fernández, S., & Oller, K. (1993). Lexical development in bilingual infants and toddlers: Comparison to monolingual norms. *Language Learning 43*, 93–120.

Pedersen, P. B. (1989). *Counseling across cultures*. Honolulu: University of Hawaii Press.

Penfield, J. (1989). *The Hispanic student: Questions and answers*. Highland Park: Penfield Associates.

Perry, T. (1998). "I 'no know why they be tripping'": Reflections on the Ebonics debate. In T. Perry. & L. Delpit (Eds.), *The real Ebonics debate: Power, language, and the education of African-American children* (pp. 3–16). Boston: Beacon Press.

Perry, T., & Delpit. L. (Eds.). (1998a). Holding on to a language of our own: An interview with linguist John Rickford. In T. Perry & L. Delpit (Eds.), *The real Ebonics debate: Power, language, and the education of African-American children* (pp. 58–70). Boston: Beacon Press.

Perry, T., & Delpit. L. (Eds.). (1998b). Embracing Ebonics and teaching Standard English: An interview with Oakland teacher Carrie Secret. In T. Perry & L. Delpit (Eds.), *The real Ebonics debate: Power, language, and the education of African-American children* (pp. 79–88). Boston: Beacon Press.

Phelps-Terasaki, D., & Phelps-Dunn. T. (1992). *Test of Pragmatic Language*. San Antonio, TX: The Psychological Corporation.

Pitres, A. (1985). Etude sur l'aphasie chez les polyglotes. *Revue Médicale, 15*, 873.

Pollack, M. D. (1980). *The effects of testwiseness, language of test administration, and language competence on the readiness and test performance of low-socioeconomic-level, Spanish-speaking children* (Microfilms International Microfiche #80-16031). Ann Arbor: University of Michigan.

Pollock, K., Bailey, G., Berni, M., Fletcher, D., Hinton, L., Johnson, I., & Weaver, R. (1998, November). *Phonological characteristics of African-American English Vernacular (AAVE): An updated feature list*. Seminar presented at the convention of the American Speech-Language-Hearing Association, San Antonio, TX.

Pope, C. (2005). Ethnolinguistic variations in communication with elderly persons who have Alzheimer's disease. *Perspectives on Communication Disorders and Sciences in Culturally and Linguistically Diverse Populations, 12*(3), 14–21.

Poplack, S. (1979). Sometimes I start a sentence in Spanish Y TERMINO EN ESPANOL: Towards a typology of code-switching. *Centro de Estudios Puertorriqueños, 4,* 1–79.

Porch, B. E. (1981). Therapy subsequent to the PICA. In R. Chapey (Ed.), *Language intervention strategies for adult aphasia.* Baltimore: Williams & Wilkins.

Proposition 227. (1998). [Text of the California law banning native language instruction]. Last retrieved April 15, 2007, from http://primary98.ss.ca.gov/VoterGuide/Propositions/227text.htm

Prutting, E. (1983). Assessing communicative behavior using a language sample. In D. R. Omark & J. G. Erickson (Eds.), *The bilingual exceptional child* (pp. 89–99). San Diego, CA: College Hill Press.

Puerto Rico. Last retrieved May 20, 2007 from http://welcome.topuertorico.org/people.shtm

Purcell-Gates, V. (1989). What oral/written language differences can tell us about beginning instruction. *Reading Teacher, 42,* 290–294.

Puyuelo, S. M., Rondal, J. A., & Wiig, E. (2000). *Evaluación del lenguaje.* Barcelona, Spain: Masson.

Queralt, M. (1984). Understanding Cuban immigrants: A cultural perspective. *Social Work, 29,* 115–121.

Radford, N., & Wiig, E. H. (2005). *AQT cognitive-screening criteria for Hispanics in the Southwest.* Working Paper, Jackson State University, Mississippi.

Ramírez, R. (2004). *We the people: Hispanics in the United States.* Washington, DC: U.S. Census Bureau.

Ramos, F. (2005). Spanish teachers' opinions about the use of Spanish in mainstream English classrooms before and after their first year in California. *Bilingual Research Journal, 29,* 411–433.

Ratner, N. B. (2004). Fluency and stuttering in bilingual children. In B. Goldstein (Ed.), *Bilingual language development and disorders in Spanish-English speakers* (pp. 287–308). Baltimore: Brookes.

Restrepo, A. (1998). Identifiers of predominantly Spanish-speaking children with language impairment. *Journal of Speech, Language, and Hearing Research, 41,* 1398–1411.

Restrepo, A. (2003). Spanish language skills in bilingual children with specific language impairment. In S. Montrul & F. Ordóñez (Eds.), *Linguistic theory and language development in Hispanic languages* (pp. 365–374). Papers from the 5th Hispanic Linguistics Symposium and the 2001 Acquisition of Spanish and Portuguese Conference, Sommerville, MA: Cascadilla Press.

Restrepo, M. A., & Gutiérrez-Clellen, V. F. (2004). Grammatical impairments in Spanish-English bilingual children. In B. Goldstein (Ed.), *Bilingual language development and disorders in Spanish-English speakers* (pp. 213–234). Baltimore: Brookes.

Ribot, T. (1882). *Disease of memory: An essay in the positive psychology.* London: Paul.

Riccio, C., Imhoff, B., Hasbrouck, J., & Davis, N. (2004). *Test of Phonological Awareness Ability in Spanish-Speaking Children* [TPAS]. Austin, TX: Pro-Ed.

Riley, D. W. (1995). The complete Kwanzaa: Celebrating our cultural heritage. New York: HarperCollins.

Riley, G. (1994). *Stuttering severity instrument for children and adults* (3rd ed.). Austin, TX: Pro-Ed.

Roberts, P. (2001). Aphasia assessment and treatment for bilingual and culturally diverse patients. In R. Chapey (Ed.), *Language intervention strategies in aphasia and related neurogenic communication disorders* (4th ed., pp. 208–232). Philadelphia: Lippincott Williams & Wilkins.

Rodríguez, B. L., & Olswang, L. B. (2003). Mexican-American and Anglo-American mothers' beliefs and values about childrearing, education, and language impairment. *American Journal of Speech-Language Pathology, 12,* 452–462.

Rodríguez, J. (1983). Mexican-Americans: Factors influencing health practices. *The Journal of School Health* (Special Issue), 136–139.

Rodríguez, R. (1982). *Hunger of memory. The education of Richard Rodríguez.* Boston: David R. Godine.

Roffey, M. (2004). *Animal ABCs: A book with fabulous flaps.* New York: Reader's Digest Children's Books.

Romaine, S. (1995). *Bilingualism.* New York: Blackwell.

Romo, H. (1984). The Mexican origin population's differing perceptions of their children's schooling. *Social Science Quarterly, 65,* 635–649.

Ronjat, J. (1913). *Le développement du language observé chez un enfant bilingue.* Paris: Champion.

Roseberry-McKibbin, C. (2002). *Multicultural students with special language needs: Practical strategies for assessment and intervention.* Oceanside, CA: Academic Communication Associates.

Roseberry-Mc.Kibbin, C., Brice, A., & O'Hanlon, L. (2005). Serving English-language learners in public school settings: A national survey. *Language, Speech, and Hearing Services in Schools, 16*(1), 48–61.

Rosenthal, M., Griffith, E., Kreutzer, J., et al. (1999). *Rehabilitation of the adult and child with traumatic brain injury* (3rd ed., pp. 8–9). Philadelphia: F. A. Davis.

Rossetti, L. (1990). *The Rossetti Infant-Toddler Scale (Spanish).* Moline, IL: LinguiSystems.

Roy, C. B. (2000). *Interpreting as a discourse process.* New York: Oxford University Press.

Ruiz, N. (1988). *Language for learning in a bilingual special education classroom.* Unpublished doctoral dissertation, Stanford University, Palo Alto, CA.

Rumberger, R. W. (2000). *Educational outcomes and opportunities for English-language learners* (Document No. 141). Working paper, Linguistic Minority Research Institute, University of California, Santa Barbara.

Russell, J. (1994). Is there a universal recognition of emotion from facial expression? A review of cross-cultural studies. *Psychological Bulletin, 115,* 102–141.

Saer, D. (1924). The effect of bilingualism on intelligence. *British Journal of Psychology, 14,* 25–38.

Salas-Provence, M. (2005). From the coordinator. *Perspectives on Communication Disorders and Sciences in Culturally and Linguistically Diverse Populations, 12*(3), 1.

Saltibañez, L., Vernez, G., & Razquin, P. (2005). *Education in Mexico: Challenges and opportunities (Summary).* Santa Monica, CA: RAND Corporation.

Samovar, L.A., & Porter, R. E. (1994). *Intercultural communication: A reader.* Belmont, CA: Wadsworth.

Sandberg, N. (1986). *Jewish life in Los Angeles*. Landham, MD: University Press of America.

Sarno, M. T. (1969). *The functional communication profile: Manual of directions; rehabilitation monograph 32*. New York: New York Institute of Rehabilitative Medicine.

Sarno, M. T., Silverman, M., & Sands, E. (1970). Speech therapy and language recovery in severe aphasia. *Journal of Speech and Hearing Research, 13*, 607–623.

Scarborough, H. S. (1998). Early identification of children at risk of reading disabilities: Phonological awareness and some other promising predictors. In B. K. Shapiro, P. J. Accardo, & A. J. Capute (Eds.), *Specific reading disabilities: A view of the spectrum* (pp. 75–119). Timonium, MD: York Press.

Schuell, H., Jenkins, K., & Jiménez-Pabón, E. (1964). *Aphasia in adults*. New York: Harper & Row.

Schwartz-Cowley, R., & Stepanic, J. J. (1989). Communication disorder and treatment in the acute trauma center setting. *Topics in Language Disorders, 9*(2), 1–14.

Semel, E., Wiig, E. H., & Secord, W. (2005). *Clinical Evaluation of Language Fundamentals* [CELF-4] [Spanish]. San Antonio, TX: The Psychological Corporation.

Seymour H. N., & Roeper, T. W. (1999). Grammatical acquisition of African-American English. In O. Taylor & L. Leonard (Eds.), *Language acquisition across North America: Cross-cultural and cross-linguistic perspectives* (pp. 109–152). San Diego, CA: Singular.

Seymour, H. N., Roeper, T. W., De Villiers, J., & De Villiers, P. (2003). *Diagnostic Evaluation of Language Variation Screening Test* [DELV]. San Antonio, TX: The Psychological Corporation.

Seymour, H. N., Roeper, T. W., De Villiers, J., & De Villiers, P. (2005). *Diagnostic Evaluation of Language Variation (DELV)—Norm Referenced*. San Antonio, TX: The Psychological Corporation.

Seymour, H., & Seymour, C. (1981). Black English and Standard American English contrasts in consonantal development of four- and five-year-old children. *Journal of Speech and Hearing Disorders, 46*, 274–280.

Shin, R. B., & Bruno, R. (2003). *Language use and English-speaking ability, 2000. Census 2000. Brief*. Washington, DC: U.S. Census Bureau.

Short, D. (1994). Expanding middle-school horizons: Integrating language, culture, and social studies. *TESOL Quarterly, 28*(3), 581–608.

Silver, J. (Ed.). (1995). *Profile of effective teaching in a multilingual classroom: Featuring Robin Liten-Tejada* [Video]. Santa Cruz, CA: The National Center for Research on Cultural Diversity and Second-Language Learning, University of California at Santa Cruz.

Singer, A. (2004, December). The Changing face of America. *e-Journal USA: Society & Values*. Retrieved April 15, 2007, from http://usinfo.state.gov/journals/itsv/1204/ijse/singer.htm

Singleton, D. (1989). *Language acquisition: The age factor*. Clevedon, UK: Multilingual Matters.

Smith, M. (1923). Bilingualism and mental development. *British Journal of Psychology, 13*, 271–282.

Smith, M. (1931). A study of five bilingual children from the same family. *Child Development, 2*, 184–187.

Smith, M. (1939). Some light on the problem of bilingualism as found from a study of the progress in mastery of English among preschool children of non-American ancestry in Hawaii. *Genetic Psychology Monographs, 21,* 119–284.

Smith-De Mateo, R. (1987, February). *Multicultural considerations: Working with families of developmentally disabled and high risk children.* Paper presented in the Conference of the National Center for Clinical Indian Programs, Los Angeles.

Smythe I., & Everatt, J. (2002). Dyslexia and the multilingual child: Policy into practice. *Topics in Language Disorders, 22*(5), 71–80.

Smythe, I., Everatt, J., & Salter, R. (2004). *International book of dyslexia: A cross-language comparison and practice guide.* Hoboken, NJ: John Wiley & Sons.

Snow, C., Burns, M., & Griffin, P. (Eds.). (1998). *Preventing reading difficulties in young children.* Washington, DC: National Academy Press.

Snow, C., Scarborough, H., & Burns, M. (1999). What speech-language pathologists need to know about early reading. *Topics in Language Disorders, 20*(1), 48–58.

Snyder L., Dabasinkas, C., & O'Connor, E. (2002). An information-processing perspective on language impairment in children: Looking at both sides of the coin. *Topics in Language Disorders, 22,* 1–14.

Sobel, J. (2006). *Shiver me letters: A pirate ABC.* New York: Harcourt.

Spanish Assessment of Basic Education (2nd ed.) (SABE/2). (2000). Monterey, CA: McGraw Hill Company.

Springer, L., Miller, N., & Bürk, F. (1998). A cross-language analysis of conversation in a trilingual speaker with aphasia. *Journal of Neurolinguistics, 11,* 223–241.

Stark, J., and Wallach, G. P. (1980). The path to a concept of language learning disabilities. *Topics in Language Disorders, 1*(1), 1–14.

Steele, R. D., Weinrich, M., Wertz, R. T., Kleczewska, M. K., & Carlson, G. S. (1989). Computer-based visual communication in aphasia. *Neuropshychologia, 27,* 409–427.

Stein, S. (1986). Medical management of cerebrovascular accidents. In R. Chapey (Ed.), *Language intervention strategies in adult aphasia* (2nd ed.). Baltimore: Williams & Wilkins.

Stockman, I. (1996). The promises and pitfalls of language sample analysis as an assessment tool for linguistic minority children. *Language, Speech, and Hearing Services in Schools, 27,* 355–366.

Stryker, S. (1985). *El habla después de una embalia.* Miami, FL: Stryker Illustrations.

Suárez-Orozco, M. (1987). Towards a psychosocial understanding of Hispanic adaptation to American schooling. In H. T. Trueba (Ed.), *Success or failure? Learning and the language minority student* (pp. 156–168). Cambridge, MA: Newbury House.

Suárez-Orozco, M., & Suárez-Orozco, C. (1996). *Transformations: Immigration, family life, and achievement motivation among Latino adolescents.* Palo Alto, CA: Stanford University Press.

Swain, M., & Cummins, J. (1982). Bilingualism, cognitive functioning and education. In V. Kinsella (Ed.), *Surveys 1.* Cambridge, UK: Cambridge University Press.

Swan, M., & Smith, B. (2004). *Learner English: A teacher's guide to interference and other problems.* Cambridge, UK: Cambridge University Press.

Swanson, E. N., and De Blassie, R. R. (1979). Interpreter and Spanish administration effects on the WISC-R performance of Mexican-American children. *Journal of School Psychology, 17,* 231–236.

Swanson, T., Hodson, B., & Aikins, M. S. (2005). An examination of phonological awareness treatment outcomes for seventh-grade poor readers from a bilingual community. *Language, Speech, and Hearing Services in Schools, 36,* 336–345.

Tabor, N. (1992). *Albertina anda arriba: El abecedario.* Watertown, MA: Charlesbridge.

Taylor, O., & Leonard, L. (1999). *Language acquisition across North America: Cross-cultural and cross-linguistic perspectives.* San Diego, CA: Singular.

Tellis, G. M. (2002). Multicultural aspects of stuttering. *Perspectives on Communication Disorders and Sciences in Culturally and Linguistically Diverse Populations, 8*(3), 8–11.

Tellis, G. M., & Blood, G. W. (2000). Stuttering inventory for Hispanic-Americans. In G. M. Tellis, *Hispanic-American college students' perceptions about stuttering, Dissertation Abstracts International, 60*(8), 3898B.

Tharp, R., & Gallimore, R. (1988). *Rousing minds to life: Teaching, learning, and schooling in a social context.* New York: Cambridge University Press.

Tharp, R. G, & Yamauchi, L. V. (1994). *Effective instructional conversation in Native American classrooms.* Santa Cruz, CA: National Center for Research on Cultural Diversity and Second Language Acquisition. Retrieved October 14, 2005, from http://www.ncela.gwu.edu/pubs/ncredsll/epr10.htm

Thomas, H. (1998). *The slave trade: The history of the Atlantic slave trade 1440–1870.* Basingstoke: Macmillan.

Thomas, W., & Collier, V. (1997). *School effectiveness for language minority students* [NCBE Resource Collection Series No. 9]. Washington, DC: National Clearinghouse for Bilingual Education. Retrieved April 14, 2007, from http://www.ncela.bwu.edu/nchepubs/resource/effectiveness

Thomas, W., & Collier, V (2002). *A national study of school effectiveness for language minority students' long-term academic achievement.* Santa Cruz. CA: Center for Research on Education, Diversity, and Excellence. Retrieved April 15, 2007, from http://www.crede.ucsc.edu/research/llaa/1.1_final.html

Threats, T. (2005). Cultural sensitivity in health care settings. *Perspectives on Communication Disorders and Sciences in Culturally and Linguistically Diverse Populations, 12*(3), 3–6.

Thurman, D. J., & Guerrrero, J. (1999). Trends in traumatic brain injury-related hospitalizations—United States, 1980–1995. In *Report of the Consensus Development Conference on the rehabilitation of persons with traumatic brain injury.* Bethesda, MD: National Institutes of Health.

Tomlin, K. J. (2006a). *Workbook of Activities for Language and Cognition* [WALC-1] [Spanish version]. Moline, IL: LinguiSystems.

Tomlin, K. J. (2006b). *Workbook of Activities for Language and Cognition* [WALC-2] [Spanish version]. Moline, IL: LinguiSystems.

Torgeson, J. K., Otaiba, S. A., & Grek, M. L. (2005). Assessment and instruction for phonemic awareness and word-recognition skills. In H. W. Catts & A. G. Kamhi (Eds.), *Language and reading disabilities* (2nd ed., pp. 127–156). Boston: Pearson.

Toronto, A. S. (1973). *Screening Test of Spanish Grammar* [STSG]. Evanston, IL: Northwestern University Press.

Toronto, A. S., Leverman, D., Hanna. C., Rozenzweig, P., & Maldonado, A. (1975). *Del Rio Language Screening Test.* Austin, TX: National Educational Laboratory.

Trueba, H. T. (1989). Raising silent voices: Educating the linguistic minorities for the 21st century. Cambridge, MA: Newbury House.

Trumbull, E., & Farr, B. (2005). *Language and learning: What teachers need to know*. Norwood, MA: Christopher Gordon.

Trumbull, E., Rothstein-Fisch, C., Greenfield, P. M., & Quiroz, B. (2001). *Bridging cultures*. Mahwah, NJ: Lawrence Erlbaum Associates.

Ukrainetz, T. A., & Fresquez, E. F. (2003). What is not language? A qualitative study of the role of the school speech-language pathologist. *Language, Speech, and Hearing Services in Schools, 35*, 284–298.

Ulatowska, H., & Bond, S. A. (1983). Aphasia: Discourse considerations. *Topics in Language Disorders, 3*(4), 21–34.

Umbel, V., & Oller, K. (1994). Developmental changes in receptive vocabulary in Hispanic bilingual school children. *Language Learning, 44*, 221–242.

Universidad Nacional Autónoma de Mexico. [Official Web site of the University of Mexico]. Retrieved April 15, 2007, from http://www.unam.mx/

U.S. Census Bureau. (2000). Census Briefs. Retrieved May 27, 2007, from http://www.census.gov/population/www/cen2000/briefs.html

U.S. Census Bureau. (2003). *Language use and English-speaking ability (2000)*. Washington, DC: U.S. Department of Commerce.

U.S. Census Bureau. (2004). *U.S. interim projections by age, sex, race, and Hispanic origin*. Retrieved April 15, 2007, from http://www.census.gov/ipc/www/usinterimproj/

U.S. Census Bureau (2005). *Population*. Retrieved May 23, 2007, from http://www.census.gov/prod/www/statistical-abstract.html

U.S. Department of Education. (2001). *Twenty-fourth annual report to congress on the implementation of the Individuals with Disabilities Education Act* (Table 11–5, pp. 11–22). Washington, DC: Author.

Valdés. G. (1996). *Con respeto: Bridging the differences between culturally diverse families and schools*. New York: Teachers College Press.

Van Kleeck, A., & Schuele, C. M. (1987). Precursors to literacy: Normal development. *Topics in Language Disorders, 7*(2), 13–31.

Vaughn, D., Gersten, T., & Chard, F. J. (2000). The underlying message in LD intervention research: Findings from research syntheses. *Exceptional Children, 67*, 99–114.

Veltman, C. J. (1988). *The future of the Spanish language in the United States*. Washington, DC: Population Reference Bureau.

Vigil, D. B., & Hwa-Froelich, D. A. (2004). Interactional styles in minority caregivers. Implications for intervention. *Communication Disorders Quarterly, 25*(3), 119–126.

Villa, R. A., Tac, L. V., Muc, P. M., Ryan, S., Thuy, N. T. M., Weill, C., & Thousand, J. (2003, Spring). Inclusion in Viet Nam: More than a decade of implementation. Research and Practice for Persons with Serve Disabilities, 28(1), 23–32.

Vista.com. (2004). *Languages in the United States*. Retrieved April 14, 2007, from http://www.vistawide.com/languages/us_languages.htm

Von Borsel, J., Maes, E., & Foulon, S. (2001). Stuttering and bilingualism: A review. *Journal of Fluency Disorders, 26*, 179–206.

Vygotsky, L. (1962). *Thought and language*. Cambridge, MA: MIT Press.

Wallace, G. L. (1997a). *Multicultural neurogenics: A resource for speech-language pathologists providing services to neurologically impaired adults from culturally and linguistically and diverse backgrounds.* San Antonio, TX: The Psychological Corporation.

Wallace, G. L. (1997b). *RANBO. The reliable assessment of neurobehavioral organization.* Cincinnati, OH: University of Cincinnati Department of Communicative Disorders and Sciences.

Wallach, G. P. (2005). A conceptual framework in language learning disabilities: School-age language disorders. *Topics in Language Disorders* 25(4), 292–301.

Wallach, G. P., & Butler K. G. (Eds.). (1984). *Language and learning disabilities in school-age children.* Baltimore, MD: Williams & Wilkins.

Wallach, G. P., & Butler K. (Eds.). (1994). *Language learning disabilities in school-age children and adolescents: Some principles and applications.* Boston: Allyn & Bacon.

Wang, W. S. Y. (1983). Speech and script relations in some Asian languages. In Chu-Chang (Ed.), *Asian and Pacific-American perspectives in bilingual education: Comparative research* (pp. 56–72). New York: Teachers College Press.

Washington, J. (1996). Assessing language abilities of African-American children. In A. Kamhi, K. Pollock, & J. Harris (Eds.), *Communication development and disorders in African-American children* (pp. 35–54). Baltimore: Brookes.

Washington, J., & Craig, H. (1992). Articulation test performances of low-income African-American preschoolers with communication impairments. *Language, Speech, and Hearing Services in Schools, 23,* 201–207.

Watanabe, A. (1998). Asian-American and Pacific-Islander-American families with disabilities: A current view. In V.O. Pang & L. Cheng (Eds.), *Struggling to be heard: The unmet needs of Asian/Pacific-American children* (pp. 151–163). Albany and NY: State of New York Press.

Wechsler, D. A. (1974). *Wechsler Intelligence Scale for Children-Revised* [WISC-R]. San Antonio, TX: The Psychological Corporation.

Weddington, G. T. (1990). Cultural considerations in the treating of craniofacial malformations in African-American. *Cleft Palate Journal, 27,* 289–293.

Wei, L., & Milroy, L. (2003). Markets, hierarchies, and networks in language maintenance and shift. In J. Dewaele, A. Housen, & L. Wei (Eds.), *Bilingualism: Beyond basic principles* (pp. 128–140). Clevedon, UK: Multilingual Matters.

Weinrich, M., Steele, R., Carlson, G. S., Kleczewka, M., Wertz, R. T., & Baker, F. H. (1989). Processing of visual syntax in a globally aphasic patient. *Brain and Language, 36,* 391–405.

Weismer, S., & Evans, J. (2002). The role of processing limitations in early identification of specific language impairment. *Topics in Language Disorders, 22,* 15–29.

Welles, E. (2004). Foreign language enrollment in United States institutions of higher education (2002, Fall). *ADFL Bulletin, 35,* 8–26.

Werner, E.O., & Kreschek, J. D. (1989). *Spanish SPELT I and II.* Sandwich, IL: Janelle Publishers.

Westby, C. (1997). There's more to passing than knowing the answers. *Language, Speech, and Hearing Services in Schools, 28,* 274–289.

Westby, C. (2004). Beyond decoding: Critical and dynamic literacy for students with dyslexia, language-learning disabilities (LLD), or attention-deficit-hyperactivity disorder (ADHD). In K. G. Butler & E. R. Silliman (Eds.), *Speaking, reading, and writing in children with language-learning disabilities: New paradigms in research and practice* (pp. 73–107). Mahwah, NJ: Lawrence Erlbaum Associates.

Westby, C., & Clauser, P. S. (2005). The right stuff for writing, assessing, and facilitating written language. In H. W. Catts & A. G. Kamhi (Eds.), *Language and reading disabilities* (2nd ed., pp. 274–345). Boston: Allyn & Bacon.

Whitmire, K. A. (2005). Language and literacy: In the age of federal initiatives. *Topics in Language Disorders, 25*(4), 302–309.

Wiig, E. H., & Langdon, H. W. (2006). *W-ABC Spanish Version.* Greenville, SC: Super-Duper Publications.

Wiig, E. H., Langdon, H. W., & Flores, N. (2001). Nominación rápida y automática en niños hispanohablantes bilingües y monolingües. *Revista de Logopedia y Foniatria, 21*(3), 106–117.

Wiig, E. H., Larson, V. L., & Olson, J. (2003). *S-Maps: Rubrics for curriculum-based assessment and intervention.* Eau Claire, WI: Thinking Publications.

Wiig, E. H., Nielsen, N. P., Minthon, L., & Warkentin, S. (2002). *Alzheimer's Quick Test.* San Antonio, TX: The Psychological Corporation.

Wiig, E., & Secord, W. (1989). *Test of Language Competence.* San Antonio, TX: The Psychological Corporation.

Wiig, E., & Wilson, C. (2000). Map it out: Visual tools for thinking, organizing, and communicating. Eau Claire, WI: Thinking Publication.

Wiig, E. H., Zureich, P., & Chan, H. W. (2000). A clinical rationale for assessing rapid naming abilities in children with language disorders. *Journal of Learning Disabilties, 33*, 359–374.

Wilcox, M. J. (1983). Aphasia: Pragmatic considerations. *Topics in Language Disorders, 3*(4), 35–48.

Williams, J. (2002, July 3). Cuban students guarantee revolutionary democracy. *Greenleft Weekly.* Retrieved September 16, 2005, from http://www.greenleft.org.aku/back/2002/498/498p12.htm

Williams, K. T. (2002). *Reading Level Indicator and Spanish Companion.* New York: Pearson.

Willig, A. (1985). A meta-analysis of selected studies on the effectiveness of bilingual education. *Review of Educational Research, 55*, 269–317.

Willis, W. (2004). Families with African-American roots. In E. Lynch & M. Hanson (Eds.), *Developing cross-cultural competence: A guide for working with children and their families* (3rd ed., pp. 141–178). Baltimore: Brookes.

Wolf, M., Bowers, P., & Biddle, K. (2000). Naming-speed processes, timing, and reading: A conceptual review. *Journal of Learning Disabilities, 33*, 387–407.

Wong-Fillmore, L. (1983). The language learner as an individual. In M. Clarke & J. Handscombe (Eds.), *TESOL, 1982, Pacific perspectives on language learning and teaching* (pp. 157–173). Washington, DC: TESOL.

Wong-Fillmore, L. (1991). Language and cultural issues in early education. In S. I. Kagan (Ed.), *The care and education of American's young children: Obstacles and opportunities* (pp. 30–40). Chicago: University Press.

Woodcock, R., Muñoz-Sandoval, A., McGrew, K., & Mather, N. (2004). *Batería III Woodcock-Muñoz.* Itasca, IL: Riverside.

Woodcock, R., Muñoz-Sandoval, A., Ruef, M., & Alvarado, C. (2004). *Woodcock-Muñoz Language Survey-Revised*. Itasca, IL: Riverside.

Worthman, C., & Kaplan, L. (2001). Literacy education and dialogical exchange: Impressions of Cuban education in one classroom. *The Reading Teacher, 54*(7), 648–656.

Wren, C. (1985). Collecting language samples from children with syntax problems. *Language, Speech, and Hearing Services in Schools, 16*, 83–105.

Wright, W. D. (2002). *Black history and black identity: A call for a new historiography*. Westport, CT: Praeger/Greenwood.

Yavas, M., & Goldstein, B. (1998). Phonological assessment and treatment of bilingual speakers. *American Journal of Speech-Language Pathology, 7*, 49–60.

Yelland, G., Pollard, J., & Mercuri, A. (1993). The metalinguistic benefits of limited contact with a second language. *Applied Psycholinguistics 14*, 423–444.

Ylvisaker, M., Szekeres, S. F., & Feeney, T. (2001). Communication disorders associated with traumatic brain injury. In R. Chapey (Ed.), *Language intervention strategies in aphasia and related neurogenic communication disorders* (4th ed., pp.745–808). Philadelphia: Lippincott Williams & Wilkins.

Yoshioka, J. G. (1929). A study of bilingualism. *Journal of Genetic Psychology, 36*, 473–479.

Yum, J. O. (1987). Korean philosophy and communication. In D. I. Kincaid (Ed.), *Communication theory: Eastern and Western perspectives* (pp. 71–86). San Diego, CA: Academic Press.

Zachman, L., Barrett, M., Huisingh, R., & Jorgensen, C. (1992). *Test of Problem Solving* [TOPS]. Moline, IL: LinguiSystems.

Zachman, L., Huisingh, R., Barrett, M., Blagden, C., Orman, J., & Monson, S. (1990). *Elementary Tasks of Problem Solving*. Moline, IL: LinguiSystems.

Zehler, A. M., Fleischman, H. L., Hopstock, P. J., Pendzick, M. L., & Stephenson, T. G. (2003). *Descriptive study of services to LEP students and LEP students with disabilities. Special topic report #4: Findings on special-education LEP students.* Submitted to U.S. Department of Education, OELA. Arlington VA: Development Associates.

Zhou, M., & Bankston, C. L. (1998). *Growing up American: How Vietnamese children adapt to life in the United States*. New York: Russell Sage Foundation.

Zúñiga, M. (1988). Chicano self-concept: A proactive stance. In C. Jacobs & D. Bowles (Eds.), *Ethnicity and race: Critical concepts in social work* (pp. 71–83). Silver Spring, MD: National Association of Social Workers.

AUTHOR INDEX

NOTE: Page numbers accompanied by *b* refer to material in a box; those with an *f* indicate a figure; and those with a *t* indicate a table.

A

Acosta, D., 72
Adamovich, B. L., 215
Administration on Aging, 216
Aftonomos, L. B., 230
Albert, M., 215
Al-Halees, Y., 221
Allen, M. B., 64
Alvarado, C., 36, 123*t*
Ambert, A., 54, 160
American Educational Research
    Association, 119
American Speech-Language-Hearing
    Association, 3, 14, 17*t*, 18–20,
    19*b*, 119, 152, 178, 212–14*f*
Anderson, N., 28, 112
Anderson, R., 41–42, 42*f*, 125
Arámbula, G., 101*b*, 228*t*
Ardila, A., 220
August, A., 62

B

Bailey, G., 112
Bain, B., 44
Baker, C., 9, 22, 23, 24, 31, 49,
    56, 59–60
Baker, F. H., 230
Baker, K., 55
Ballard, W. S., 123*t*
Bankston, C. L., 87
Barik, H., 44

Barrett, M., 122, 129, 130*t*
Bashir, A. S., 144
Bassetti, B., 32, 155, 156*t*, 157
Bates, E., 79, 123*t*, 196
Battle, D., 112
Beaumont, C., 64, 65, 66, 67, 178,
    181*f*, 182, 187, 191–92
Bedore, L. M., 160
Bellert, A., 150
Ben-Zeev, S., 44
Beringer, M., 123*t*
Berman, P. B., 62
Berni, M., 112
Bhatnagar, J., 200
Bialystok, E., xvii, 24, 25, 29, 43, 44,
    49, 190
Biber, D., 60
Biddle, K., 139
Bilodeau, L., 28
Birdwhistell, R. L., 5
Blagden, C., 129, 130*t*
Blood, G. W., 100–101
Bloom, L., 79
Bollinger, R. L., 227
Bond, M., 217
Bond, S. A., 228
Bonder, B., 81, 95, 103, 107
Bosh, L., 28
Bourgeois, M. S., 224–25
Bowers, P., 121, 139
Brice, A., 18, 20

SUBJECT INDEX

NOTE: Page numbers accompanied by *b* refer to material in a box; those with an *f* indicate a figure; and those with a *t* indicate a table.